PATHOLOGY for Gynaecologists

PATHOLOGY *for* Gynaecologists

SECOND EDITION

H. Fox MD, FRCPath

Professor of Reproductive Pathology, University of Manchester; Honary Consultant Pathologist, Manchester Royal Infirmary and St Mary's Hospital, Manchester

C. H. Buckley MD, MRCPath

Senior Lecturer in Pathology, University of Manchester; Honary Consultant Pathologist, St Mary's Hospital, Manchester

Edward Arnold
A division of Hodder & Stoughton
LONDON MELBOURNE AUCKLAND

© 1991 H Fox and C H Buckley

First published in Great Britain 1982
Second edition 1991

British Library Cataloguing in Publication Data
Fox, H. (Harold)
  Pathology for gynaecologists.–2nd. ed.
  1. Women. Reproductive system. Diseases
  I. Title   II. Buckley, C. H. (Cathryn Hilary)
  618.1

  ISBN 0–340–54444 9

Typeset in 10/12 pt Bembo by
Butler & Tanner Ltd, Frome and London
Printed and bound in Great Britain for Edward Arnold, a division of
Hodder and Stoughton Limited, Mill Road, Dunton Green, Sevenoaks,
Kent TN13 2YA
by Butler & Tanner Ltd, Frome, Somerset

Preface to the first edition

In few fields of medical practice is collaboration between the diagnostic histopathologist and those with direct clinical responsibility for the care of patients more necessary and potentially more fruitful than in gynaecology. It has long been recognized that a thorough understanding of the pathology of the female genital tract provides an essential foundation for the practice of gynaecological surgery and medicine, and acquirement of the knowledge necessary for this is considered to be an important component of the training and education of the gynaecological surgeon. The gynaecologist, whether established or in training, does, however, face a dilemma when attempting to gain a knowledge of female genital pathology, for clinical texts tend to deal with the pathological aspects of disease in a rather perfunctory and unsatisfactory manner: pathological tomes, on the other hand, usually dwell at length on the finer points of accurate histological diagnosis and provide details of differential histological diagnosis which fall outside the province, though not necessarily the interest, of the clinical gynaecologist.

This book has been written in an attempt to fill the gap between these extremes of excess and poverty and it is hoped that it will provide the gynaecologist with a comprehensive account of the pathology of the female genital tract and ovaries. We would stress, however, that it is purely an account and that no attempt has been made to discuss the finer histological points, to detail the minutiae of differential histological diagnosis or to expound upon the traps into which the unwary pathologist may fall. The account is, however, a full one and no concessions have been made in terms of excluding pathological entities because of their rarity: it is indeed hoped that any diagnosis which the gynaecologist may encounter in a pathological report is discussed in the text.

The outline of the book is perhaps slightly unusual for we have described, as far as possible, the various conditions in terms of pathological processes rather than detailing the pathology of each organ in turn. We have adopted this approach partly because we consider that pathology is particularly concerned with processes and partly because we feel it to be clinically more practical and useful than is the traditional format.

We have not felt it necessary to provide extensive references but have contented ourselves with listing a small number of key articles which it is thought will be useful to those seeking greater detail of a particular topic: where possible, reviews rather than individual papers have been cited.

It is hoped that this book will prove of value to gynaecologists in training, to the established gynaecologist in his daily practice and to those responsible for training gynaecologists. Pathologists wishing for a straightforward account of this fascinating branch of human pathology may, it is hoped, also find this volume of some interest.

Manchester 1982   HF
                                                                                                        CHB

Preface to the second edition

The aim of this book remains unchanged in its second edition, namely to provide for clinical gynaecologists a comprehensive account of the pathology of the female genital tract without dwelling on the niceties of histological diagnosis or the complexities of differential histopathological diagnosis.

In the years that have elapsed since the first edition new entities have been described, new nomenclatures have been introduced and new concepts have evolved. We have attempted a thorough update of the text and references and have tried to incorporate all these advances and changes. Some chapters, particularly those on epithelial abnormalities, malignant neoplasms, ovarian tumours, ectopic pregnancy, abortion and trophoblastic disease have been extensively rewritten.

We hope that this book will again prove of value to clinical gynaecologists and that those medical oncologists and radiotherapists involved in treating gynaecological disease may also find this account of value. Junior pathologists wishing for a straightforward and relatively short description of the diseases that may affect the female genital tract may find this volume a useful preparation before embarking on the larger texts of gynaecological pathology.

H Fox
C H Buckley   Manchester, 1990

Acknowledgements

We are indebted to Asha K Dube for making the line drawings used in chapter 1 and are most grateful to Dr E Blanche Butler (London) for providing us with Figure 5.6 and to Dr Hilary Lavery (Belfast) for providing us with Figure 5.3.

Figure 8.2 is a black and white photograph of a print which occurs in colour in V R Tindall's *A Colour Atlas of Clinical Gynaecology* (Wolfe Medical Publications, 1981) and we are grateful to both Professor V R Tindall and Wolfe Medical Publical Publications Ltd for their permission to use this print.

Figure 11.1 has been reproduced from *Muir's Textbook of Pathology (Eleventh Edition)* by kind permission of the editor, Professor J R Anderson.

Figures 17.1 and 17.8 were kindly supplied to us by Dr C W Elston (Nottingham). They have been previously published in *Pathology of the Placenta*, by H Fox, and are reproduced here by kind permission of W B Saunders Ltd.

Figures 4.1 and 10.23 have been previously published in *Biopsy Pathology of the Endometrium* (1989) by C H Buckley and H Fox and are reproduced here by kind permission of Chapman and Hall.

We are indebted to Professor D O'B Hourihane (Dublin) for Figure 17.6 and to Grune and Stratton for their kind permission to use both this illustration and Figure 17.7. These have previously appeared in *A Textbook of Gynaecological Oncology*, Edited by G R P Blackledge, J A Jordan and H Singleton.

We wish to express our appreciation and thanks to Mr Richard Pope, who was responsible for taking most of the photographs of gross specimens and to Mrs L Chawner for her invaluable assistance in the preparation of the photomicrographs.

Contents

I

Malformations of the female genital tract

By convention, the term 'malformation', when applied to the female genital tract, refers to anatomical abnormalities of the tract in women who otherwise have no phenotypic, sex chromosomal, gonadal or endocrinological abnormality. Such malformations probably arise as a result of relatively minor abnormalities of motility or fusion during embryogenesis and it is therefore necessary to consider in brief outline the normal development of the female genital tract. Consideration of the factors controlling and directing this development will be deferred until the next chapter.

Development of the female genital tract

The primordial gonads appear, at about the fourth week of embryonic life, as a pair of longitudinal ridges, formed by a proliferation of the coelomic epithelium and a condensation of the underlying mesenchyme. They are situated just caudal and lateral to the developing mesonephroi, which are connected to the cloaca by the wolffian (or 'mesonephric') ducts. By the sixth week of development the müllerian (or 'paramesonephric') ducts are formed, these arising as a longitudinal invagination of the coelomic epithelium on the anterolateral surface of the genital ridge. These ducts run parallel to the mesonephric ducts for much of their course and, indeed, the wolffian ducts appear to act almost as a scaffolding for the later development of the müllerian ducts. The cranial parts of the two müllerian ducts remain separate, but caudally they grow medially, the two ducts from each side coming into contact in the midline and, after being initially separated by a septum, they eventually fuse to form the uterine canal. Further caudal growth of the fused müllerian ducts brings them into contact with the posterior wall of the urogenital sinus, where they produce a small swelling known as the müllerian tubercle. The two wolffian ducts, which remain separate from each other, open into the urogenital sinus on either side of the tubercle. The cranial non-fused portions of the müllerian ducts form the fallopian tubes whilst the caudal fused portions develop into the uterus. The embryology of the vagina is still a matter of dispute and the relative contributions made to this organ by the müllerian ducts and the urogenital sinus are still undecided. It is certain that the vagina is initially a solid cylindrical structure which assumes its hollow form by a process of canalization, but whether the solid precursor of the vagina, known as the vaginal plate, results from a cellular proliferation of the caudal end of the müllerian ducts or from cells arising in the originally bifid urogenital sinus is uncertain. The belief that the definitive vagina is entirely formed from the urogenital sinus is one that is now winning wider acceptance, but there must almost certainly be an interplay between müllerian and urogenital tissues during embryogenesis. Studies of the anomalies arising in girls receiving prenatal diethystilboestrol suggest that the initial hollowing of the cylinder is probably a müllerian function and that urogenital sinus epithelium then grows upwards to replace müllerian tissue in the wall of the cylinder.

Classification and types of malformation

Female genital tract malformations can be divided into four main groups:

(i) aplasias,
(ii) fusion defects,
(iii) failures of septum dissolution,
(iv) failures of canalization.

This is a somewhat artificial classification and it is often difficult to know into which particular category a specific anomaly should be placed. Indeed, it is possible that any individual abnormality may be the end result of varying forms of developmental failure.

Aplasia

Total aplasia of the müllerian ductal system is extremely rare and is virtually confined to cases of sympodia. Unilateral aplasia of the müllerian system results in a hemiuterus (uterus unicornis unicollis) (Fig. 1.1) and is also uncommon. The most common form of aplasia is vaginal aplasia (also known as 'vaginal atresia'). In an organ with a complex and poorly understood mode of development it is impossible to classify with any degree of accuracy the various forms of aplasia and their differing pathogeneses, but by far the most common variety of vaginal aplasia is that which is associated with either an absent uterus and vestigial tubes or with a rudimentary uterus and normal tubes. This anomaly, known as the Rokitansky–Küster–Hauser syndrome, is clearly due to a failure of development of the caudal portions of the müllerian ductal system. There is a high accompanying incidence of abnormalities of the urinary tract, such as renal agenesis or single fused kidney, and this suggests that the basic defect may be in wolffian duct formation, the absence, or inadequate development, of this structure resulting in the lack of a scaffolding for subsequent müllerian duct development. Skeletal abnormalities are also commonly found in this syndrome.

A less common type of vaginal atresia is that which is associated with a normal uterus. This may be due either to a failure of fusion of the caudal fused müllerian ducts with the urogenital sinus or to a defect in urogenital sinus formation. Vaginal aplasia associated with a normal uterus is sometimes segmental rather than complete and this abnormality, known also as persistent vaginal plate, is probably better regarded as a failure of canalization rather than as a type of aplasia.

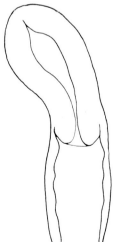

Fig. 1.1   A schematic representation of uterus unicornis unicollis (hemiuterus).

Fusion defects

Partial or complete failure of fusion of the two müllerian ducts produces a variety of malformations which are often regarded as being of an atavistic nature, it being argued that the further down the evolutionary scale a mammal is placed the greater is the degree of separation of müllerian ductal structures. However, this view is untenable, if only because some very primitive animals, such as the armadillo, have a single uterus.

Total failure of the two müllerian ducts to fuse results in the formation of two uterine bodies, two cervices and two vaginas, this anomaly being known as a *uterus didelphys* (Figs. 1.2 and 1.3).

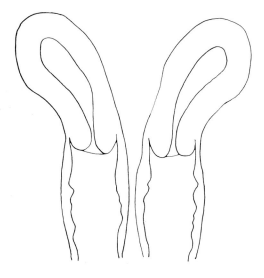

Fig. 1.2   A schematic representation of uterus didelphys with double vagina.

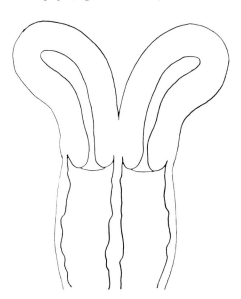

Fig. 1.3   A schematic representation of uterus didelphys with septate vagina.

However, it is possible that some examples of this anomaly are due to a reduplication rather than a fusion defect, for some cases are associated with duplication of other pelvic organs such as the colon or bladder. Progressively lesser degrees of müllerian duct failure result in a *uterus bicornis bicollis* (Fig. 1.4) in which there are two uterine bodies and cervices but only one vagina (which is, however, often septate), or a *uterus bicornis unicollis* (bicornuate uterus) (Fig. 1.5) characterized by the presence of two uterine bodies with a single cervix and vagina. The most minor form of fusion defect is the *arcuate uterus* in which the fundus of the uterine body is flatter than normal and has a mid-line notch, the uterus having a shape which resembles the heart as it is portrayed on a playing card (Fig. 1.6).

It will be remarked that a fusion defect is always most marked cranially and it should also be noted that variations on this relatively simple theme of fusion defect are quite common. Thus, in a bicornuate uterus, one horn may be rudimentary, solid or detached and sometimes does not communicate with the main uterine cavity (Fig. 1.7). Communicating variants of fusion defects, in which there is a lower uterine communication between otherwise separate uterocervical cavities, have also been described.

Failures of septum dissolution

These can result in a fully or partially septate uterus (Fig. 1.8), a septate cervix or a septate vagina, the first two anomalies being due to a failure of dissolution of the septae between the two müllerian ducts

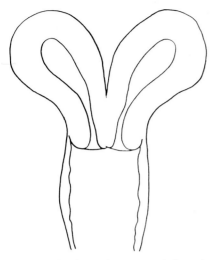

Fig. 1.4   A schematic representation of a uterus bicornis bicollis.

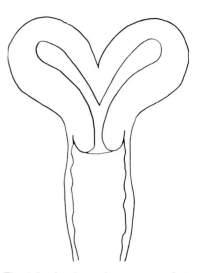

Fig. 1.5   A schematic representation of uterus bicornis unicollis.

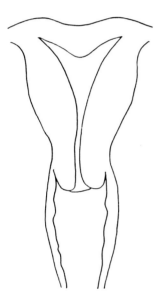

Fig. 1.6   A schematic representation of an arcuate uterus.

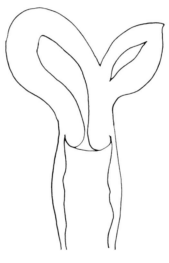

Fig. 1.7   A schematic representation of a bicornuate uterus with a non-communicating rudimentary horn.

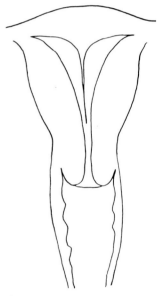

Fig. 1.8   A schematic representation of a septate uterus.

and the latter probably being the result of a similar failure of septal dissolution between the two arms of the early urogenital sinus.

Failures of canalization

A persistent vaginal plate (or segmental vaginal aplasia) is probably due to a partial failure of canalization of the originally solid vagina because of inadequate upgrowth of the urogenital sinus. An anomaly of this type should be distinguished from an imperforate hymen, which is due to the persistence of a urogenital membrane and is analogous to an imperforate anus.

Aetiology and pathogenesis of genital tract malformation

Genetic factors may play a role in the development of some anomalies, for there have been a number of reports of familial müllerian duct fusion defects and of familial Rokitansky–Küster–Hauser syndrome. Familial hydrometrocolpos, due to a persistent vaginal plate, has been fully documented in a number of Amish families, whilst an association between this condition and the Ellis–van Creveld syndrome (genetically determined chondrodystrophy and polydactyly) has also been noted. Uterine fusion defects are an integral component of the hand–foot–uterus syndrome, a genetic disorder characterized by malformations of the hands, feet and uterus.

There is no association between sex chromosomal abnormalities and genital tract malformations, but trisomy 13 is characteristically accompanied by uterine fusion defects whilst occasional genital tract abnormalities have been noted in cases of trisomy 18. The only identified teratogen known to produce genital tract abnormalities is thalidomide.

It has been suggested that müllerian duct fusion defects closely resemble craniofacial fusion abnormalities and are probably similarly also the end result of an interaction of genetic and environmental factors. A plausible suggestion has been that a fusion defect results from a slight physical separation of the müllerian ducts at a critical stage of development, possibly because of a genetically-determined altered shape of the embryonic pelvis.

Incidence and clinical features

The exact incidence of genital tract malformations is unknown but a reasonable estimate is that a malformation of greater or lesser degree is found in between 0.25 per cent and 0.5 per cent of all women. In a proportion of such women, the malformation is of no clinical significance but the majority suffer either major or minor symptoms. A persistent vaginal plate may result in a hydrocolpos in early life whilst vaginal atresia commonly presents as primary amenorrhoea which may or may not be accompanied by a haematocolpos. Fusion defects are associated with a high incidence of menorrhagia, dysmenorrhoea and infertility, whilst a septate or atretic vagina will cause dyspareunia or apareunia. Endometriosis is particularly common in those women who have an obstruction to the free drainage of menstrual blood from the uterus. About a third of women with fusion defects have a normal reproductive history, but the remainder have an unduly high incidence of abortion, premature labour, abnormal birth presentation, incoordinate labour and uterine rupture. A particular danger is that of implantation in a rudimentary horn, a form of pregnancy that will invariably result in uterine rupture at a relatively early stage of pregnancy.

Key references

Buttram V C Jr. (1983) Müllerian anomalies and their management. *Fertility and Sterility* **40**, 159–63.
Elias S, Simpson J L, Carson S A, Malinak L R and Buttram V C Jr. (1984) Genetic studies in incomplete Müllerian fusion. *Obstetrics and Gynecology* **63**, 276–9.
Golan A, Langer R, Bukovsky I and Caspi E. (1989) Congenital anomalies of Müllerian system. *Fertility and Sterility* **51**, 747–55.

Green L K and Harris R E. (1976) Uterine anomalies: frequency of diagnosis and associated obstetric complications. *Obstetrics and Gynecology* **47**, 427–9.

Heinonen P K, Saarikoski S and Pystynen P. (1982) Reproductive performance of women with uterine anomalies. *Acta Obstetrica et Gynecologica Scandinavica* **61**, 157–62.

Jarcho J. (1946) Malformations of the uterus. *American Journal of Surgery* **73**, 106–66.

Pinsonneault O and Goldstein D P. (1985) Obstructing malformations of the uterus and vagina. *Fertility and Sterility* **44**, 241–7.

Rock J A and Schlaff W D. (1986) The obstetric consequences of utero-vaginal anomalies. *Fertility and Sterility* **43**, 681–92.

Tarry W F, Duckett J W and Stephens F D. (1986) The Mayer–Rokitansky syndrome: pathogenesis, classification and management. *Journal of Urology* **136**, 648–52.

2

Abnormalities of sexual development

Patients with an abnormality of sexual development show a spectrum of external appearances (or 'phenotypes') ranging from an individual who is an apparently normal female to one who appears fully masculinized: the gynaecologist will tend only to encounter those individuals whose phenotypes lie largely on the female side of this spectrum, and hence this account will be concerned principally with those abnormalities associated with a fully, or predominantly, female phenotype and gender identity.

Normal sexual development

During early embryonic life, the gonad is of an indifferent nature and capable of developing into either an ovary or a testis. Differentiation along one or other of these alternative pathways is determined by the sex chromosomal constitution of the embryo: if the embryo is XY, the germ cells, which migrate to the gonad from the yolk sac at about the third week of development, will carry a nuclear membrane antigen, known as H-Y antigen, which will induce differentiation of the gonad into a testis. The H-Y antigen is under the control of the Y chromosome and embryos that lack a Y chromosome also lack H-Y antigen. Germ cells which do not carry the H-Y antigen will not stimulate testicular differentiation and the gonad containing such germ cells will develop into an ovary.

The Sertoli cells of the developing testis secrete a protein, known as 'müllerian inhibiting factor' (MIF), which acts locally to inhibit ipsilateral müllerian duct development: thus, MIF secreted from a left gonad inhibits duct development only on the left side and has no effect on the müllerian duct system of the right side. Müllerian inhibiting factor is not secreted by a developing ovary and in the absence of this substance there is a passive development of the müllerian duct system, no stimulatory factor being required.

The embryonic testis begins to secrete testosterone at about the 65th day of life and this hormone acts locally on the ipsilateral wolffian duct to induce differentiation into epididymis, vas deferens and seminal vesicle: in the absence of testosterone the wolffian duct system will regress and atrophy. Testosterone is also responsible for masculinization of the external genitalia, though for this action to occur testosterone must first be converted in the target tissues to dihydrotestosterone by the enzyme 5-α-reductase: in the absence of dihydrotestosterone, the external genitalia will develop along female lines.

Consideration of the control mechanisms of sexual development allows for the defining of two general principles.

1. Control of sexual development is hierarchical, with chromosomal sex determining gonadal sex and gonadal sex controlling somatic sex.
2. The ovary does not play any role in normal sexual development and a neuter embryo will always develop along female lines, deviation into a male pattern of somatic development being dependent upon testicular secretion of MIF and testosterone.

Classification of abnormalities of sexual development

Sex can be defined in terms of chromosomal constitution, gonadal structure, phenotypic form or gender identity and therefore abnormalities of sexual development can be defined and categorized at many different levels. However, because the fundamental determinant of sex is the remit of the X and Y chromosomes, it seems logical to regard the chromosomal constitution as a basis for the primary classification of these abnormalities, further subclassification being dependent on the type of gonad present and, to a lesser degree, phenotype.

1. Disorders associated with normal sex chromosomes:
   (a) *With macroscopically normal gonads*
      (i) XX chromosomal constitution with bilateral macroscopically normal ovaries:
         congenital adrenal hyperplasia
         administration of androgens or progestagens to mother during pregnancy
         maternal virilizing tumour
      (ii) XY chromosomal constitution with bilateral macroscopically normal testes:
         CNS defect
         Leydig cell agenesis
         defective testosterone synthesis
         defective MIF secretion
         androgen resistance syndromes
   (b) *With macroscopically abnormal gonads*
      (i) XX chromosomal constitution with streak gonads:
         pure gonadal dysgenesis
      (ii) XX chromosomal constitution with ovary and testis:
         hermaphroditism
      (iii) XY chromosomal constitution with streak gonads:
         testicular regression syndrome
      (iv) XY chromosomal constitution with ovary and testis:
         hermaphroditism

2. Disorders associated with abnormal sex chromosomes:
   (a) *Non-mosaic forms*
      (i) XO chromosomal constitution with streak gonads:
         Turner's syndrome
      (ii) XXY chromosomal constitution with hypoplastic testes:
         Klinefelter's syndrome
   (b) *Mosaic forms*
      (i) XO/XX chromosomal constitution with streak gonads:
         Turner's syndrome
      (ii) XO/XY chromosomal constitution with streak gonad and testis:
         mixed gonadal dysgenesis
      (iii) XO/XY chromosomal constitution with ovary and testis:
         hermaphroditism
      (iv) XX/XY chromosomal constitution with ovary and testis:
         hermaphroditism

It will be realized that this classification simplifies, but not unduly, a very complex subject and does not cover all eventualities: this applies particularly to the chromosomal mosaic abnormalities which are extremely numerous and only the most common are included above.

Disorders associated with normal sex chromosomes

With macroscopically normal gonads

XX chromosomal pattern and bilateral macroscopically normal ovaries
Individuals with a 46XX chromosomal constitution and two normal ovaries but who have been exposed to androgen excess during fetal life, will show partial masculinization of their external genitalia: the term 'female pseudohermaphroditism' is often applied to this syndrome.

The most common cause of female pseudohermaphroditism is *congenital adrenal hyperplasia*, a condition in which there is a congenital deficiency of one or other of the chain of enzymes necessary for the synthesis of adrenal corticosteroids, with a consequent accumulation of androgenic intermediary metabolites. In the vast majority of cases the deficiency is of the enzyme 21-hydroxylase, an absence of which will lead to an accumulation of 17-hydroxyprogesterone which is transformed into androstenedione and, eventually, into testosterone, with consequent virilization of the external genitalia. A minority of cases are due to $11\text{-}\beta$-hydroxylase deficiency, this defect resulting in an excess production of both deoxycortiscosterone and androstenedione, with a resulting combination of hypertension and masculinized external genitalia. A very rare deficiency is of $3\text{-}\beta$-hydroxysteroid-dehydrogenase, which results in mild masculinization due to an accumulation of dihydroepiandrosterone and which is manifest by clitoromegaly, together with a marked, and often fatal, tendency to lose salt because of defective synthesis of aldosterone precursors. Treatment of the common form of congenital adrenal hyperplasia is with cortisone, and prompt therapy will arrest the otherwise progressive masculinization of the external genitalia.

Administration of androgens or progestagens to the mother of a female infant during pregnancy will also induce masculinization of the external genitalia, though the degree of virilization is usually less profound than that found in congenital adrenal hyperplasia and there is no progression in the degree of genital abnormality after birth.

The presence during pregnancy of a maternal virilizing tumour is a rare cause of female pseudo-hermaphroditism. Most women with an androblastoma fail to conceive but some have achieved pregnancy, and there have been a few reports of rather mild masculinization of the external genitalia of female children resulting from such pregnancies. The least rare virilizing lesion occurring during gestation is the luteoma of pregnancy (see Chapter 12) which, in a small number of cases, is accompanied by mild virilization of the mother and some degree of masculinization of the external genitalia of a female child, this being due to the ability of the luteoma to secrete a variety of androgenic substances.

XY chromosomal pattern and bilateral macroscopically normal testes
Individuals with a 46XY chromosomal constitution and bilateral macroscopically normal testes who, because of a relative or absolute androgen deficiency during fetal life, have poorly masculinized or female external genitalia, are often grouped together as examples of 'male pseudohermaphroditism'. Uncommon causes of this syndrome include *Leydig cell agenesis*, *deficient synthesis of MIF* and *defective testosterone synthesis*, this last deficiency being due to a variety of congenital enzyme deficiencies.

The *androgen resistance syndromes* are the most common cause of male pseudohermaphroditism and are of particular importance because they are usually associated with a fully female phenotype and gender identity. Nevertheless, most patients not only have a 46XY chromosomal constitution and bilateral testes but also high or normal plasma testosterone levels, and it has become clear that the failure of their external genitalia to masculinize is due to an end organ insensitivity to the effects of androgens. It will be recalled that testosterone is partially converted peripherally to dihydrotestosterone by the enzyme $5\text{-}\alpha$-reductase: both hormones bind to the same receptor protein in the cytosol of target cells and the hormone–receptor complexes diffuse into the nucleus. The testosterone–receptor complex is believed to regulate wolffian duct development, gonadotrophin secretion and spermatogenesis, whilst the dihydrotestosterone–receptor

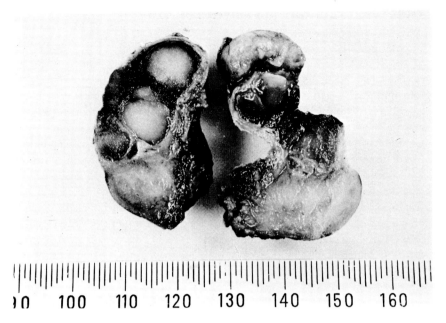

Fig. 2.1   Gonads removed from a 17-year-old patient with testicular feminization syndrome. The nodular appearance of the cut surface of the testes is quite characteristic.

complex is responsible for external virilization during embryogenesis and for much of the development of secondary sex characteristics at puberty. This system can break down if there is a deficiency of 5-α-reductase, an abnormality of the androgen receptor protein or a failure of the cells to respond to the receptor–hormone complex.

An androgen–receptor protein defect is responsible for the clinical syndrome of *testicular feminization*. Patients with this abnormality have an XY karyotype and female external genitalia: the vagina is short and blind whilst internal genitalia are absent, apart from bilateral testes which may lie in the abdomen, inguinal canal or labia majora (Figs. 2.1 and 2.2). At puberty, affected individuals undergo breast development and feminization: their fully female appearance is combined with a complete gender identity and patients present either because of primary amenorrhoea or with bilateral inguinal swellings that are often thought to be hernias. These clinical features suggest a complete absence of androgens (but not of MIF) but, nevertheless, plasma levels of both testosterone and dihydrotestosterone are either normal or high; the patients are also completely refractory to exogenous androgens and it is now clear that this syndrome is due to a familial defect or deficiency of androgen–receptor protein. Because the receptor deficiency also involves the hypothalamic centres, the androgen feedback mechanism is inoperative and luteinizing hormone (LH) levels are elevated: synthesis of oestrogens is therefore increased and the high levels of these hormones are responsible for the complete pubertal feminization and for the well marked breast development. The testes of these patients are particularly prone to develop a neoplasm, most importantly a seminoma, but there is virtually no risk of this occurring before the age of puberty and it is usual to delay castration until after the patient has undergone pubertal feminization.

An incomplete or partial form of testicular feminization is sometimes encountered: this differs from the complete form of the syndrome in that there is a variable degree of masculinization of the external genitalia and some degree of wolffian duct development; these patients tend to both masculinize and feminize at puberty and hence gonadectomy is performed in the prepubertal years. Although there is

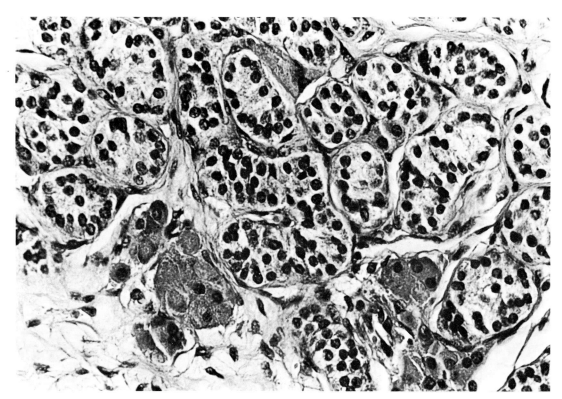

Fig. 2.2 The histological features of the testes shown in Fig. 2.1. There are fetal-like seminiferous tubules lined by Sertoli cells between which there are groups of large, darkly staining Leydig cells (H. & E. × 270).

some sensitivity to androgens the basic defect, an androgen–receptor deficiency, appears to be very similar to that found in the complete testicular feminization syndrome.

A small proportion of patients with an androgen–receptor deficiency have a predominantly male phenotype and present as inadequately virilized males: the range of abnormalities in such individuals is collectively known as the *Reifenstein syndrome*, and appears to be due to a partial deficiency of androgen–receptor protein.

A rare condition is that of *receptor positive androgen resistance*, in which patients with all the clinical features of the complete testicular feminization syndrome are found to have normal amounts of androgen receptor and normal nuclear localization of the receptor–hormone complex. This condition may be due to a nuclear unresponsiveness to the receptor–hormone complex.

The final form of androgen resistance is that due to *5-α-reductase deficiency*. This is a rare condition in which XY males with bilateral inguinal or labial testes are of female phenotype at birth but have fully developed wolffian duct structures (epididymis, vas deferens, seminal vesicles) that terminate in the vagina. At the time of puberty there is a degree of virilization of the external genitalia, some growth of pubic and axillary, but not facial, hair and, occasionally, a switch in gender identity from female to male. These abnormalities are those which would be expected if there were a deficiency of dihydrotestosterone, but not of testosterone, during development and indeed these individuals have been shown to have high plasma testosterone values and low levels of plasma dihydrotestosterone. It has been clearly demonstrated that this condition is due to a deficiency of 5-α-reductase, this deficiency leading to an inability of target tissues to convert testosterone to dihydrotestosterone and being due to the homozygous state of an autosomal recessive gene.

With macroscopically abnormal gonads

Individuals with normal XX chromosomal patterns but with either bilateral streak gonads or both an ovary and a testis are occasionally encountered. The latter group is one variant of hermaphrodite (a condition discussed later) whilst the former are classed as examples of *pure gonadal dysgenesis*. Patients with pure gonadal dysgenesis have normal, but infantile, internal and external genitalia, are of normal stature and have none of the physical stigmata of Turner's syndrome. These cases are sometimes familial, do not have any predisposition to gonadal neoplasia and may be due to a specific failure of a hypothetical gonadal 'inductor' substance.

Individuals with a 46XY chromosomal constitution may have bilateral streak gonads or even completely absent gonads. Such cases were previously referred to as 'pure XY gonadal dysgenesis', 'anorchia' or 'Swyer's syndrome' but are now thought to represent the *testicular regression syndrome*, in which, for reasons as yet unknown, the testes regress at some stage of fetal life. This results in a very wide spectrum of abnormalities, the nature of which depends upon the timing of gonadal regression in relationship to the secretion of MIF and testosterone. At one end of this spectrum the external genitalia are female in type, the internal organs are absent and the gonads are either absent or are streaks, this condition being due to gonadal regression at a very early stage of embryogenesis before differentiation of the wolffian and müllerian duct systems. At the other extreme are phenotypic males with normal internal genitalia and infantile or nearly normal external genitalia, such cases being due to testicular regression in late fetal life.

Individuals of 46XY type with both an ovary and a testis represent yet another form of true hermaphroditism (see page 14).

Disorders associated with abnormal sex chromosomes

Individuals with a sex chromosomal abnormality may have a pure karyotype, e.g. 45XO, or may be chromosomal mosaics e.g. 45XO/46XX. The possible chromosomal and clinical permutations are many but, in very general terms, most cases of sex chromosomal abnormality fall into one of four clinical groups, namely Turner's syndrome, Klinefelter's syndrome, mixed gonadal dysgenesis or true hermaphroditism.

Turner's syndrome

The vast majority of patients with this syndrome have a 45XO chromosomal constitution, although a small minority are XO mosaics (usually either 45XO/46XX or 45XO/47XXX). In its classic form, the syndrome consists of sexual infantilism and streak gonads in a phenotypic female of short stature, but a number of other physical abnormalities, collectively known as Turner's stigmata, may or may not be present. These include neck webbing, lymphoedema, high palate, shield chest, increased cubital carrying angle, coarctation of the aorta etc.

The internal genitalia are of normal female form, though infantile, and the gonads are represented by white fibrous streaks, 2–3 cm long and about 0.5 cm in diameter, in the site normally occupied by the ovaries (Fig. 2.3). The gonad of an XO individual contains a normal complement of germ cells during embryonic life, but these rapidly degenerate, are almost all lost by the time of birth and have completely disappeared well before puberty. It has been suggested, therefore, that two X chromosomes are necessary for the control of granulosa cell development and that in the absence of two such chromosomes the granulosa cells will fail to differentiate, with subsequent degeneration of the germ cells. Patients with an XO mosaicism may retain a few germ cells into adult life (Fig. 2.4) and occasionally menstruate, some

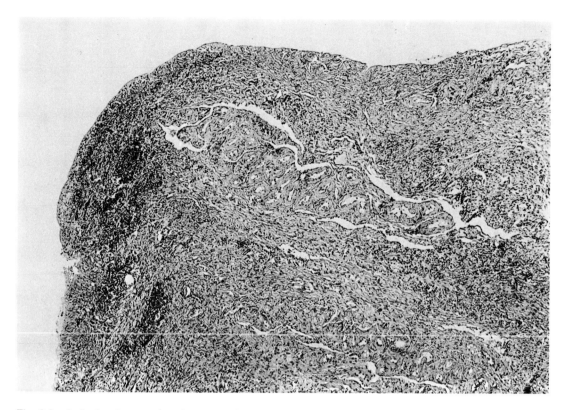

Fig. 2.3 A single micrograph at low magnification includes almost an entire streak gonad. A thin rim of stroma representing the medulla and cortex surrounds a vascular core (H. & E. × 45).

even becoming pregnant. Patients with Turner's syndrome do not have any tendency to develop gonadal neoplasms.

Klinefelter's syndrome

Patients with this condition are phenotypic males with a 47XXY chromosomal constitution: exceptionally, there is an XXY mosaicism. The syndrome is characterized by azoospermia, gynaecomastia and atrophic testes: most patients have sparse body and facial hair, unduly long legs and, often but not invariably, are of rather low intelligence. The testes rarely exceed 2 cm in diameter and show marked hyalinization and degeneration of the seminiferous tubules with a relative increase in the number of Leydig cells.

Mixed gonadal dysgenesis

Patients with this abnormality have asymmetrical sexual development, usually having a streak gonad on one side and a testis, albeit one often showing some degree of immaturity and disorganization, on the other side. The chromosomal constitution is variable but is most commonly a 45XO/46XY mosaicism. There is a considerable range of development of internal and external genitalia but most patients present as phenotypic females with partially masculinized external genitalia. Both müllerian and wolffian duct structures are commonly present and the gender identity is more often female than male. These patients

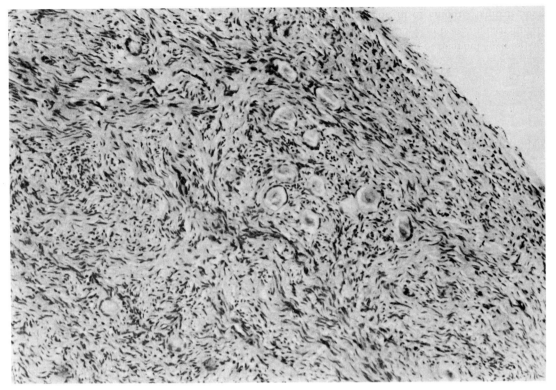

Fig. 2.4   A section of ovary from a patient with 45XO/46XX mosaicism. A small number of primordial follicles are present (H. & E. × 108).

tend to virilize at puberty and run a high risk of developing germ cell neoplasms of their gonads: hence gonadectomy before the time of puberty is usually advised.

True hermaphroditism

Patients with this condition have both ovarian and testicular tissue and the term is applied independently of chromosomal constitution. The majority of patients (about 60 per cent) have a 46XX chromosomal constitution but a minority have a 46XY chromosomal pattern or are either 46XX/46XY or 45XO/46XY mosaics: there may be an ovary on one side and a testis on the other or, most commonly, there may be bilateral combined ovotestes. The patients most often present as predominantly phenotypic males with ambiguous external genitalia, though a minority have a predominantly female phenotype. A variety of complex combinations of internal duct development may be encountered but most true hermaphrodites will have a uterus, a minority menstruating and even, on rare occasions, becoming pregnant.

The basic abnormality in most cases of hermaphroditism, particularly those with an XX chromosomal pattern, is unknown, but it has recently been shown that XX hermaphrodites are often H-Y antigen positive. Indeed, the ovarian tissue may be H-Y antigen negative whilst the testicular tissue is H-Y antigen positive, this suggesting that there may be a mosaic primordium irrespective of apparent karyotype.

The gonads of a true hermaphrodite have some tendency to develop germ cell neoplasms, though the risk is much lower than in cases of mixed gonadal dysgenesis. Gonadectomy is therefore generally recommended and, in those individuals brought up as females, this operation should be performed before puberty so as to prevent pubertal virilization.

Key references

Bercu B B and Schulman J D. (1980) Genetics of sexual differentiation and of female reproductive failure. *Obstetrical and Gynecological Survey* **35**, 1–11.

Dewhurst J. (1987) Abnormal sexual development: a clinical overview. In: *Haines and Taylor, Obstetrical and Gynaecological Pathology, 3rd edn.* pp. 56–63. Edited by H Fox, Churchill Livingstone, Edinburgh.

Edman C D. (1983) Testicular regression syndrome. *Seminars in Reproductive Endocrinology* **1**, 129–137.

Gerald P S. (1978) Current concepts in genetics: sex chromosome disorders. *New England Journal of Medicine* **294**, 706–8.

Griffin J E and Wilson J D. (1980) The syndrome of androgen resistance. *New England Journal of Medicine* **302**, 198–209.

Robboy S J, Welch W R and Cunha C R. (1987) Pathological basis of intersex. In: *Haines and Taylor, Obstetrical and Gynaecological Pathology, 3rd edn.* pp. 928–43. Edited by H Fox, Churchill Livingstone, Edinburgh.

Scott J S. (1978) Intersex and sex chromosome abnormalities. In: *Scientific Basis of Obstetrics and Gynaecology, 2nd edn.* pp. 310–44. Edited by R R MacDonald, Churchill Livingstone, Edinburgh.

Wachtel S S. (1979) The genetics of intersexuality, clinical and therapeutic perspectives. *Obstetrics and Gynecology* **54**, 671–85.

3

Cyclical changes in the female genital tract: physiological and pathological aspects

Physiological aspects

The morphology of the female genital tract is not static but, during the years from the menarche to the menopause, undergoes repetitive cyclical changes which are a consequence, and a reflection, of the recurring fluctuation in ovarian hormone production that is an essential component of the ovulatory cycle. During a woman's reproductive life, ovulation occurs at approximately monthly intervals. Each month about twenty ovarian primordial follicles begin to mature but usually only one develops into a mature ovum, the remainder undergoing spontaneous atresia. This follicular, or preovulatory, stage of the cycle is stimulated by rising follicle stimulating hormone (FSH) levels and the developing follicle secretes large quantities of oestrogens. Ovulation occurs at approximately mid-cycle in response to a surge of LH, which is provoked by a critical oestrogen level. The ovum is expelled from the follicle, which then undergoes conversion into a corpus luteum. Under the influence of LH, the corpus luteum secretes considerable amounts of both oestrogens and progesterone but, in the absence of pregnancy, the corpus luteum degenerates after approximately fourteen days, luteolysis being accompanied by a sharp decline in oestrogen and progesterone levels. The tissues of the female genital tract possess steroid hormone receptors and are therefore capable of responding to these cyclical hormonal changes, the changes in these tissues representing a recurrent priming for a potential pregnancy. It is, however, worth remarking that menstruation is not an essential component of this recurrent cycle, for certain primates have similar cycles but do not menstruate. Necrosis of the endometrium, and hence menstrual loss, is a consequence of very rapid regression of the endometrium at the end of the cycle, the abruptness of this change being due to the very rapid decline in circulating oestrogen and progesterone levels as the corpus luteum degenerates. If these levels declined more slowly, as is the case in certain other species, endometrial regression would be more gradual and necrosis and menstrual loss avoided, but only at the cost of prolonging the cycle and thus reducing the number of ovulations during the limited period of female reproductive capacity.

Although all of the female genital tract shows cyclical changes in structure, these are most apparent in the endometrium and a carefully timed biopsy of this tissue provides information, albeit of an indirect nature, of ovulation and of the response of the tissues to hormonal stimulation.

Endometrium

In the prepubertal child the endometrium is shallow, with a compact stroma and small inactive glands. At the menarche the endometrium grows and increases in depth in response to the increased ovarian production of oestrogens which precedes the establishment of ovulation. With the commencement of ovulation, a regular pattern of growth, differentiation and menstrual shedding is established, though this sequence is confined to the more superficial functional layer of the endometrium, the deeper basal layer being relatively unresponsive to ovarian hormones.

In this account, the first day of menstruation is taken as being day 1 of the menstrual cycle. This is the traditional view, although reasoned arguments have been made for regarding the day of ovulation as day

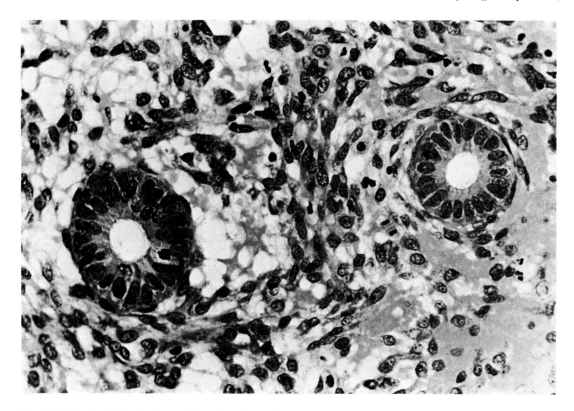

Fig. 3.1 Endometrium in the proliferative phase showing narrow glands lined by multilayered non-secretory epithelium. Mitoses are present in both the glandular epithelium and stroma (H. & E. × 270).

1, the most cogent of these being that the time interval between ovulation and menstruation is fairly constant, variations in cycle length being generally due to alterations in the preovulatory phase.

Following menstruation there may be a resting, or interval, phase lasting for a day or two but it is not unusual to observe regenerative changes in both glands and stroma as early as the third day of the cycle, this early regenerative phase possibly being independent of hormonal stimuli. During the preovulatory follicular phase, when oestrogen levels are high, the various elements of the functional layer proliferate and grow synchronously, the endometrium thus being said to be in the proliferative phase (Fig. 3.1). The glands are at first straight and narrow but both they and the vessels become somewhat tortuous in the latter part of this phase as their growth rate outstrips that of the stroma. The gland-to-stromal ratio is low during the preovulatory stage and the glands are lined by columnar cells with basally situated nuclei, there often being some degree of multilayering towards the later part of this phase. Mitotic figures are seen throughout the follicular phase, both in glands and in stroma and the stroma, which is originally compact, becomes somewhat oedematous towards the middle of the phase, only to become compact again in the immediately preovulatory stage.

In the average cycle, ovulation occurs at about the fourteenth day but there are normally fertile women in whom ovulation occurs as late as the twenty-first day. Following ovulation there are high levels of both oestrogens and progesterone, and the endometrium is now in the secretory phase which is characterized by the twin processes of glandular secretion and stromal differentiation. The morphological changes that identify the early secretory phase take 24 to 36 hours to develop (Fig. 3.2). This phase normally lasts for about four days and during this time the glands increase in diameter and become more tortuous. The defining feature of the early secretory phase is, however, the appearance of glycogen-containing subnuclear

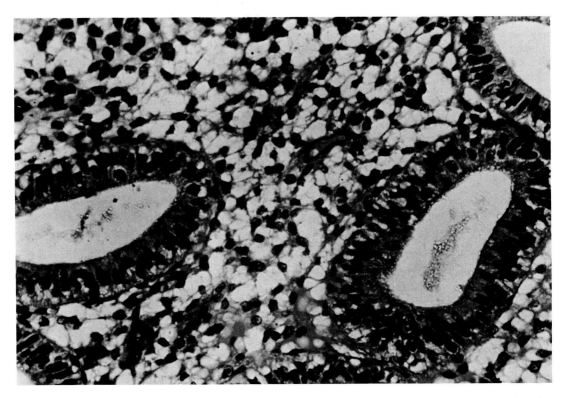

Fig. 3.2   Endometrium in transition from proliferative to early secretory phase. The glandular epithelium is still multilayered and contains mitoses but in addition subnuclear vacuoles are forming (H. & E. × 270).

vacuoles in the glandular epithelium (Fig. 3.3), the presence of such vacuoles being presumptive evidence that ovulation has occurred. This presumption is, however, only valid if subnuclear vacuoles are present in virtually all of the cells of at least 50 per cent of the glands, for scattered small subnuclear vacuoles can develop in anovulatory cycles. Occasional mitotic figures may still be seen within both glands and stroma throughout the early secretory phase. On the fifth postovulatory day the endometrium enters the mid-secretory phase (Fig. 3.4), which persists until the ninth day after ovulation. In this phase the subnuclear vacuoles move to a supranuclear position and their contents are secreted into the lumen, the nuclei of the glands resuming a basal position. Glandular secretion reaches a peak at this stage and the epithelium of the increasingly tortuous glands becomes pale, eosinophilic and somewhat granular. During the mid-secretory phase the stroma is markedly oedematous .

On the tenth postovulatory day (i.e. normally the twenty-fourth day of the cycle) the endometrium enters the late secretory phase, in which still further tortuosity of the glands throws their lining epithelium into folds, imparting to them a 'saw-tooth' appearance (Fig. 3.5). Glandular secretion is less marked than in the mid-secretory phase. The stromal oedema regresses rapidly after the tenth postovulatory day and the stromal cells then take on a predecidual appearance (Fig. 3.6), becoming plump and acidophilic with finely granular cytoplasm and small round nuclei. The predecidual cells appear first as a mantle around the spiral arterioles which, after being previously inconspicuous, are now well developed and prominent. Later, predecidual change is seen in cells around glands and below the surface epithelium. Towards the latter part of the late secretory phase the stroma consists of solid sheets of predecidual cells which are infiltrated by K cells (granulated lymphocytes). Neutrophil polymorphonuclear cells are also present in the stroma and these increase in number as the endometrium enters the menstrual phase (Fig. 3.7), which

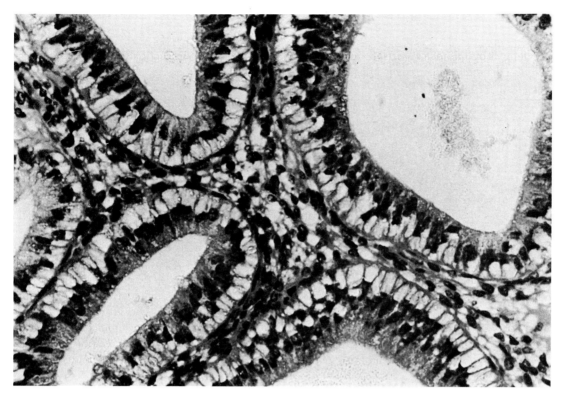

Fig. 3.3 Endometrium in the early secretory phase, twenty-four hours later than Fig. 3.2. The glandular epithelium now shows well-marked subnuclear vacuolation and the epithelial cytoplasm is less basophilic and hence paler in this section (H. & E. × 270).

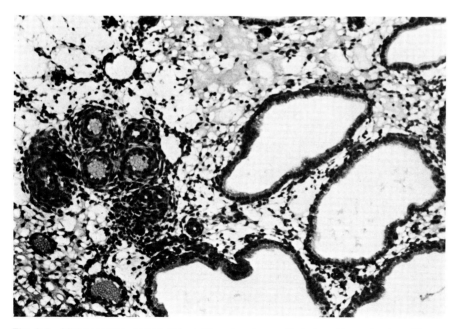

Fig. 3.4 Mid-secretory endometrium. The glands are dilated and irregular in outline, contain secretion and are lined by a single layer of secretory columnar cells with pale, eosinophilic cytoplasm. The stroma is oedomatous and spiral artery development can be seen (H. & E. × 87.5).

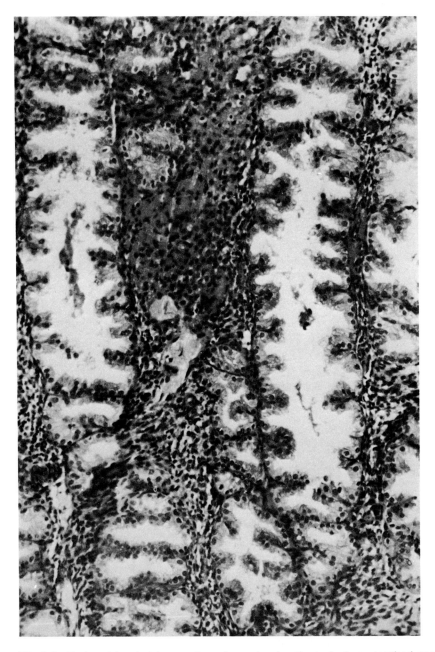

Fig. 3.5   Endometrium in late secretory phase showing the typical saw-toothed appearance of the glands (H. & E. × 120).

is characterized by haemorrhage, crumbling, glandular collapse and necrosis. Shedding of much of the functional layer is complete in two or three days, although shedding is not total and some of the functional layer is retained to enter a fresh proliferative phase during the next ovulatory cycle.

It will be appreciated from this account that, during the preovulatory phase of the cycle, the endometrial changes show a rather constant pattern throughout and that accurate 'dating' of the endometrium is

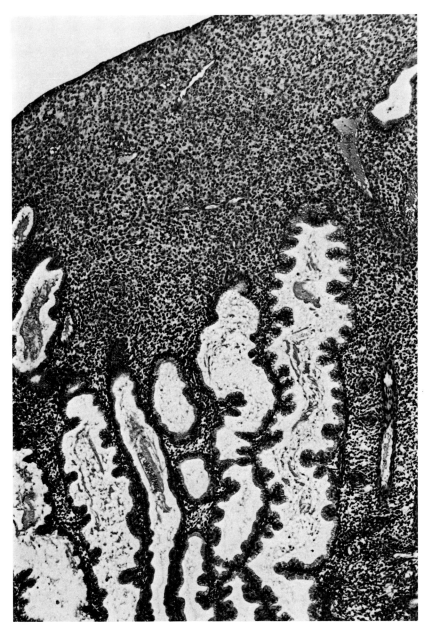

Fig. 3.6 Late secretory endometrium showing the decidual change in the superficial compact layer of the endometrial stroma (H. & E. × 50).

difficult, if not impossible. During the postovulatory phase, however, the endometrium shows an ordered pattern of time-related changes that allow the specific stage of the ovulatory cycle to be accurately identified.

It will also be recognized that the changes described above are those seen in a cycle in which pregnancy does not occur. If a conceptus forms during a cycle, the corpus luteum persists, the oestrogen and progesterone levels remain high and the morphological changes which normally precede menstruation

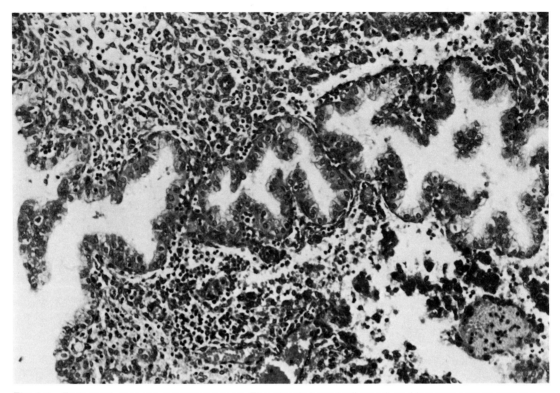

Fig. 3.7   Endometrium in the menstrual phase. The glands have 'collapsed' and become stellate and the stroma is crumbling and becoming fragmented (H. & E. × 108).

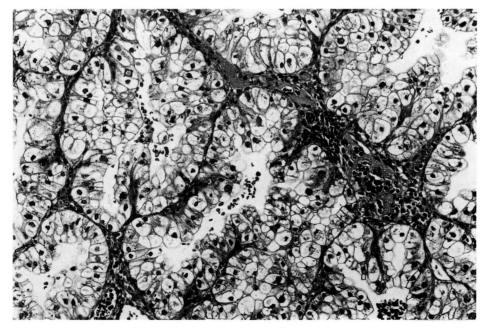

Fig. 3.8   Endometrium showing Arias–Stella change. There is glandular enlargement and hypersecretory activity, as shown by the cellular enlargement and vacuolation of the cytoplasm (H. & E. × 186).

do not occur. Glandular secretion persists undiminished and the stroma remains oedematous even though the stromal cells show a florid predecidual change. Later, the decidual change becomes more marked, the endometrium thickens, the spiral arterioles dilate and a true decidua is formed. In some women the glandular epithelium become hypersecretory, with vacuolated cytoplasm and enlarged, pleomorphic nuclei; intraglandular tufting of the lining epithelium may be conspicuous (Fig. 3.8). This appearance, known as the Arias–Stella change, is usually a focal one and occurs not only in normal intrauterine pregnancy but in any patient in whom trophoblast, whether normal or abnormal, is present in either a uterine or an ectopic site.

Cervix

The cyclical changes in the cervix are less well defined than those in the endometrium. Oestrogens stimulate the squamous epithelium of the ectocervix to become fully mature, hence this appearance is seen during the follicular phase of the cycle. However, progesterone inhibits full squamous maturation, and hence fully mature squamous epithelium is not seen during the luteal phase. The cyclical changes in the endocervical epithelium are extremely subtle but a peak of cellular growth and secretion occurs at the time of ovulation and declines thereafter.

Fallopian tube

The normal tube is lined by an epithelium containing ciliated, secretory and intercalary cells. The epithelium increases in height during the follicular phase but declines somewhat in the luteal phase and reaches its lowest level during menstruation. During the luteal phase, the ciliated cells become broader and relatively low, whilst the secretory cells, inactive during the follicular phase, become taller and project above the surface level of the ciliated cells, often forming a dome or cupula. The ciliated cells reach their greatest degree of development at the time of ovulation and their cilia beat synchronously in waves towards the uterus.

Vagina

The squamous epithelium of the vagina is hormonally responsive. During the follicular phase of the cycle, the epithelium thickens and matures, cellular maturation being at a peak just prior to ovulation when oestrogen levels are at their highest. The rising progesterone level during the luteal phase leads to inhibition of squamous maturation at the intermediate stage and to marked exfoliation of cells.

Pathological aspects

Pathological aspects of the ovulatory cycle are manifest entirely in the endometrium.

Anovulatory cycles

Most women have occasional anovulatory cycles but these occur principally at the time of the menarche and in the perimenopausal years. A follicle matures in such cycles but no ovum is shed and a corpus luteum is not formed. The endometrium remains under the influence of oestrogen until such time, usually five or six weeks, as the follicle degenerates and undergoes atresia. During the first few anovulatory cycles, the endometrium shows only a proliferative pattern, although focal subnuclear vacuolation of the glandular epithelium is sometimes seen. After two or three anovulatory cycles there may be some multilayering of the glandular epithelium and an unusual degree of variability of glandular diameter, and after five or six such cycles a simple endometrial hyperplasia (see Chapter 9) usually develops.

Luteal phase insufficiency

This abnormality, also known as corpus luteum defect, short luteal phase or luteal inadequacy, can be due to a variety of causes in which the common denominator is a diminished production of progesterone by the corpus luteum. Thus, the normal abrupt rise of progesterone levels which follows ovulation either does not occur or occurs in a gradual and step-like manner, with subsequent impairment of endometrial secretory transformation, a factor that may lead to either failure of blastocyst implantation or to early unrecognized abortion. There is no single aetiological factor for this insufficiency of progesterone secretion, which may be due to inadequate follicular development because of low FSH levels, inadequate luteinization of the granulosa cells due to the preovulatory peak of LH being too low or too short lasting, a primary defect in the ability of the ova to organize the developing follicle or suppression of progesterone

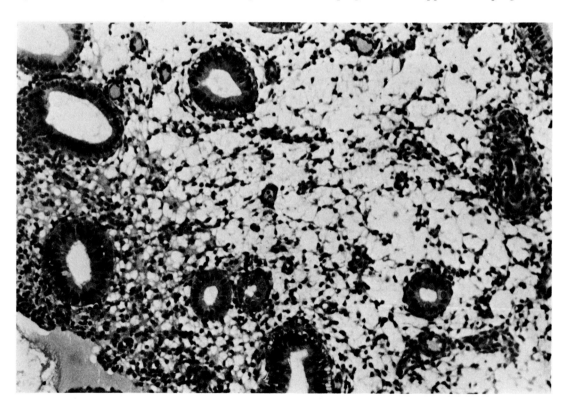

Fig. 3.9 Endometrium from the twenty-second day of the cycle in a woman with infertility. It shows the poor glandular development with rather variable secretory activity and poor stromal maturation characteristic of inadequate secretory transformation (H. & E. × 108).

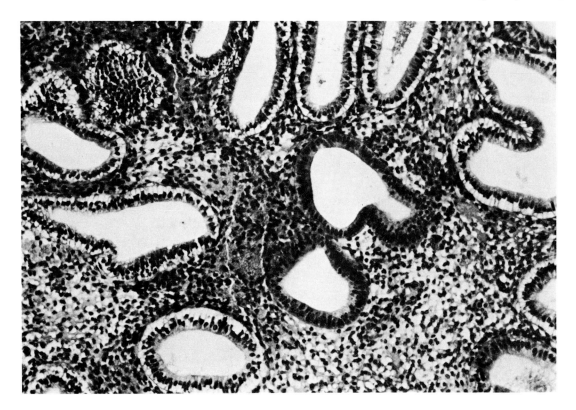

Fig. 3.10 Endometrium showing irregular ripening. Glands can be seen both in proliferative and well-established early secretory phase (H. & E. × 108).

release by elevated prolactin levels. Irrespective of cause, the condition can be diagnosed by endometrial biopsy, which should preferably be performed between the twenty-second and the twenty-sixth day of the cycle, when the full effects of the progestational stimulation of the endometrium are normally at their most apparent. In the most typical form, that of *inadequate secretory transformation* (Fig. 3.9), the glands, instead of being closely packed, dilated and highly convoluted, will, if corpus luteum function is impaired, be widely spaced, narrow and lacking in tortuosity. Secretory activity is diminished, stromal oedema does not develop well and predecidual changes may not occur. In other cases, glandular and stromal maturation is asynchronous, the stroma, for example, showing the features of the late secretory phase whilst the glands have an appearance more typical of the mid-secretory phase. On the other hand, glandular and stromal maturation may be synchronous but delayed, the secretory changes seen in the endometrium lagging three or four days behind those expected for the stage of the menstrual cycle. A further morphological facet of this condition occurs when the glands do not mature synchronously. Thus glands in the proliferative, early secretory and established secretory phases co-exist in the same endometrium. This is known as *irregular ripening* (Fig. 3.10) and in such cases the glands showing the most advanced secretory change are those nearest to the spiral arterioles, i.e. those exposed to the highest concentration of progesterone.

A state of luteal insufficiency occurs sporadically in normal women but persistent inadequacy is of considerable importance in the aetiology of dysfunctional uterine bleeding, early abortion and infertility.

Delayed endometrial shedding

Menstrual endometrium is normally shed in two or three days, but in some women there is prolonged menstruation and secretory glands may still be identified in curettings taken as late as the tenth day after the onset of bleeding. This phenomenon of delayed endometrial shedding has been attributed to an undue persistence of the corpus luteum but in fact this is only true in so far as the time interval between ovulation and menstruation is unduly short in such patients, the endometrium breaking down despite the presence of a corpus luteum. This is probably due to a malfunction of the corpus luteum, which is unable to provide adequate support for a secretory endometrium, and this condition is therefore probably another manifestation of the luteal insufficiency syndrome.

Key references

Buckley C H and Fox H. (1989) *Biopsy Pathology of the Endometrium*. Chapman and Hall, London.

Dallenbach-Hellweg G. (1987) *Histopathology of the Endometrium, 4th edn*. Springer-Verlag, Berlin.

Hendrickson M R and Kempson R L. (1980) *Surgical Pathology of the Uterine Corpus*. W B Saunders, Philadelphia.

More I A R. (1987) The normal human endometrium. In: *Haines and Taylor, Obstetrical and Gynaecological Pathology, 3rd edn*. pp. 302–19. Edited by H Fox, Churchill Livingstone, Edinburgh.

Noyes R W and Haman J O. (1953) The accuracy of endometrial dating. *Fertility and Sterility* **4**, 504–17.

Noyes R W, Hertig A T and Rolk J. (1950) Dating the endometrial biopsy. *Fertility and Sterility* **1**, 3–25.

4

Postmenopausal changes in the female genital tract and ovary: physiological and pathological aspects

Following the cessation of ovarian hormonal secretion, cyclical changes cease in the genital tract and all the constituent tissues of the tract undergo some degree of atrophy.

Endometrium

Anovulatory cycles are common during the perimenopausal period, for reasons discussed later, and hence a degree of simple hyperplasia of the endometrium is not infrequently encountered at this stage. The reduction in oestrogen levels at the time of the menopause may be quite abrupt and this is followed by endometrial atrophy, the endometrium becoming shallow, the glands small and inactive and the stroma compact (Fig. 4.1); the differentiation between functional and basal layers is lost. In other instances the decline in oestrogen levels is more gradual and there may be a rather irregular pattern of proliferation, with mitotic activity being discernible for one or two years after cessation of ovulation. Gradually, however, even this low grade stimulation ceases and, if mitotic figures are seen in the endometrium more

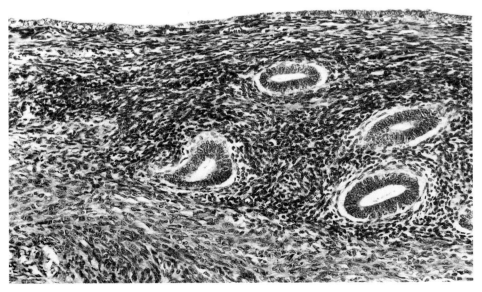

Fig. 4.1 Endometrium from a postmenopausal woman. The endometrium is thin, the glands few and inactive and the stroma is compact (H. & E. × 120).

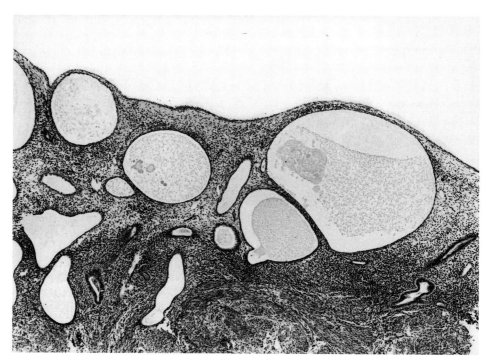

Fig. 4.2 Cystically dilated glands in the atrophic endometrium of a postmenopausal woman (H. & E. × 60).

than three years after the menopause, this can be taken as a clear indication of either an abnormal source of endogeneous oestrogens or the administration of exogenous oestrogens.

In a high proportion of postmenopausal women the endometrial glands are, either focally or diffusely, cystically dilated (Fig. 4.2). Such glands are lined by a single layer of flattened cuboidal epithelial cells and mitotic figures are not seen. The incidence of such cystic change in the postmenopausal endometrium increases progressively with advancing age and it is clear that this is because of blockage of the gland ducts during the process of endometrial atrophy and condensation, there being no evidence to suggest that this change is indicative of a 'regressed' simple endometrial hyperplasia.

An intense lymphocytic infiltration occurs in the atrophic endometrium in some patients, but the cells usually form aggregates and are not a consequence of infection. Endometrial polypi can occur after the menopause and it has been suggested that their incidence in postmenopausal women is increasing. However, it may be that such polypi are more frequently detected than in the past because of the greater awareness of the significance of postmenopausal bleeding in women receiving hormonal replacement therapy.

Total squamous metaplasia (see Chapter 6) of the endometrium occurs in a small proportion of elderly women and the aetiology of this is usually thoroughly obscure.

Myometrium

The postmenopausal myometrium shows a marked reduction in bulk and, because this is mainly the result of a decrease in cell cytoplasm, a picture of increased nuclear density is imparted. Leiomyomata also assume a condensed appearance similar to that seen in the rest of the myometrium, and degenerative changes are common in these tumours.

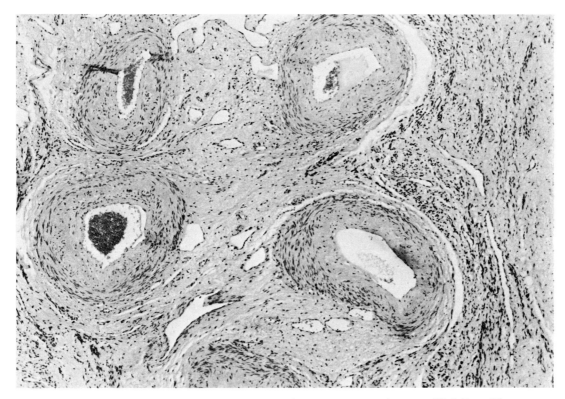

Fig. 4.3   Prominent myometrial arteries in the uterus of a postmenopausal woman (H. & E. × 45).

The myometrial arteries show degenerative changes, hyalinization, fibrosis, reduplication of the internal elastic lamina and calcification and, because they undergo less atrophy than the adjacent myometrium, they become unduly prominent, particularly in the parous woman (Fig. 4.3).

Fallopian tube

After the menopause there is a tendency for the epithelium to become cuboidal or cubocolumnar throughout the tube and the plical complexity is diminished. Many years after the menopause there is epithelial deciliation and the mucosal stroma becomes more fibrous.

Cervix and vagina

The depth and maturity of the cervical and vaginal squamous epithelium depend upon an adequate level of circulating oestrogen. After the menopause it becomes shallow and maturation is arrested at the mid- or upper mid-zone (Fig. 4.4). It is also common to find up to three layers of basal or parabasal cells imparting a somewhat spurious appearance of intraepithelial neoplasia. This atrophic mucosa is particularly susceptible to infection (see Chapter 5) and, when it is inflamed, there may be not only an artificially induced maturation or epithelial keratinization but also reactive cellular changes in the squamous epi-

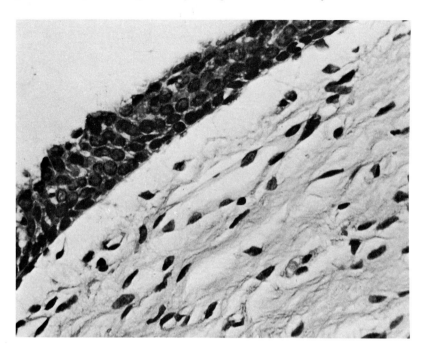

Fig. 4.4 Atrophic ectocervical squamous epithelium in a postmenopausal woman. Maturation is arrested at the mid-zone (H. & E. × 300).

thelium which may, superficially, resemble intraepithelial neoplasia. The vagina becomes reduced in length and calibre, distensibility and elasticity are lost and rugae diminished or absent.

There is a marked reduction in secretion in the endocervix and in most women the squamocolumnar junction becomes withdrawn into the endocervical canal. The inflammation and eversion of the endocervical canal, which may occur in the patient who develops a prolapse after the menopause, are associated with active squamous metaplasia which would normally not be expected in patients of this age group.

Ovary

As the total number of primordial follicles decreases, the number available to transform from primary to secondary follicles each month declines and, as the development of tertiary follicles depends, among other factors, on the presence of an adequate number of developing follicles, fertility and corpus luteum formation diminish and anovulatory cycles become increasingly common in the perimenopausal years.

The cessation of cyclical hormonal changes marks the completion of the menopause.

The postmenopausal ovary is small and lacks follicular activity. The cortex usually involutes, although in some patients it remains broad and scalloped, due to the presence of whorled hyperplastic nodules of stromal cells.

Epithelium inclusion cysts are commonly seen in the postmenopausal ovary and appear to increase in frequency with age.

Key references

Buckley C H and Fox H. (1989) *Biopsy Pathology of the Endometrium.* Chapman and Hall, London.

Coleman D V and Evans D M D. (1988) *Biopsy Pathology and Cytology of the Cervix.* Chapman and Hall, London.

Crompton A C. (1976) The cervical epithelium during the menopause. In: *The Cervix*, pp. 128–33. Edited by J A Jordan and A Singer, W B Saunders, London.

Lang W R and Aponte G E. (1967) Gross and microscopic anatomy of the aged female reproductive organs. *Clinical Obstetrics and Gynecology* **10**, 454–65.

McBride J H. (1954) Normal postmenopausal endometrium. *Journal of Obstetrics and Gynaecology of the British Empire* **61**, 691–7.

McClean J M. (1988) Anatomy and physiology of the vulval areas. In: *The Vulva*, pp. 39–65. Edited by C M Ridley, Churchill Livingstone, Edinburgh.

Steger, R W and Hefez E S E. (1978) Age associated changes in the vagina. In: *The Human Vagina*, pp. 95–106. Edited by E S E Hefez and T N Evans, North Holland, Amsterdam.

5

Inflammatory disease

It is convenient, when describing inflammatory lesions of the female genital tract, to discuss each anatomical zone in turn, but it must be remembered that such a division is quite artificial, for an inflammatory lesion often affects two or more sites simultaneously or spreads to involve different areas in succession. It has also to be borne in mind that inflammation is not synonymous with infection, many inflammatory lesions of the genital tract being of non-infective origin. Furthermore, many clearly infective lesions are of a non-specific polymicrobial nature.

Vulva

Non-infective inflammation

Non-infective vulvitis may be provoked by irritants such as soaps, scents or deodorants, whilst excessive washing, particularly if combined with the liberal use of antiseptics, may cause or aggravate inflammation rather than alleviate it. A non-infective inflammation may also accompany any condition which causes maceration of the skin, such as incontinence of urine, excessive sweating, occlusive clothing or copious vaginal discharge. A vulvitis of this nature tends to be perpetuated by scratching and there is not uncommonly secondary bacterial or fungal infection.

Histologically, the acute stage is characterized by oedema and congestion, whilst if the inflammation subsides into a chronic phase there is hyperkeratosis, acanthosis and a non-specific chronic inflammatory cell infiltration of the dermis, these latter changes often being called 'lichenification'. A variant of this histological picture, regarded by some as a discrete entity but probably non-specific in nature, is the so-called *plasma-cell vulvitis*, in which the dermis contains a heavy plasma-cell infiltrate and deposits of haemosiderin.

A *Lipschütz ulcer* is an acute, self-limiting, painful ulcer of the labia minora and is associated with local lymphadenopathy and fever. The histological features are non-specific, the floor of the ulcer being formed by granulation tissue which is heavily infiltrated with neutrophil polymorphs and plasma cells. The condition is of unknown aetiology and is an entity distinct from aphthous ulceration (see below) and the vulval ulceration of Behçet's syndrome (see Chapter 18).

Aphthous ulcers affect the labia majora, where they appear as grey macules which ulcerate to leave a yellow base with a red margin. The histological appearances are those of a non-specific inflammation. The aetiology is unknown but some patients develop symptoms suggestive of Behçet's syndrome.

The term *vulval dermatitis* is applied to a particular form of inflammatory reaction which can be caused by repeated application of an irritant (primary irritant dermatitis) or may be due to a hypersensitivity (allergic contact dermatitis) and develop only after exposure to a specific allergen. The histological appearances of the two types are identical and both may extend to involve the vagina. Histologically, the early phase is characterized by epidermal oedema with the formation of bullae or vesicles. There is a mononuclear cell infiltrate of the epidermis and around the capillaries of the upper dermis. If the condition becomes chronic, the vesicles tend to disappear and there is acanthosis, parakeratosis and hyperkeratosis. The perivascular mononuclear infiltrate persists in the upper dermis which is hypervascular and may show fibrosis.

Seborrhoeic dermatitis presents as well defined areas of reddening in the folds of the vulva, being seen particularly in obese women. The histological picture is similar to that of a chronic dermatitis, although dermal inflammation is mild.

Vulval tissues are relatively sensitive to radiation and a *radiodermatitis*, characterized by atrophy, pigmentary changes, telangiectasis and sometimes ulceration, may develop after radiation damage.

On rare occasions, a deep seated folliculitis of the vulval apocrine glands occurs, this being known as *suppurative hidradenitis*. This is a disease of the reproductive years which worsens premenstrually and is of unknown aetiology. Suggested causes include an antigen–antibody reaction and an abnormal response to hormonal stimulation, but the only clear fact is that it is not due to a bacterial infection. The early lesions are red, tender nodules that become fluctuant and eventually discharge pus, this tending to lead to sinus formation and scarring. Histologically, the early lesions are characterized by dilatation of the apocrine gland ducts and an active non-specific inflammatory reaction around the follicle. The dilated ducts contain inflammatory cells and bacteria, these probably being secondary invaders. Later there is a progressive inflammatory destruction of the epithelial appendages with granuloma formation, the appearance of foreign body-type giant cells, development of sinuses and fibrosis.

Fox–Fordyce disease, in which tiny, firm pruritic papules are found on the mons and labia and in the axillae, may be a related apocrine abnormality. In this condition, which tends to appear at puberty, the primary event is obstruction of the apocrine duct by a plug of keratin. There is subsequent formation of an apocrine retention vesicle and development of a perifolliculitis.

Infective inflammation

Viral infections

A *herpetic vulvitis*, usually due to infection with herpesvirus hominis type II but occasionally with type I, is not uncommon; it is acquired through sexual contact and is seen particularly in teenagers or young adults. The condition presents as a painful, sharply marginated, ulcerative vulvitis and lesions may also be present in the urethra, bladder, cervix and vagina. The initial lesion is vesicular and usually painless, there often being no local symptoms: viraemia at this stage may, however, cause malaise and fever. Histological examination of an early lesion shows an intraepidermal vesicle which occasionally extends to become subepidermal. The cells surrounding the vesicle show a ballooning-type of degeneration, are often multinucleated and contain eosinophilic intranuclear inclusions. After the lesion ulcerates, these characteristic features are lost and a rather non-specific picture, accompanied by a variable degree of dermal inflammation, is seen. The diagnosis of this disease can be made with certainty only by serological means, although examination of fluid from a vesicle will often demonstrate cells showing ballooning and nuclear abnormalities.

Herpes zoster of the vulva is rare, but typical vesicular eruptions and pain may occur in the area of cutaneous distribution of the pudendal nerve. The histological features of the lesions are identical to those of herpes simplex infection.

The lesions of *molluscum contagiosum* are transmitted by a DNA pox virus and present as multiple, or occasionally single, umbilicated, pearly cutaneous nodules or papules: these may be asymptomatic or cause slight itching. The characteristic histological appearances are of a well demarcated nest of lobulated acanthotic squamous epithelial cells in which the maturing squamous cells contain intracytoplasmic viral inclusions (Fig. 5.1a and b). In the deeper parts of the lesion these are small and eosinophilic but as the surface is approached they become larger and basophilic. The surrounding dermis shows little or no inflammation unless, as happens rarely, the lesion ruptures and discharges molluscum bodies into the

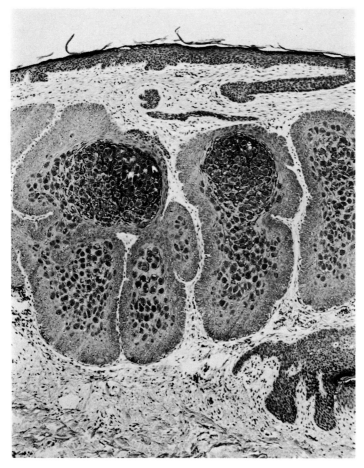

Fig. 5.1(a) Molluscum contagiosum of the vulva. The lobulated acanthotic squamous epithelium is seen centrally (H. & E. × 40).

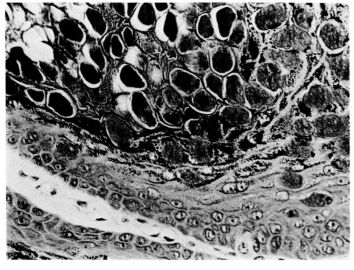

Fig. 5.1(b) Molluscum contagiosum. At higher magnification the intracytoplasmic viral aggregates can be seen as pale-staining granular 'molluscum' bodies (H. & E. × 174).

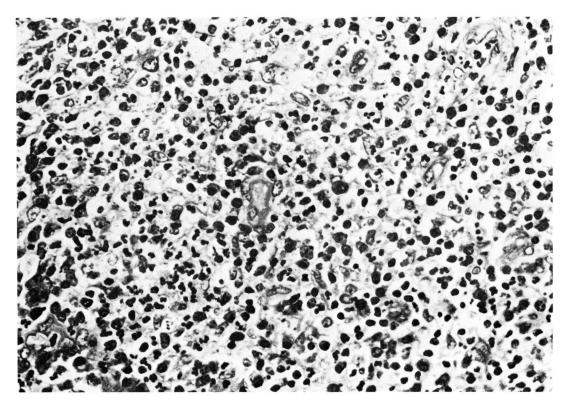

Fig. 5.2 Vulval granuloma inguinale. There is non-specific granulation tissue with an infiltrate of plasma cells and histiocytes (H. & E. × 270).

tissues, these provoking an inflammatory cell response in which foreign body giant cells may be present. The lesions commonly regress spontaneously but occasionally persist, and remain infective, for many years.

Bacterial infections
Granuloma inguinale is due to infection with the Gram-negative organism *Donovania granulomatis*, a member of the Enterobacteriaceae, and is largely a disease of tropical or subtropical countries; the prediliction of the infection for the genitalia suggests that it may be sexually transmitted but this has not been proven. Primary lesions occur on the mons or labia minora as painful papules or nodules which break down to form a spreading ulcer that may extend to involve the inguinal or pubic areas. Abundant granulation tissue formation in the base of the ulcer imparts to it a beefy-red velvety appearance. At a later stage the infection may also spread via the lymphatics to involve the inguinal nodes and other sites in the genital tract. Healing of the lesion is characterized by dense fibrosis which can lead to extensive keloid scarring and lymphatic obstruction. A brawny oedema of the vulva is not uncommon and can occur independently of lymphatic blockage. The typical histological picture is of a luxurious production of non-specific granulation tissue with an infiltrate of plasma cells and histiocytes (Fig. 5.2). The latter are large and foamy and contain large numbers of the rounded or rod-like Donovan bodies which appear purplish on haematoxylin and eosin staining and red with Giemsa stain. The adjacent squamous epithelium often shows marked pseudoepitheliomatous hyperplasia and, very occasionally, a squamous carcinoma supervenes.

Chancroid, or 'soft sore', is an acute sexually transmitted infection with *Haemophilus ducreyi*. The primary lesions develop on the labia as painless nodules or papules, single or multiple, which break down into ulcers measuring only a few millimetres in diameter. Later these tend to coalesce and form ulcerated areas as large as 3 cm across. The ulcers have a ragged, rather irregular appearance with an excavated margin; there is little or no induration. The infection tends to spread to the inguinal nodes to produce a painful lymphadenitis that may evolve into large fluctuant masses which discharge through the skin. Histologically, the floor of the vulvar ulcer is seen to be formed by a narrow zone of neutrophil polymorphs, fibrin, red blood cells and necrotic tissue, whilst deep to this is a wide band of non-specific granulation tissue in which the numerous vessels often show marked endothelial proliferation and intramural degenerative changes. Deeper still is a heavy infiltrate of plasma cells and lymphocytes.

Tuberculosis of the vulva is very rare and is usually associated with tuberculous infection elsewhere in the genital tract, spread to the vulva being either via the bloodstream or by direct extension. A tuberculous lesion begins as a semitranslucent 'apple-jelly' nodule on the labia or in the vestibule which later breaks down to form a shallow ragged ulcer. Microscopy shows the typical caseating epithelioid granulomata which contain Langhans giant cells.

A *gonococcal vulvitis* occurs as a component of a vulvovaginitis in infants and preadolescent girls. It usually results from direct contact with infected adults and is rarely sexually transmitted. The vulvitis is often transitory but the organisms tend to persist in the periurethral glands.

Erysipelas is a superficial cellulitis which is usually due to haemolytic streptococcus. Vulval erysipelas tends to recur and is often preceded by a pharyngitis. A necrotizing vulvitis due to Gram-positive organisms has always been rare and is now virtually extinct.

Chlamydial infections

Lymphogranuloma venereum is a venereal infection with a chlamydia, an obligatory intracellular parasite. The primary lesion, developing three to thirty days after exposure, is a small papule or shallow ulcer on the vulva. This tends to heal spontaneously in a few days, only to be followed by a suppurative inguinal lymphadenitis, which is usually painful. The enlarged nodes tend to become matted together and liquefy to form fluctuant buboes which discharge through the skin via indolent sinuses. In a proportion of patients the disease progresses to a chronic destructive ulceration which may involve the vulva, vagina and rectum and is associated with rectal and vaginal fibrosis, fistulae formation and chronic lymphoedema. Spontaneous resolution may occur but more commonly the disease persists if untreated.

In the early lesion, histological examination shows infiltration of the tissues by mononuclear cells, plasma cells and occasional eosinophil. Later, pseudotubercles may form and the later stages are dominated by lymphatic dilatation and fibrosis. In long standing cases, the epidermis may show a florid pseudo-epitheliomatous hyperplasia and, rarely, a squamous carcinoma develops. Within the lymph nodes the characteristic, but not pathognomonic, lesion of the early stage is the formation of stellate abscesses. Later, acellular necrosis is seen and large numbers of plasma cells are present.

Treponemal infections

The causative organism of *syphilis* is the *Treponema pallidum*, which is transmitted sexually, the vulva being the usual site for the primary lesion (or 'chancre'). The primary lesion takes the form of a hard, brownish-red nodule or plaque with surface erosion or punched out ulceration (Fig. 5.3). The chancre is painless unless secondary infection supervenes, heals spontaneously within a few weeks and often passes unnoticed. There may be an associated painless, rubbery inguinal lymphadenopathy.

Secondary lesions appear at any time from six weeks to six months after the primary episode. Diffuse brownish-red macular or papular rashes may affect the skin and mucous membranes and in some individuals papules in the anogenital area enlarge to form elevated moist plaques known as condylomata lata. These can involve not only the vulva but also the adjacent perineum, perianal region and the thighs.

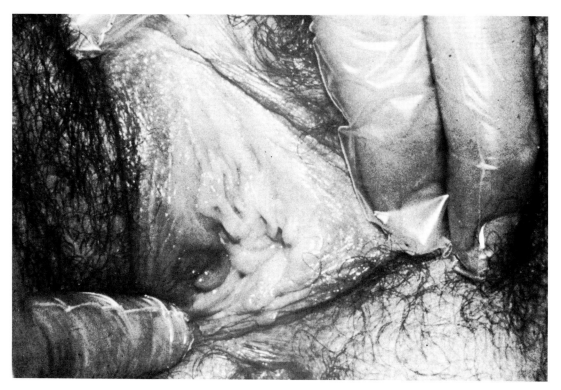

Fig. 5.3 Chancre of the vulva. An ulcerated dark nodule is seen on the inner surface of the right labium minor at the introitus.

Snail track ulcers, with their characteristic silvery base, are sometimes seen on the vulva during the secondary stage. The tertiary lesion of syphilis, the gumma, rarely involves the vulva.

Histologically, the typical chancre shows a dense infiltrate of chronic inflammatory cells amongst which plasma cells predominate. The infiltrate is often perivascular and the vessels show a marked endothelial proliferation. Necrosis, of a rather bland type, usually supervenes and there may be a few scattered multinucleated giant cells. Chancres are, however, rarely biopsied for they team with spirochaetes which can be readily identified in fluid from the lesion by dark ground illumination microscopy.

Fungal infections
The overwhelming majority (98 per cent) of cases of mycotic vulvitis are due to *Candida albicans*. This organism is present in the mouth, gastrointestinal tract and vagina of normal individuals, where it leads a saprophytic existence. In certain circumstances, however, the organisms become pathogenic, a *monilial vulvitis* tending to occur in diabetics, during pregnancy, in individuals with congenital immunodeficiency, in patients being treated with immunosuppressives, corticosteroids or antibiotics and in women using oral contraceptives.

A monilial vulvovaginitis is nevertheless most common in young, sexually active women and presents as a severe, painful, often pruritic, inflammation of the entire vulvovaginal mucosa. The labia majora are erythematous, oedematous and covered by a white macerated layer. Fissures are common and infection often coexists in the gluteal and inguinal folds, where macerated and ulcerated plaques, having a typical white rim, are found. Histological examination reveals Periodic acid-Schiff (PAS)-positive yeast cells and pseudofilaments in the keratinized layer of the epithelium and hair follicles and subcorneal pustules develop. The diagnosis is, however, usually established not by biopsy but by examination of scrapings from the surface of the lesions.

Parasitic and metazoan infections
The vulva may be involved in *scabies* and the bites of the pubic louse in this site may become secondarily infected.

Vulval involvement in *schistosomiasis* is by no means rare in areas in which this disease is endemic. Vulval lesions are found most commonly in prepubertal girls and are characterized by pain and swelling, with the formation of papules or plaques that may coalesce and occasionally ulcerate. Histologically a granulomatous reaction is seen around ova.

Vulval lesions may accompany vaginal or cervical infection by *Trichomonas vaginalis*.

Bartholin's gland

Acute inflammation of Bartholin's gland often progresses to an abscess and is usually caused by Staphylococci or faecal organisms. However, it should be noted that Bartholin's gland does not share the resistance offered to gonococcal infection by the adult vaginal mucosa, and *Neisseria gonorrhoea* is an important cause of a Bartholin's gland abscess. *Mycoplasma hominis* has been implicated in some cases of acute inflammation of the gland. The histological appearances are simply those of an acute inflammation (Fig. 5.4) and this usually subsides with antibiotics and adequate drainage. The inflammation may, however, leave a residue in the form of a ductal cyst or may sink into a chronic stage.

A chronic Bartholin's adenitis may be a sequel to an inadequately treated acute infection and is often asymptomatic, presenting only as a nodule or an area of induration in the lateral wall of the introitus. However, there may be repeated episodes of acute flare-up of the infection which can lead to an abscess or to cyst formation.

Occasionally, Bartholin's gland is infected by *Mycobacterium tuberculosis*. Whilst the gland alone is sometimes involved, it is more usual to find evidence of tuberculosis elsewhere in the genital tract.

Vagina

Inflammatory disease of the vagina rarely exists in isolation, usually being associated with either vulval or cervical inflammation.

Non-infective inflammation

A non-infective vaginitis often follows trauma or surgery. This is particularly evident in the vault following a hysterectomy when non-specific granulation tissue may form and can be perpetuated by the presence of foreign material. Inflammation is sometimes seen in patients with a prolapse where the exposed vaginal mucosa is subject to trauma and may complicate the wearing of a pessary, or a tampon, the introduction of foreign bodies or irritant chemical substances. A post-irradiation vaginitis is

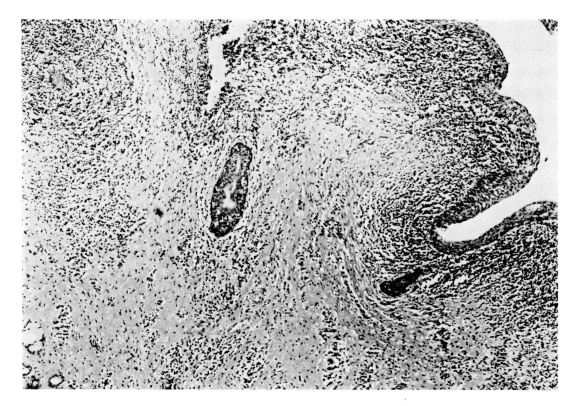

Fig. 5.4 Bartholin's gland abscess. The lumen of the distended, thick-walled, inflamed duct lies to the right and glandular acini can be seen in the lower left corner (H. & E. × 45).

characterized by a plasma cell infiltrate, obliterative endarteritis, atypia of stromal fibroblasts and hyalinization of vaginal collagen; it may be complicated by the development of vesicovaginal or rectovaginal fistulae.

A particular form of non-infective inflammation is the rare condition of *desquamative inflammatory vaginitis* in which the vaginal mucosa is thin and red, resembling that of the postmenopausal woman. Histological examination shows oedema, congestion and a heavy chronic inflammatory cell infiltrate. Plasma oestrogen levels, are normal in this condition, the aetiology of which is currently unknown.

Infective inflammation

Many infections of the vagina are classed as *non-specific*, these tending to occur prepubertally or postmenopausally when the low oestrogen levels are associated with a high vaginal pH and poor cornification of the epithelium. A rather similar state of affairs exists in the puerperium and a non-specific vaginitis is also common at this time. Histological examination reveals a thin atrophic epithelium, which is often focally ulcerated, and a subepithelial lymphoplasmacytic infiltrate. It is now believed that many cases of non-specific vaginitis are due to infection with *Gardnerella vaginalis*, which is sexually transmitted. However, the role of mycoplasma, chlamydia and viruses in the aetiology of this condition is not yet fully determined and these organisms may eventually be recognized as important factors.

Viral infections

Herpes hominis virus vaginitis is present in nearly all patients with a herpetic vulvitis but is often over-shadowed by the vulval lesions and hence overlooked. The macroscopic and histological features are similar to those already described in the vulva, but occasionally the lesions may form large excavated ulcers which mimic a carcinoma.

Bacterial infections

Gonorrhoea may cause some slight oedema and congestion of the vagina in adults but does not produce a true vaginitis, the epithelium being resistant to infection by *N. gonorrhoea*. In childhood, however, the thinner mucosa is permeable to the organism, which is able to enter the stroma and produce oedema, hyperaemia and a chronic inflammatory cell infiltrate. Infection tends to be persistent and may resolve only if oestrogens are given. *Chancroid* and *granuloma inguinale* can involve the vagina and produce a destructive ulceration which may be confused clinically with a neoplasm. Vaginal *tuberculosis* is extremely rare and, although usually due to spread from elsewhere in the genital tract may, very exceptionally, be sexually transmitted. *Malakoplakia* of the vagina is a rare condition characterized by an infiltrate of foamy histiocytes in which laminated calcispheroids or Michaelis–Guttman bodies can be found. The condition is believed to represent an abnormal response to infection by *Escherichia coli*.

Spirochaetal infections

The chancre of primary *syphilis* rarely occurs in the vagina but the mucous snail track ulcers and condylomata lata of the secondary stage of the disease are occasionally found in the lower vagina.

Chlamydial infection

Lymphogranuloma venereum not infrequently involves the vagina and can lead to extensive ulceration which heals by marked fibrosis to produce a vaginal stricture or deformity. A non-specific vaginitis due to *Chlamydia trachomatis* may occur in the postmenopausal woman in whom the epithelium is atrophic.

Fungal infections

These are usually due to *C. albicans* and are often associated with a vulvitis. It should be noted, however, that most women who harbour this fungus in their vagina do not have any clinical evidence of a vaginitis. When a vaginitis does occur it is characterized by the presence of easily removed white patches and histological examination reveals fungal hyphae and an inflammatory exudate on the epithelial surface with an accompanying inflammatory cell infiltrate of the underlying tissues.

Protozoal infections

Trichomonal infection of the vagina is common during the reproductive years and is due to the flagellate protozoan *T. vaginalis*; infection is usually, but not invariably, transmitted sexually. In the acute stage there is vaginal discharge and the mucosa is reddened and granular. Oedema, erythema and a lymphoplasmocytic infiltrate of the stroma, which may extend into the epithelium to form pseudoabscesses, are the typical histological features; there may be focal ulceration. In a proportion of patients, following an acute episode, the infection passes into a chronic phase, this being associated with a malodorous vaginal discharge and a persistence of the inflammatory process, although in a somewhat damped down manner, in the vagina. Other patients become asymptomatic carriers, the organism persisting in the vagina but not eliciting any inflammatory reaction.

Schistosomiasis of the vagina occurs in areas in which this disease is endemic.

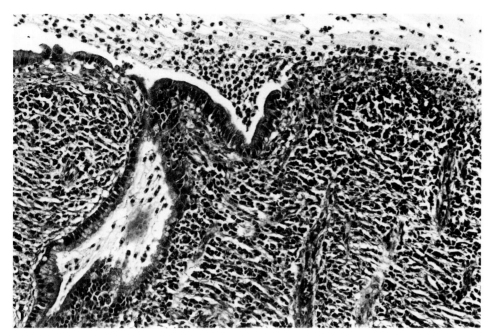

Fig. 5.5 Active chronic non-specific cervicitis. The stroma is heavily infiltrated by chronic inflammatory cells and, to the right, there is a purulent exudate where the surface is ulcerated (H. & E. × 186).

Cervix

A cervicitis can occur as an isolated lesion or may be part of a more widespread inflammatory process in the genital tract. However, there has been, and indeed still is, a tendency to diagnose cervicitis, particularly the chronic form, with undue and unwarranted frequency. The cervix has a normal population of lymphocytes and plasma cells, particularly in the area adjacent to the squamocolumnar junction, and the presence of such cells in relatively small or moderate numbers does not justify a diagnosis of inflammation in the absence of other features of an inflammatory process. The cervix has, in fact, a rather stereotyped and non-specific response to inflammatory agents, whether these be of an infective or non-infective nature. Thus, acute inflammation is characterized by stromal oedema and congestion, together with a polymorph infiltration of the epithelium, stroma and crypts. In severe cases there may be loss of secretory activity by the epithelial cells, degenerative changes in the columnar epithelium and focal ulceration (Fig. 5.5). If inflammation persists and enters a chronic phase, the cellular infiltrate becomes predominantly lymphoplasmacytic and histiocytic, although polymorphs may persist in the crypts and surface epithelium. There may be formation of non-specific granulation tissue and gradual fibrosis. In some instances granulomata may be seen, whilst in others lymphoid follicles with prominent germinal centres develop in the upper part of the stroma (follicular cervicitis).

Non-infective inflammation

An acute cervical inflammation may follow the use of douches, ointments or abortifacients, obstetric trauma, surgery, cryosurgery or diathermy. A chronic inflammatory cell infiltrate is also commonly seen in women using an IUCD or ICD, whilst bleeding from cervical endometriosis may elicit a similar response. Exposure of the columnar epithelium of an ectopy to the acid pH of the vagina may result in an acute or chronic inflammation, whilst ulceration of a prolapsed cervix will similarly be accompanied by an inflammatory infiltrate. Irradiation of the cervix is generally followed by a plasmacytic inflammatory response.

An *inflammatory pseudotumour* or *lymphoma-like lesion* of the cervix may develop when there is chronic inflammation. It is characterized by the presence of a dense infiltrate of large, mitotically active lymphoid cells and is distinguished from a lymphoma by its superficial nature, the frequent presence of surface ulceration and the presence, within the infiltrate, of neutrophil polymorphonuclear leucocytes, polyclonal plasma cells and small lymphocytes. It is rare for such infiltrates to form a clinically significant mass and their importance lies in their possible misinterpretation as a neoplasm.

A *necrotizing granulomatous cervicitis* is sometimes found following cervical surgery or in the presence of endometriosis. Its cause is uncertain but its behaviour is benign and the condition is usually diagnosed only following examination of a cervix removed for unrelated purposes.

Infective inflammation

Many infections of the cervix are of a non-specific polymicrobial nature. Bacterial infections tend to involve the endocervix in particular, partly because the deep crypts afford a safe harbour to bacteria and other organisms and partly because the columnar epithelium of the endocervix offers less resistance to infection than does the stratified squamous epithelium of the ectocervix. Chronic cervical inflammation occurs when there is obstruction to, and stasis of, cervical secretions and is therefore encountered when the vagina is obstructed by a foreign body or tumour or when the endocervical canal is blocked by a polyp, neoplasm or stricture. The resultant scarring and fibrosis lead to further crypt distortion, increasing obstruction and perpetuation of the inflammatory process. The organisms commonly isolated from inflamed cervices under these circumstances include coliforms, commensals, mycoplasma, *G. vaginalis* and chlamydiae, but the role of these organisms as initiators of an inflammatory process is not yet proven.

The post-partum or postabortive state may be complicated by an acute or chronic cervicitis, the causative organisms of which have usually been identified as Gram-positive cocci or fecal organisms. The inflammation associated with an IUCD, although usually of an irritative, sterile nature, is sometimes due to a polymicrobial infection.

Viral infections

Herpes hominis virus infection of the cervix is often associated with vaginal and vulval infection. Herpetic lesions of the cervix usually take the form of shallow ulcers with a necrotic base and raised margins; rarely, there may be a gross necrotizing cervicitis. The histological changes (Fig. 5.6) are similar to those already described for vulval herpetic lesions.

There is an epidemiological association between intraepithelial and invasive neoplasia of the cervix and herpes infection, but a true causal relationship between the two has not yet been established.

Bacterial infections

The cervix is an important site of localization of *gonorrhoea* but, because the squamous epithelium of the ectocervix is relatively impermeable to *N. gonorrhoea*, infection with this highly contagious sexually transmitted organism initially causes an acute exudative endocervicitis, characterized by stromal congestion and oedema with a seropurulent exudate. The surface columnar epithelium shows patchy degeneration and focal ulceration. The infection spreads into the endocervical crypts from which it may clear, become chronic, or spread to the endometrium and fallopian tubes. An asymptomatic carrier state supervenes in a proportion of patients. A chronic gonococcal cervicitis is associated with pericryptal fibrosis, crypt distortion and stasis of cervical secretions, all factors which not only tend to perpetuate the disease but also predispose to secondary infection.

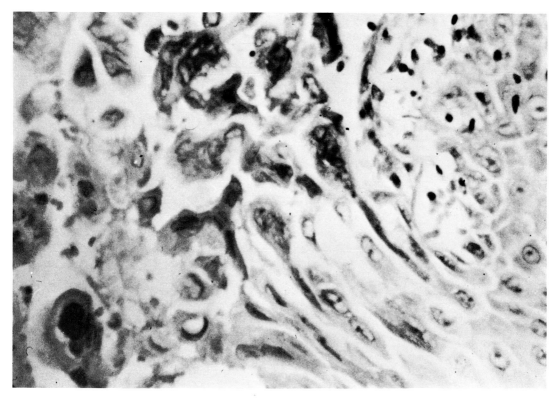

Fig. 5.6 Herpes simplex. The margin of a cervical herpetic ulcer shows a viral inclusion with surrounding halo in the lower left corner and multinucleated epithelial cells are present in the centre (H. & E. × 300).

Chancroid occasionally affects the cervix, as does *granuloma inguinale*. *Tuberculosis* of the cervix is rare and usually due to spread from elsewhere in the genital tract. However, very exceptional instances of sexual transmission of cervical tuberculosis have been recorded. The cervix affected by tuberculosis often has a rather non-specific gross appearance but is sometimes bulky, friable and extensively ulcerated, an appearance that may lead to an unfounded suspicion of a carcinoma. The diagnosis is established histologically by the presence of caseating granulomata.

Infection with *Actinomyces israelii* may follow surgical instrumentation or criminal abortion, is sometimes encountered in women wearing an IUCD and may be a consequence of direct spread from an intestinal or parametrial infection.

Chlamydial infections
Primary cervical lesions of *lymphogranuloma venereum* may pass unnoticed but the destructive ulceration and extensive scarring characteristic of the chronic stage of this disease can result in marked cervical distortion. Spread of the inflammatory process into the parametrium may fix the cervix and produce a mass that is easily mistaken for a carcinoma. The histological appearances are identical to those seen in the vulva (see above).

Other members of the chlamydial group of organisms have been isolated from cervices showing a non-specific chronic inflammation, this often having a follicular pattern.

Spirochaetal infections

The primary lesion of *syphilis* occurs in the cervix in approximately 40 per cent of genital infections with *T. pallidum*. The lesions may be small or form the typical hard, ulcerated chancre. Occasionally, multiple small ulcers, resembling those seen in a herpetic cervicitis, are seen, whilst the chancre may have a hypertrophic fungating appearance suggestive of a carcinoma. When the endocervix is infected, the whole *portio vaginalis* may become indurated and oedematous. The histological features of a cervical chancre are identical to those of a vulval primary lesion (see above). The mucous patches of the secondary stage can occur on the cervix but condyloma lata are not seen and the cervix is a most exceptional site for the development of a gumma.

Mycotic infections

Infection of the cervix by *C. albicans* usually occurs as a complication of a monilial vulvovaginitis. White patches are seen on the cervix and removal of these leaves either an area of erythema or a shallow ulcer.

Protozoal infections

Infections of the vagina and cervix by *T. vaginalis* are inseparable. In the acute phase, the cervix is erythematous and has a 'strawberry' appearance, the red spots on the cervix corresponding to congested ectatic capillaries in the epithelial papillae. The squamous epithelium shows superficial degeneration and is infiltrated by acute inflammatory cells, whilst there is usually a mild chronic inflammatory cell infiltrate of the stroma. Trichomonads may be seen in cervical smears, but in about one-third of cases in which these organisms are detected in this manner, the cervix shows no histological abnormality.

Schistosomiasis not infrequently involves the cervix to produce a bulky induration which is sometimes associated with the formation of polypoidal masses and with ulceration. The typical histological picture is of a severe granulomatous reaction to the presence of ova, but there is sometimes a more diffuse inflammatory infiltrate of plasma cells, histiocytes and eosinophils, whilst occasional focal eosinophilic abscesses may be formed. Progressive fibrosis may lead to the formation of a firm mass and to gross cervical distortion. The squamous epithelium of the cervix often shows a pseudoepitheliomatous hyperplasia and this, in association with the gross appearances, can lead to an erroneous diagnosis of carcinoma. Carcinoma of the cervix is, in fact, common in areas where schistosomiasis is rife and hence the two conditions may coexist, almost certainly fortuitously, in the same cervix.

Endometrium

The endometrium has a normal complement of lymphocytes, lymphoid follicles and polymorphonuclear-like cells (K cells) whilst oedema, congestion, polymorph infiltration and necrosis are all normal features of the luteal phase of the cycle. Hence, endometritis is difficult to define in precise histological terms, although the presence of microabscesses which disrupt the stroma and glands is taken as a diagnostic criterion of acute endometritis. The presence of plasma cells in the endometrium is usually regarded as the hallmark of a chronic endometritis but, in practice, an increase in the stromal population of lymphocytes and histiocytes is usually also present (Fig. 5.7). The presence of granulomata is, of course, clear evidence of an inflammatory process.

In many cases of endometritis the cyclical activity of the endometrium continues normally, but some severe infections appear to induce a resistance to ovarian hormones with consequent loss of the normal pattern of cyclic activity.

Any severe or long standing endometritis may result in fibrosis with the formation of synechiae. This condition, known as Asherman's syndrome, is discussed in Chapter 14.

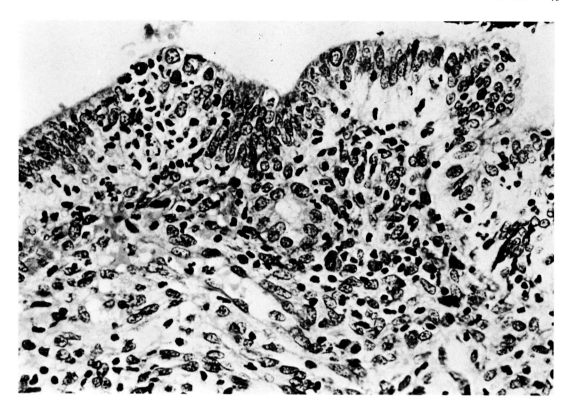

Fig. 5.7 Active chronic non-specific endometritis. A cellular infiltrate of polymorphs and occasional plasma cells is present in the endometrial stroma and epithelium (H. & E. × 270).

Non-infective inflammation

The introduction of chemical irritants into the uterine cavity, e.g. in attempting to procure an abortion, causes an acute endometritis whilst the presence of a foreign body, such as an IUCD, will also elicit an inflammatory response. A non-specific inflammation of the endometrium, which is predominantly plasmacytic and is associated with tissue necrosis and obliterative lesions of the vessels, may follow irradiation. In early pregnancy, remodelling of the decidua is associated with focal necrosis and an acute inflammatory cell infiltrate, changes which are physiological and should not be interpreted as indicative of infection. Similarly, there may be a quite well marked lymphoplasmacytic infiltrate of the mature decidua, which may persist for some time after delivery.

Cervical stenosis, due either to neoplasm or to postoperative fibrosis, sometimes results in a pyometra in which sterile purulent material fills and distends the uterine cavity. This is often associated with extensive squamous metaplasia of the endometrium and is occasionally complicated by a squamous cell carcinoma. Cervical obstruction may also be associated with an unusual form of *histiocytic endometritis*, in which the uterine cavity is partially or completely lined by sheets of foamy histiocytic cells. Focal collections of plasma cells and lymphocytes are usually present. The histiocytes contain lipid, and often iron, and it is thought that this condition represents the end stage of an absorbed pyometra.

Infective inflammation

Infection occurs less commonly in the endometrium than elsewhere in the genital tract, this being attributable to the combination of an effective cervical mucus barrier, excellent natural drainage and regular endometrial shedding.

Instrumentation or the insertion of an IUCD may introduce vaginal or cervical organisms into the normally sterile endometrial cavity, whilst trauma to the cervix by obstetrical damage or deep cone biopsy may disrupt the cervical barrier and allow for the ascent of similar organisms. Some organisms, such as *N. gonorrhoea*, can penetrate the normal cervical barrier, whilst others descend from the tubes. Only occasionally does infection reach the endometrium via the bloodstream. Certain intrauterine factors predispose to the establishment of an infection; these include the postpartum state, the retention of products of conception, endometrial neoplasm and the presence of infarcted tissues such as twisted endometrial polypi or pedunculated submucous leiomyomata. The infection complicating such conditions is of a non-specific nature and commonly polymicrobial, faecal organisms being isolated with greatest frequency.

Viral infections
Herpes infection is recognized much less commonly in the endometrium than in the lower genital tract. This infection does, however, produce characteristic changes, which include nuclear enlargement with a typical 'ground glass' appearance, epithelial multinucleation and viral inclusion bodies.

Cytomegalovirus endometritis is unusual but can be recognized by the presence of very large haematoxyphilic intranuclear inclusions and small basophilic cytoplasmic inclusions in the same cell.

Bacterial infections
A *gonococcal endometritis* is usually a transient, acute asymptomatic infection which is rarely recognized histologically. In the very unusual cases of chronic gonococcal endometritis, the appearances are quite non-specific and are characterized only by a lymphoplasmacytic infiltrate.

Tuberculosis of the endometrium is now uncommon in Western countries but is still frequently encountered in other parts of the world. It occurs most commonly during the reproductive years, is rare after the menopause and is almost invariably associated with, and is secondary to, tuberculous salpingitis. The facts that infection of the endometrium occurs by direct transluminal spread to the zona superficialis, that the infection takes fifteen to twenty days to become established and that the functional layer of the endometrium is regularly shed in premenopausal women have three important bearings on diagnosis. First, infection of the basal layer and of the myometrium is very uncommon because the infected, more superficial, layer is shed before the disease can penetrate to that depth. Second, unless a biopsy is taken late in the cycle there may have been insufficient time for the development of the typical granulomata and the histological findings may thus be totally non-specific. Third, there may be little or no caseation. The persistence of endometrial tuberculosis despite the regular shedding of the reproductive years suggests that constant reinfection probably occurs from the tubes.

In premenopausal women, a biopsy taken late in the menstrual cycle will often reveal caseating or, more commonly, non-caseating granulomata formed of epithelioid cells, Langhans giant cells and a perigranulomatous cuff of lymphocytes (Fig. 5.8). Intraglandular polymorphs are often also present. However, in some cases, tuberculosis masquerades as a non-specific chronic endometritis characterized by an infiltrate of lymphocytes and plasma cells. In such cases, a clue to the true nature of the infection is sometimes given by the presence of intraglandular polymorphs or of isolated cystically dilated glands containing inflammatory debris. In all cases a diagnosis of tuberculosis should be confirmed by culture, the finding of tubercle bacilli in histological sections (using the Ziehl–Neelsen technique) being notoriously difficult and unreliable.

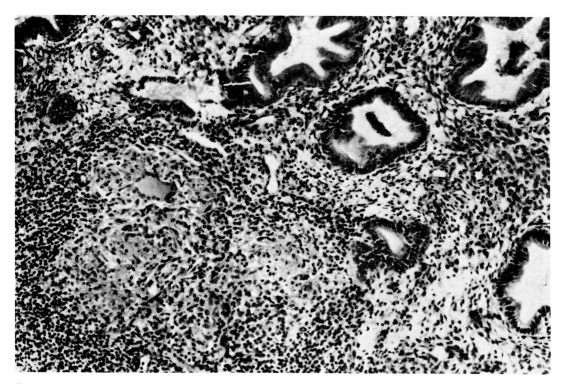

Fig. 5.8 Tuberculosis of the endometrium in a premenopausal woman. Two small non-caseating granulomata are present in the lower left of the illustration and one contains a Langhan's giant cell (H. & E. × 108).

Tuberculous endometritis is rare in postmenopausal women, possibly because of the decreased vascularity of the tissue. However, the lack of regular endometrial shedding in such patients means that there is no bar to the establishment of the infection and to its progression to caseation (Fig. 5.9). The uterine lining is shaggy and yellow-white, whilst the lumen may contain caseous material. Histological examination shows multiple granulomata, which are often confluent, extensive caseation and a variable degree of fibrosis. In contrast to the premenopausal patient, in whom tuberculosis is most often associated with infertility because of the presence of tubal disease, tuberculosis presenting in the postmenopausal years often causes bleeding and there may be a history of past normal fertility.

Actinomycosis of the endometrium is rare but has an increased incidence in patients wearing an IUCD; the infection is usually ascending. The histological picture is one of combined suppuration and granulomatous inflammation. Abscesses, which contain a dense core of neutrophil polymorphs and a surrounding rim of granulation tissue, form. The purulent exudate contains the stellate aggregates of the organism, these form the sulphur granules characteristic of this disease. The infection may be asymptomatic but can extend to produce a tubo-ovarian abscess. It should be stressed that the finding of *Actinomyces* in the endometrium of an IUCD wearer does not, in the absence of a typical inflammatory response, necessarily indicate an infection, for it is believed that the organism can behave as a commensal.

Malakoplakia of the endometrium is exceptionally rare. It is similar in many ways to a histiocytic endometritis, for example in that the lesions are characterized by aggregates of foamy histiocytic cells, but differs in that small iron- and calcium-containing bodies, known as Michaelis–Gutmann bodies, are present both within and outside the cells. The histiocytes contain partially digested bacteria and it is thought that the condition is usually due to an abnormal and inadequate histiocytic response to *E. coli*.

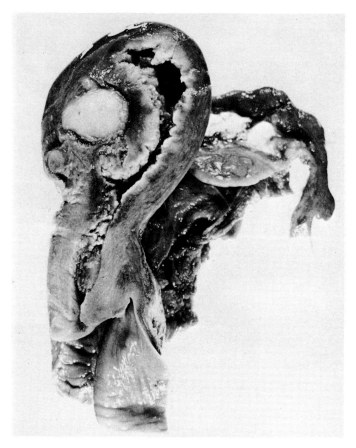

Fig. 5.9   Tuberculosis in the uterus of a postmenopausal woman. It is lined by a shaggy layer of caseous material.

Chlamydial infection
Chlamydiae have been isolated from cases of active chronic and non-specific chronic endometritis and their presence has been implicated in infertility.

Mycoplasmal infection
The morphological characteristics of a mycoplasmal endometritis are often rather subtle and there may be only a focal infiltrate of lymphocytes, neutrophil polymorphs and histiocytes. However, mycoplasma can also produce a typical chronic endometritis.

Fungal infections
A mycotic endometritis is extremely rare but very occasional lesions due to *Blastomyces*, *Cryptococcus*, *Aspergillus* and *Coccidioides* have been reported as occurring during the course of disseminated disease.

Protozoan and metazoan infections
Toxoplasma gondii has been isolated from some cases of chronic endometritis and cyst forms may be found in the uteri of chronically infected women. The histological appearances are otherwise quite non-specific.
   Schistosomiasis (Fig. 5.10) involves the endometrium less commonly than it does the vagina or cervix,

but the presence of ova elicits a granulomatous response and eosinophilic abscesses may develop. The effect of this infection on the endometrium can be very destructive.

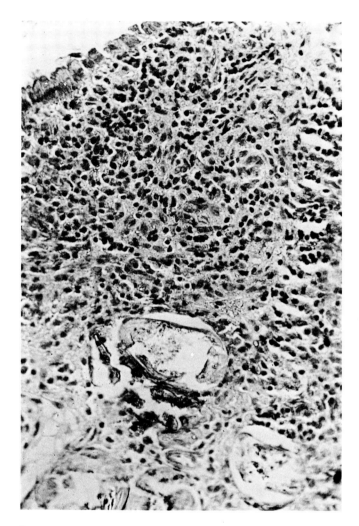

Fig. 5.10 Schistosomiasis. Degenerate ova in the endometrium of an East African patient, the inflammatory response is non-specific (H. & E. × 240).

Myometrium

Inflammatory disease of the myometrium is distinctly uncommon. In an acute inflammation the uterus is swollen and hyperaemic. Histologically, there is oedema, congestion and a neutrophil polymorph infiltrate. In a chronic myometritis there may be little or no macroscopic evidence of the disease but histological examination reveals a variable degree of plasmalymphocytic infiltrate and fibrosis.

Non-infective inflammation

This may occur as a response to degenerative changes in a leiomyoma, haemorrhage from adenomyosis or irradiation. Following an endometrial or cervical biopsy, a diffuse *eosinophilis myometritis* occasionally develops. The eosinophils probably represent a tissue response to trauma and their presence is of no pathological or clinical significance. A non-specific chronic myometritis characterized by aggregates of lymphocytes, lying particularly in relation to the lymphatics and veins of the myometrium, is also described and, on rare occasions, chronic inflammation may lead to the development of an *inflammatory pseudotumour* of the myometrium. This has been reported in childhood and in the reproductive years and is characterized by the presence of a solid, non-encapsulated but well-circumscribed, tumour-like mass of interweaving bundles of myofibroblastic spindle cells interspersed with mixed inflammatory cells. The prognosis for these benign lesions is excellent and their removal is usually associated with resolution of any systemic disturbances.

Infective inflammation

Myometrial infection occurs almost without exception as a consequence of spread from a severe endometritis and is seen occasionally in the puerperium, after an abortion and in IUCD wearers. An acute myometritis sometimes complicates gonorrhoea, whilst in postmenopausal women, endometrial tuberculosis may extend into the myometrium.

Fallopian tube

The term pelvic inflammatory disease refers to an all-embracing clinical concept which encompasses inflammatory lesions in the fallopian tubes, ovary, uterine ligaments and parametrial tissues. However, the use of this expression as a pathological diagnosis is insufficiently precise. It is true that, because of the close proximity of the tubes and ovaries, infection in one often leads to adhesions between the two organs and spread of infection to produce *tubo-ovarian disease* and, indeed, pelvic inflammation may be so extensive at the time of diagnosis that it may be impossible to recognize a primary focus. However, such cases are in the minority and inflammation is usually limited to one organ or site, most commonly to the fallopian tube.

Non-infective inflammation

Inflammation is sometimes noted in tubes removed during the menstrual phase or in the immediate postpartum period. This is known as *physiological salpingitis* and is often thought to represent a reaction to the presence of blood and fragments of necrotic endometrium that have entered the tube as a result of uterotubal reflux. The inconsistency and low incidence of inflammatory change, together with its absence in some cases in which tissue fragments are clearly visible, suggest that this may not be the whole story, although it must be admitted that no infective cause for this not uncommon lesion has been established.

The presence of foreign bodies, either on the tubal serosa, e.g. starch granules or a sterilizing clip, or within the wall of the tube, e.g. suture material, will provoke a granulomatous response. Oily substances are no longer used for radiological studies because they were also prone to cause the development of granulomatous inflammation. From time to time, however, this abnormality is encountered in a patient who had studies undertaken many years previously.

Infective inflammation

Organisms may enter the tube by direct ascent through the uterine cavity, or alternatively, reach the tube via lymphatics or blood vessels. Transluminal spread will lead to an infection which predominantly involves the mucosa, and which will thus result in an *endosalpingitis*, whilst organisms reaching the tube via the lymphatics will localize principally in the wall and thus produce an *interstitial salpingitis*.

In practice, most cases of tubal infection seen today are of the endosalpingeal type. It was traditionally thought that *N. gonorrhoea* was the prime cause of such an infection: however, it is now recognized that many, probably most, such infections are of a non-specific polymicrobial nature, with organisms such as *Bacteroides* species, *E. coli*, chlamydiae, viruses and *Mycoplasma* species playing an aetiological role. In a proportion of cases, *N. gonorrhoea* may well have initiated the inflammatory episode but the ability of this organism to produce an established salpingitis is now doubted by many, perpetuation of inflammation being due to a secondary infection of the damaged tube by a variety of organisms. In an acute endosalpingitis (Fig. 5.11a and b), the tube is congested and thickened, the mucosa being swollen, hyperaemic and focally haemorrhagic. The lining epithelium undergoes focal necrosis and the lumen becomes filled and distended with cellular debris and an exudate of neutrophil polymorphs. In very severe infections there may be spread to the tubal wall, a transmural polymorph infiltration with production of a local peritonitis or extension to the ovary to produce an oöphoritis or a tubo-ovarian abscess. Pus may leak from the fimbrial end of the tube and this can lead to a pelvic abscess, a subphrenic abscess or a generalized peritonitis. More commonly, although pus is spilled in small amounts from the tube, the fibropurulent exudate causes fimbrial agglutination and obstruction, the pus accumulating within a progressively distended tube to produce a *pyosalpinx*. However, this is an unusual complication of an acute endosalpingitis, occurring more commonly in subacute, progressive or recurrent infections.

The sequelae of an acute endosalpingitis vary with the degree of tubal damage incurred in the acute phase. Mild inflammation may resolve completely or result only in a minor degree of mucosal scarring. However, if inflammation has been associated with marked epithelial necrosis and a fibropurulent exudate there may be total obliteration of the lumen in the isthmus, where it is narrow, and in the ampulla, where the lumen is wider, the plicae tend to fuse as healing occurs and this results in a subdivision of the lumen into a honeycomb by a meshwork of epithelial strands covering fine fibrovascular cores (Fig. 5.12). A *follicular salpingitis* is indicative of severe tubal damage and there are associated functional disturbances which include the development, in the isthmus, of diverticula. These are sometimes known by the descriptive term *salpingitis isthmica nodosa* (Fig. 5.13). Both follicular salpingitis and salpingitis isthmica nodosa predispose to tubal pregnancy. If there has also been a local peritonitis, fibrous adhesions may form between the tube and ovary or between adjacent loops of the tube. Fimbrial agglutination during the acute stage may result in permanent tubal occlusion.

In other cases, the end result of a tubal inflammation may be a *hydrosalpinx*, in which the tube becomes distended with watery fluid (Fig. 5.14). The wall is thin and translucent and the tubal lumen may be loculated (follicular hydrosalpinx). Histologically, the epithelium is flattened but otherwise well preserved, and occasional shallow plicae are found (Fig. 5.15); the mural muscle may be partially fibrosed. A hydrosalpinx is traditionally thought to be an end result of a pyosalpinx but this is unlikely and, indeed, it is not known with certainty whether a hydrosalpinx is a consequence of infection and acute inflammation. In many cases there is certainly no preceding history of pelvic inflammation. It also has to be noted that, although the fimbrial ostium of a hydrosalpinx is occluded, the uterine ostia are patent and the medial portion of the tube little, if at all, dilated. This suggests that the basic damage may well have been to the muscle wall with a consequent failure of tubal motility.

An interstitial salpingitis is extremely rare nowadays but used to occur with some frequency in the pre-antibiotic era as a result of streptococcal spread to the tube, via the lymphatic vessels, from a puerperal uterine sepsis. The inflammation under such circumstances is largely confined to the tubal wall, which is

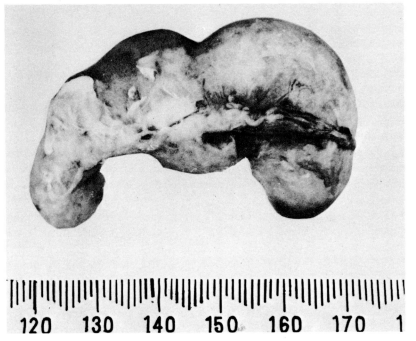

Fig. 5.11(a) Acute salpingitis. The tube is distended, the ostium occluded and the serosa is covered by a pale, purulent exudate.

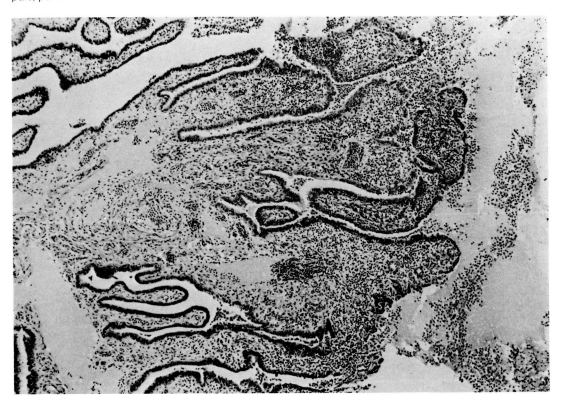

Fig. 5.11(b) Acute endosalpingitis. The plicae are swollen and infiltrated by polymorphs. The covering epithelium is focally ulcerated and the lumen contains pus (H. & E. × 45).

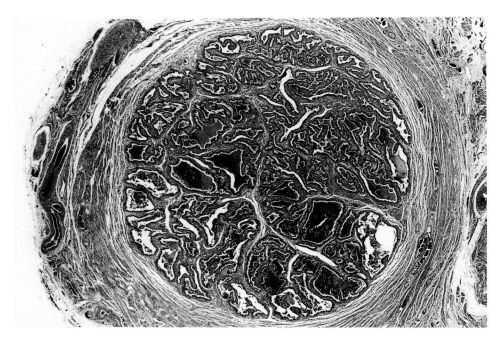

Fig. 5.12 Follicular salpingitis. The lumen is traversed by bands formed by plical fusion but there is minimal residual active inflammation (H. & E. × 18.5).

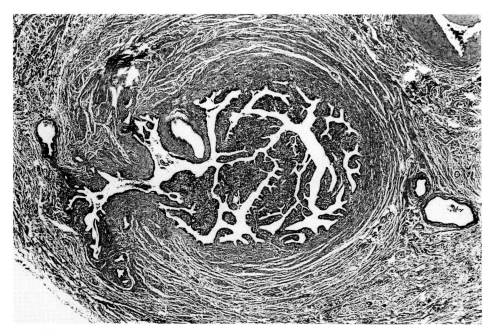

Fig. 5.13 Salpingitis isthmica nodosa. A diverticulum extends from the lumen of the fallopian tube (left) and several other diverticula can be seen, within the wall, cut in transverse section (H. & E. × 37).

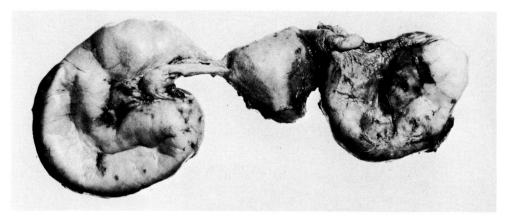

Fig. 5.14   Hydrosalpinx. Both fallopian tubes are occluded distally and distended, their general appearance being 'retort-shaped'.

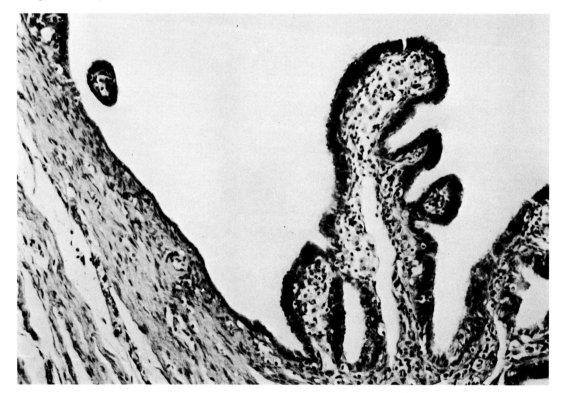

Fig. 5.15   The wall of a hydrosalpinx. Although the tube is greatly distended, shallow plicae persist. The mucosal stroma contains foamy macrophages and occasional lymphocytes indicative of chronic inflammation (H. & E. × 108).

thickened by an infiltrate of acute inflammatory cells. Because of the relative, or absolute, sparing of the epithelium, subsidence of this type of salpingitis may leave a functionally normal tube.

Bacterial infections

Tuberculosis of the tube is invariably secondary to a focus of infection elsewhere in the body, the organisms

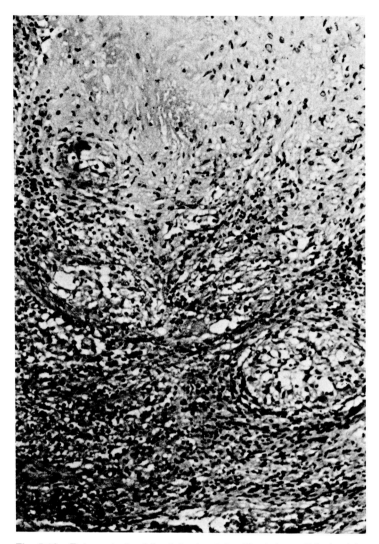

Fig. 5.16 Tuberculosis of the fallopian tube. The tube wall (below) is completely replaced by fibrous tissue, granulomata and a chronic inflammatory cell infiltrate. The mucosa is destroyed and the lumen (above) contains caseous material (H. & E. × 108).

reaching the tube via the bloodstream from a pulmonary focus, by lymphatic spread from an intestinal lesion or by direct spread from the genitourinary tract, gastrointestinal tract or peritoneum. Tubal lesions are found in approximately 20 per cent of women dying from tuberculosis, are associated with endometrial tuberculosis in about 50 per cent of cases, are frequently asymptomatic and are now an uncommon cause of infertility in Western countries.

At the time of diagnosis, the tube has often become converted into a distended retort-shaped, fibrotic sac which is focally calcified and contains caseous material. Surprisingly, the fimbria are sometimes relatively normal and the ostium patent. In some instances, the disease may cause only a little focal nodular thickening of the tube, with scanty peritoneal adhesions, whilst in other cases adhesions form between the tube and ovary and around the fimbria and ostia, with resulting complete tubal occlusion.

In the typical case, histological examination shows a chronic endosalpingitis together with caseating granulomata in the mucosa (Fig. 5.16). These may extend into, and destroy, the wall. Caseation is not invariably found and in the non-caseating form granulomata may be numerous and the giant cells frequently contain laminated Schaumann bodies. By the time a tuberculous pyosalpinx is reached, the wall is usually focally calcified and there is a lining of granulation tissue and caseous material in which occasional tuberculous granulomata may be present. The possibility of some cases of hydrosalpinx having a tuberculous origin is suggested by the finding of foci of calcification in the wall. Tubal tuberculosis may be accompanied by a marked epithelial hyperplasia, which may show some degree of atypia and thus be mistakenly considered as a carcinoma. To complicate matters still further, there have been a few reports of undoubted coexistent adenocarcinoma and tuberculosis of the tube.

Most patients with tubal tuberculosis are rendered sterile, although if treatment of the disease is undertaken at an early stage, a patent but scarred tube may result, a situation that appears to predispose to tubal gestation.

Actinomycosis of the tube is rare and usually also involves the ovary. Infection occurs via the uterine cavity or by direct spread from a focus in adjacent pelvic or abdominal organs. A multilocular fibrous mass with irregular cavities lined by shaggy, congested tissue and containing pus in which typical 'sulphur granules' may be found gradually develops. Histologically, the locules contain an acute purulent exudate and the walls are composed of granulation tissue infiltrated by plasma cells, lymphocytes and histiocytes. The histiocytes tend to be large and characteristically have a clear, slightly foamy cytoplasm. Aggregated masses of the organism are usually readily apparent. Although actinomycosis is, as already remarked, a rare infection, it has increased in incidence in recent years, this being due to the tendency for this infection to affect women wearing an IUCD.

Mycoplasmal infections

Mycoplasma hominis can cause a chronic salpingitis with a predominantly plasmalymphocytic infiltrate but with clusters of neutrophil polymorphs associated with focal epithelial necrosis.

Protozoan and metazoan infections

Schistosomiasis is a common cause of tubal disease in those parts of the world where this disease is endemic. The lesions are nodular and fibrotic and are associated with infertility and tubal pregnancy.

Ovary

Non-infective inflammation

This may occur as a consequence of bleeding from ovarian endometriosis, as a result of surgery or as a consequence of irradiation. It is often particularly marked following hysterectomy and, as a consequence, adhesions may bind the residual tube and ovary together. The subsequent accumulation of fluid within the peritoneal adhesions may mimic the development of an ovarian cyst and may give rise to pain.

Infective inflammation

Ovarian infection is uncommon and is usually due to direct spread of organisms from an adherent infected fallopian tube. In the absence of tubal disease, infection is usually related to surgery or investigative procedures. Spread of organisms from the tube may affect only the surface of the ovary and produce either an acute or a chronic *perioöphoritis* (Fig. 5.17). Often, however, the infection does extend into the ovarian substance. Histological examination at the stage of a perioöphoritis will show a fibrinous exudate

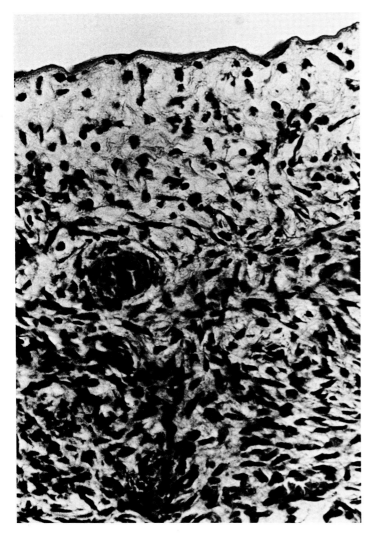

Fig. 5.17 Acute non-specific perioöphoritis. The surface of the ovary is oedematous and there is a mild acute non-specific inflammatory cell infiltrate. Focal superficial haemorrhage is present (H. & E. × 270).

on the surface but, with extension into the ovarian parenchyma, a multilocular thick-walled abscess develops. This usually involves both the ovary and tube and microscopy will show necrosis, granulation tissue formation and a neutrophil polymorph infiltration. In older lesions, dense fibrosis, a plasmalymphocytic infiltrate and the presence of foamy macrophages are characteristic features.

Viral infections
Viral infections of the ovary are seldom recognized but approximately 5 per cent of women with *mumps* develop clinically apparent oöphoritis and a greater number probably have asymptomatic involvement of the ovary. Rarely, in immunosuppressed patients, *cytomegalovirus* infection of the ovary can be detected histologically.

Bacterial infections

Tuberculosis of the ovary is uncommon and may be either secondary to tubal infection or share a common haematogenous source. The ovarian cortex may contain granulomata but caseation and abscess formation are rare.

Actinomycotic ovarian abscesses can develop by spread from an appendicular focus, but are more commonly due to an ascending infection in IUCD wearers.

Protozoan and metazoan infections

Schistosomiasis of the ovary results in the formation of multiple, small, white surface nodules which consist of granulomata formed around ova. An associated inflammatory infiltrate of histiocytes, lymphocytes and eosinophils may also be present.

Key references

Buckley C H and Fox H. (1989) *Biopsy Pathology of the Endometrium.* Chapman and Hall, London.
Chow W, Patten V and Marshall J R. (1979) Bacteriology of acute pelvic inflammatory disease. *American Journal of Obstetrics and Gynecology* **132**, 362–5.
Coleman D V and Evans D M D. (1988) *Biopsy Pathology and Cytology of the Cervix.* Chapman and Hall, London.
Eschenbach D A *et al.* (1975) Polymicrobiol etiology of acute pelvic inflammatory disease. *New England Journal of Medicine* **293**, 166–71.
Gilks C B, Taylor G P and Clement P B. (1987) Inflammatory pseudotumor of the uterus. *International Journal of Gynecological Pathology* **6**, 275–86.
Oriel J D. (1988) Infective conditions of the vulva. In: *The Vulva*, pp. 78–137. Edited by C M Ridley, Churchill Livingstone, Edinburgh.
Schmidt W A. (1987) Pathology of the vagina. In: *Haines and Taylor, Obstetrical and Gynaecological Pathology, 3rd edn.* pp. 146–217. Edited by H Fox, Churchill Livingstone, Edinburgh.
Sweet R L. (1975) Anaerobic infections of the female genital tract. *American Journal of Obstetrics and Gynecology* **122**, 891–901.
Weiner S and Wallack E E. (1974) Ovarian histology in pelvic inflammatory disease. *American Journal of Obstetrics and Gynecology* **43**, 431–7.

6

Metaplasia and heterotopia

Both metaplasia and heterotopia occur with some frequency in the female genital tract and ovaries, the changes resulting from these processes ranging in importance from mere histological curiosities to lesions of considerable clinical significance. *Metaplasia* is the term applied to the process by which a differentiated cell type changes into, or is replaced by, a quite different type of cell which is alien to that site, e.g. squamous metaplasia of the columnar epithelium of the endocervix results in the replacement of the columnar by squamous epithelium. *Heterotopia*, by contrast, refers to the displacement into an ectopic site of differentiated, non-metaplastic tissue, a classic example of this being the presence of endometrial tissue in the gastrointestinal tract. A distinction between metaplasia and heterotopia is, however, not always possible. Thus, for example, if spicules of bone are found in the endometrium it is usually impossible to tell if this is due to heterotopic bone formation or to osseous metaplasia of endometrial stromal cells. Furthermore, some abnormalities often assumed to be of a clearly heterotopic nature may in reality be the result of a metaplastic change, e.g. pelvic endometriosis may be due, not to displacement of endometrial tissue, but to endometrial metaplasia of the peritoneal mesothelium. A distinction between the processes of metaplasia and heterotopia is usually only of academic interest but, for the purposes of clarity, an attempt will be made to differentiate between the two in this chapter.

Metaplasia

Cervix

Squamous metaplasia in the cervix is a physiological process. It will be appreciated that the endocervix is lined by columnar epithelium and the ectocervix by squamous epithelium, which is in continuity with that of the vagina. The site where these two epithelia meet is known as the squamocolumnar junction and, although this varies in position, in prepubertal girls, it is usually at the margins of the external os. During puberty and, even more markedly, in pregnancy there is a considerable increase in cervical bulk and this leads to an unfolding of the cervix with a passive eversion of the distal endocervical columnar epithelium out on to what is anatomically the ectocervix, this being known as an *ectopy* (often wrongly called an erosion). The exposure of the delicate endocervical epithelium to the acid environment of the vagina results in its undergoing squamous metaplasia to produce a more robust epithelium of stratified squamous cells. In the early stages of this process, immature squamous cells are seen below, and pushing up, the columnar cells, a condition often referred to as *reserve cell hyperplasia* (Fig. 6.1). The columnar cells eventually degenerate and there is differentiation of the cells into immature and, eventually, mature squamous epithelium, the immature form differing from the mature epithelium in its lack of surface differentiation (Fig. 6.2). The end result of this process of squamous metaplasia is that the squamocolumnar junction will again be at the margin of the external os and the area of new squamous epithelium between the original squamocolumnar junction, which now lies out on the ectocervix, and the new squamocolumnar junction at the lip of the os is known as the *transformation zone*. It is in this zone that

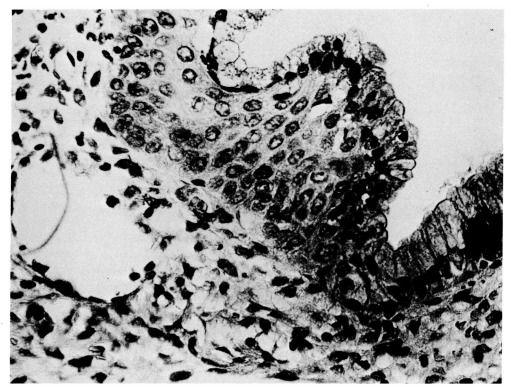

Fig. 6.1 Reserve cell hyperplasia in the cervix. Immature squamous cells (reserve cells) are seen beneath a layer of normal endocervical columnar cells (H. & E. × 270).

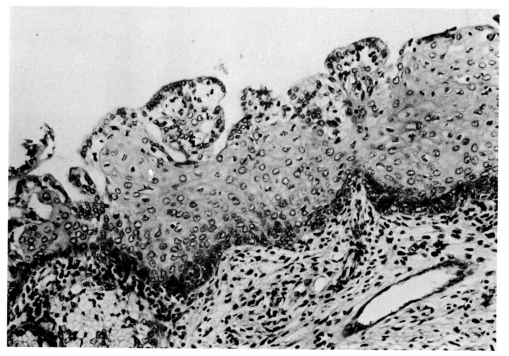

Fig. 6.2 Immature squamous metaplasia in the cervix. Although the full thickness of the epithelium is occupied by squamous cells, they show a lack of surface differentiation (H. & E. × 108).

intraepithelial neoplasia and most invasive squamous cell neoplasms of the cervix originate and it is believed that during the relatively short time, probably not more than two or three weeks, which it takes for the transformation zone to undergo squamous metaplasia, the changing epithelium is particularly susceptible to oncogenic agents.

The exact mechanism by which squamous metaplasia is initiated in the cervix is ill-understood, although it is almost certain that the newly formed squamous epithelium is derived from uncommitted cells. Earlier suggestions that the squamous cells developed from undifferentiated 'reserve cells' lying between the base of the columnar epithelium and the basement membrane, from ingrowth of the ectocervical squamous epithelium beneath the columnar epithelium or from circulating mononuclear cells have not been substantiated.

Tubal metaplasia is commonly seen in the endocervical canal in either the surface epithelium or within the crypts. Apart from the fact that it appears more darkly staining than the normal mucus-secreting epithelium and may be mistaken, by the unwary, for cervical glandular intraepithelial neoplasia, it is without clinical significance. *Endometrial metaplasia* also occurs, the term being restricted to those cases in which metaplasia affects only the epithelium, the term endometriosis being used when both endometrial stroma and glands are present.

Less common forms of metaplasia include gastrointestinal metaplasia and epidermization. *Gastrointestinal metaplasia* is recognized by the presence, within the columnar epithelium, of goblet cells and by a change in the mucus to that of intestinal type. On occasions neoplasms may develop from these areas, thus giving rise to adenocarcinomata of gastrointestinal type. The term *epidermization* or *epidermal metaplasia* is used when the non-keratinizing squamous epithelium of the ectocervix is replaced by an epidermis characterized by the presence of skin appendages, including sebaceous glands and, on rare occasions, hair.

Endometrium

This tissue has a particular propensity to undergo metaplasia and undifferentiated endometrial cells possess a latent capacity to differentiate along a variety of müllerian pathways, thus giving rise to metaplastic epithelia which mimic those of the endocervix, fallopian tube or upper part of the vagina.

Squamous metaplasia is very common and diligent search will reveal occasional foci of metaplastic squamous epithelium in the endometria of the vast majority of healthy premenopausal women. The squamous epithelium is usually intraglandular (Fig. 6.3), often growing into the lumen as an island of squamous tissue but sometimes completely replacing the gland. The squamous nature of the cells is usually clearly apparent but there may be masses of rather indifferent-appearing cells showing little overt evidence of squamous differentiation. These masses often known as *morules*, are best regarded as foci of immature squamous metaplasia. Intraglandular squamous metaplasia is often particularly prominent in hyperplastic and neoplastic endometria. Nevertheless, this form of metaplasia is not in itself of any clinical or pathological significance and its presence is neither diagnostic of hyperplasia or neoplasia nor indicative of any tendency for the endometrium to develop these abnormalities. The endometrial surface epithelium occasionally undergoes focal squamous metaplasia in women wearing an IUCD whilst, rarely, the entire endometrium is replaced by squamous epithelium to give the condition of *ichthyosis uteri* (Fig. 6.4). This can complicate a chronic pyometra but on occasion develops spontaneously in elderly women, the squamous epithelium in such cases being prone to ulceration which may cause bleeding. The very rare squamous cell carcinomata of the endometrium usually arise in an ichthyotic uterus.

Tubal metaplasia is also commonly seen in the endometrial glandular epithelium, both during the normal proliferative phase and in hyperplasia. In true tubal metaplasia, all three cell types normally present in tubal epithelium (ciliated columnar cells, secretory cells and peg cells) are found (Fig. 6.5); the presence of ciliated cells only is not indicative of metaplasia, such cells being normally present in the

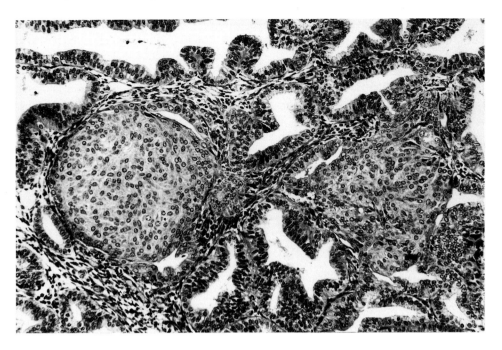

Fig. 6.3 Complex endometrial hyperplasia showing the typical intraglandular morules of squamous epithelium (H. & E. × 186).

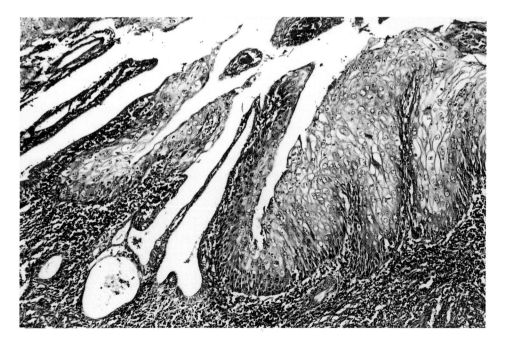

Fig. 6.4 Ichthyosis uteri. The endometrium from this elderly patient was replaced over large areas by metaplastic squamous epithelium, beneath which small foci of atrophic endometrium persist (H. & E. × 93)

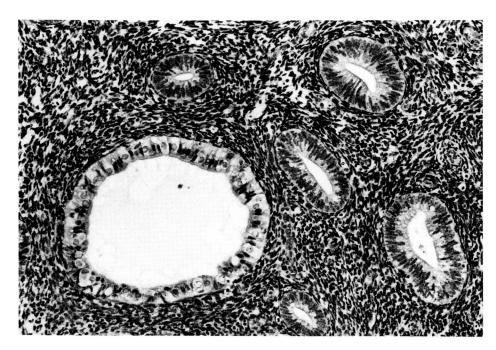

Fig. 6.5 Tubal metaplasia in the endometrium. The dilated gland (left) is lined by an epithelium in which ciliated, secretory and peg cells can be clearly seen. In contrast, the basal endometrial glands (right) are lined by a single population of cells (H. & E. × 186).

endometrium. The term *ciliated cell metaplasia* is sometimes used to describe an excess of endometrial ciliated cells but is not strictly appropriate to a tissue in which such cells are a normal component. Tubal metaplasia is, in itself, devoid of any clinical or pathological significance but it is probable that the rare serous papillary carcinoma of the endometrium is derived from metaplastic epithelium of this type.

Mucinous metaplasia, in which endometrial glandular epithelium undergoes metaplasia into columnar cells of endocervical type (Fig. 6.6) is uncommon. Single glands, or small groups of glands, are usually involved but occasionally the entire endometrium undergoes mucinous metaplasia, a change that can be accompanied by a markedly excessive accumulation of mucus in the uterine cavity.

Clear cell metaplasia and *hobnail metaplasia* are terms applied to the presence of glands lined by cuboidal cells with clear cytoplasm, these sometimes having hobnail nuclei. Glands with lining cells showing this pattern are the benign counterparts of the neoplastic glands seen in a clear cell adenocarcinoma of the endometrium, which is now considered to be of müllerian rather than mesonephric origin and which is formed of hypersecretory cells. Hence, this morphological appearance is probably due to a functional change in endometrial epithelial cells rather than to a metaplastic process. Similarly, the term *eosinophilic metaplasia* is applied to the finding of endometrial glands in which the lining cells have a strikingly acidophilic, granular cytoplasm (Fig. 6.7). Such cells are equivalent to the oncocytes seen in the thyroid and salivary glands and their unusual histological appearance is probably due to an alteration in their content of cytoplasmic organelles rather than to a metaplastic process.

Gastrointestinal metaplasia is a rare development in the endometrium. It is characterized by the presence of an epithelium composed partly or predominantly of goblet cells and may affect small or large areas of the endometrium.

Foci of mature bone or cartilage are occasionally encountered in the endometrial stroma and the presence of these alien tissues is usually attributed to *osseous* or *cartilaginous metaplasia* of endometrial

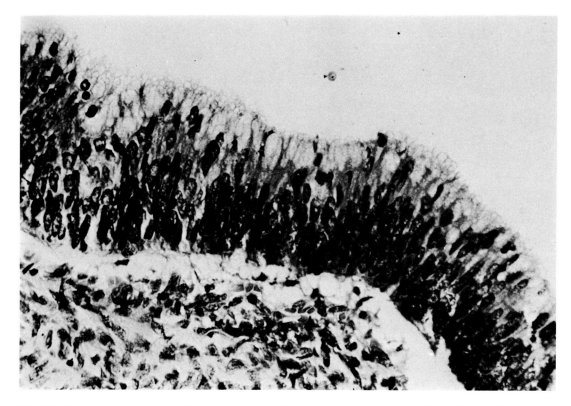

Fig. 6.6 Mucinous metaplasia of the endometrium. The entire endometrium is replaced by multilayered tall columnar cells similar in type to those seen in the cervix (H. & E. × 270).

stromal cells. This could well be true for most cases, but some examples of apparent cartilaginous or osseous metaplasia may, in fact, be due to implantation of fetal remnants following an abortion. Osseous metaplasia tends to occur particularly in chronically inflamed endometria but the only real significance of this, or of cartilaginous metaplasia, is that the finding of bone or cartilage may prompt an unfounded suspicion of mixed tumour with heterologous elements. Nodules of smooth muscle, forming so-called *intraendometrial leiomyomata*, are sometimes seen in the endometrium. Many such foci of smooth muscle probably arise from the endometrial stromal cells by a process of *leiomyomatous metaplasia* but some may develop from heterotopic smooth muscle fibres. *Fatty metaplasia* of the endometrial stroma is extremely rare and is not to be confused with an infiltration of lipid-laden macrophages.

Fallopian tube

Metaplastic changes are distinctly uncommon in the tube, although both *mucinous* and *squamous metaplasia* are occasionally encountered. However, it is by no means uncommon to find foci of endometrial tissue in, or replacing, the epithelial lining of the tube and although this could well be due to endometrial metaplasia it is usually impossible to exclude endometriosis. An endometrial-like lining to the tube is seen particularly at the isthmic end and this may simply represent an extension of the uterine endometrium into the tube.

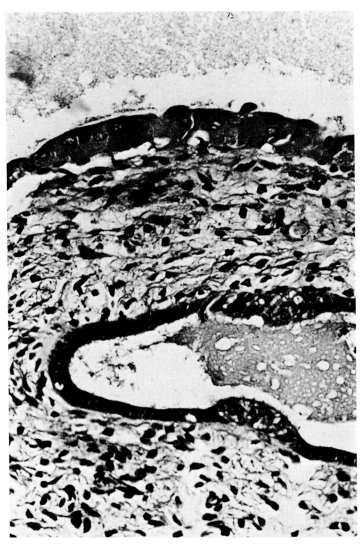

Fig. 6.7 Eosinophilic metaplasia of the endometrium. The gland at the top is lined by large eosinophilic cells with round central nuclei and abundant granular cytoplasm. In contrast, the lower gland is lined by more normal epithelium (H. & E. × 270).

Ovary

Mucinous and *tubal* (*serous*) *metaplasia* are well recognized as occurring not only in the surface epithelium of the ovary but also in simple ('germinal') inclusion cysts which were originally lined by an indifferent type of epithelium (Fig. 6.8a and b). It is probable that the cysts which have undergone these forms of metaplasia, which are an expression of the capacity of the surface epithelium for differentiation along a variety of müllerian pathways, are the source of origin of many of the mucinous and serous cysts found in the ovaries. It would be expected that, in addition to differentiating along endocervical and tubal pathways, the surface epithelium could also undergo endometrial metaplasia and this does occur.

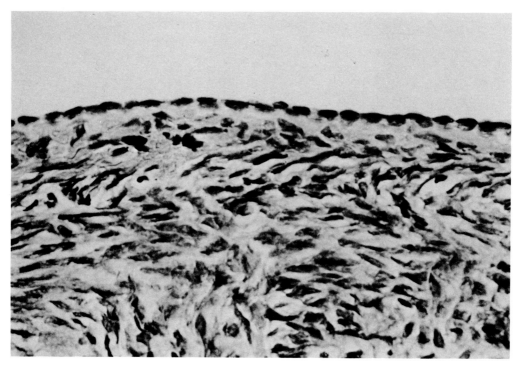

Fig. 6.8(a) The normal surface epithelium of the ovary which is flattened, cuboidal and featureless (H. & E. × 383).

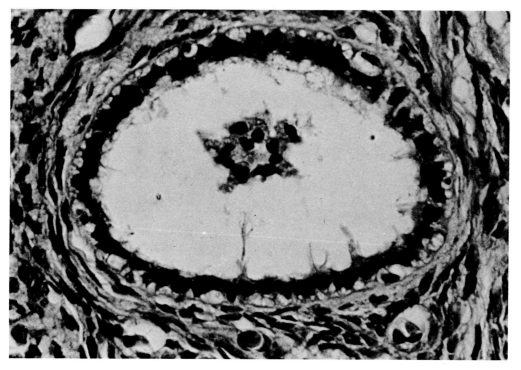

Fig. 6.8(b) A simple ('germinal') inclusion cyst of the ovary lined by epithelium showing tubal metaplasia. Ciliated and clear cells are clearly visible (H. & E. × 383).

Both *osseous* and *cartilaginous metaplasia* sometimes occur in the ovarian stromal cells, but the only significance of the presence of bland foci of ovarian cartilage or bone is, again, their propensity to arouse an unfounded suspicion of a teratoma or mixed tumour with heterologous elements. *Fatty metaplasia* of the ovarian stroma is very uncommon, the fat cells usually being in a subcapsular site.

Pelvic lymph nodes

Serial sectioning of pelvic lymph nodes from females (but not from males) will often reveal small gland-like inclusions within the cortex of the nodes. These apparent glands may be very similar to ovarian epithelial inclusion cysts but are frequently lined by an epithelium of tubal type. It seems almost certain that these inclusions are not due to lymphatic transport of tissue but to a metaplasia of the overlying pelvic mesothelium, the metaplastic foci pursuing the same course as do those in the ovarian mesothelium and sinking into the underlying tissue. In pregnancy, or in women taking a progestagen, the stroma associated with the inclusions may undergo decidualization. Very exceptionally, a tumour may arise in a lymph node inclusion.

Heterotopia

Although metaplastic lesions are best described systematically on an organ-by-organ basis, it is easier to consider heterotopia in terms of the nature of the ectopically sited tissue.

Endometrial tissue

Ectopically sited endometrial tissue is a common finding both within and outside the uterus. The presence of ectopic endometrial tissue in the myometrium is referred to as *adenomyosis* whilst, if the ectopic tissue is in an extramyometrial site, the condition is called *endometriosis*. Attempts have been made to impose a conceptual unity on these abnormalities by referring to adenomyosis as 'internal endometriosis' whilst grouping the extramyometrial lesions as 'external endometriosis'. However, there can be little justification for this form of usage, which tends to conceal the fact that adenomyosis and endometriosis are unrelated conditions of differing aetiology and pathogenesis.

Adenomyosis
Adenomyosis is a disease principally of parous women in the later years of their reproductive life and is characterized by the presence of endometrial tissue deep within the myometrium. There is almost invariably an associated hypertrophy of smooth muscle fibres around the ectopic islands of endometrium. However, the interface between normally sited endometrium and the myometrium is often irregular and tangential cutting of the basal endometrium may produce apparently isolated islands of endometrial tissue surrounded by myometrium. It is for this reason that the word 'deep' is insisted upon in the definition of adenomyosis, although there has been some dispute as to its interpretation. It has been variously suggested that, to justify a diagnosis of adenomyosis, the ectopic endometrium should be at least one high power, or alternatively, one low power microscopic field below the base of the endometrium, but these are imprecisely defined criteria which ignore myometrial thickness, and an insistence that the intramyometrial endometrial glands must be at a distance of more than one-quarter of the full thickness of the uterine wall away from the endometrial–myometrial junction has much to recommend it.

The nodules of ectopic endometrium may be distributed diffusely throughout the myometrium, in which case the uterus shows a roughly symmetrical enlargement which is usually due as much, or indeed more, to the accompanying muscle hypertrophy than to the ectopic endometrium. The cut surface has a trabeculated firm appearance with focally depressed areas corresponding to the nodules of endometrial

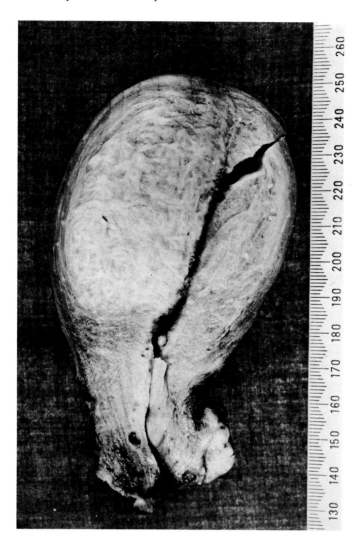

Fig. 6.9   Adenomyosis. The uterus is asymmetrically enlarged by an ill-defined mass in the posterior wall. Note the whorled appearance.

tissue. Less commonly, adenomyosis occurs focally and forms a poorly delineated tumour-like asymmetrical thickening of the myometrium (Fig. 6.9). This localized variety is often known as an *adenomyoma*, an unfortunate term because of its false connotation of neoplasia. Histologically, the foci of adenomyosis consist of both endometrial glands and stroma (Fig. 6.10). The stromal element is often formed of closely packed spindle-shaped cells and the glands are commonly of the basal type and thus do not show cyclical activity. Occasionally the glands are sensitive to oestrogens but unresponsive to progesterone, and thus tend to undergo simple hyperplasia and, occasionally, atypical hyperplasia. It is theoretically possible for the latter to progress to an adenocarcinoma but, if such a phenomenon does indeed occur, it is very rare. True cyclical changes in adenomyosis are very uncommon and, although evidence of recent or old haemorrhage is sometimes detected, this is distinctly unusual.

Adenomyosis is due to a downgrowth of the basal layer of the endometrium into the myometrium and serial sectioning will invariably demonstrate a continuity between the basal endometrium and

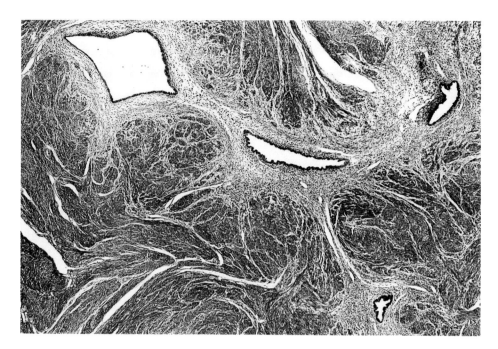

Fig. 6.10 A focus of intramyometrial adenomyosis. Endometrial glands of basal type lie in an irregular area of endometrial stroma (H. & E. × 45).

underlying foci of adenomyosis. However, the aetiology of this condition is obscure and although trauma, in the form of curettage, and oestrogenic stimulation have been postulated as causal factors, there is no real proof that either plays a significant aetiological role.

The incidence of adenomyosis in surgically resected uteri is uncertain, the reported frequency ranging from 8 to 80 per cent. This lack of agreement clearly reflects the use of differing diagnostic criteria but it is probable that the lower figure is a nearer approximation to the truth. The clinical significance of adenomyosis is also uncertain because, although menorrhagia and dysmenorrhoea are usually cited as manifestations of this disease, there is no clear relationship between the presence of adenomyotic foci and symptoms of this nature. Menorrhagia may be due to an increased uterine size but it is difficult to understand why dysmenorrhoea should complicate a condition in which cyclical changes are the exception rather than the rule.

Endometriosis
The presence of ectopic endometrial tissue in an extramyometrial location is both common and important. The ectopic tissue occurs most commonly in the ovaries, pouch of Douglas, uterine ligaments, pelvic peritoneum, rectovaginal septum, cervix, appendix, inguinal hernial sacs and the bowel. Foci of endometriosis are occasionally encountered in surgical scars, in the vulva, at the umbilicus, in the bladder or in the skin, whilst exceptional instances of lesions occurring in lymph nodes, kidney, limbs, pleura and lungs have been recorded.

The pathogenesis of endometriosis is still uncertain but one possible mechanism for its development is the reflux of endometrial tissue through the fallopian tubes as a result of retrograde menstruation, with subsequent implantation on, and growth in, the ovaries, pelvic peritoneum and uterine ligaments. It has been argued that retrograde menstruation is extremely uncommon and that the shed tissue fragments are dead and thus incapable of further growth; nevertheless, the following facts may be marshalled to support this concept:

1. Retrograde menstruation is, in fact, quite common and is frequently observed at laparoscopy.
2. The distribution of endometriosis in the pelvis is that which would be expected if the endometrial tissue were regurgitated via the tube.
3. Women with congenital obstruction of the lower genital tract tend to have severe endometriosis. In patients with a bifid uterus with drainage from only one side obstructed, endometriosis tends to occur only on that side in which outflow is dammed back.
4. Animal experiments have shown that endometrial tissue shed through an artificially created uteropelvic fistula implants and grows on the pelvic peritoneum.
5. Scar endometriosis following uterine surgery appears to be clearly an implantation phenomenon.

An alternative, but not mutually exclusive, view is that, in the pelvis at least, endometriosis arises as a result of endometrial metaplasia of the peritoneal serosa. This is a feasible hypothesis and it may well be that, in fact, such metaplasia is induced by contact with regurgitated fragments of endometrium which, after initiating the metaplastic process, subsequently die and are absorbed. The existence of endometriotic foci in lymph nodes and in distant sites, such as the lung, can clearly not be explained by this mechanism and hence lymphatic or haematogenous dissemination of endometrium must be invoked in such cases. It is indeed almost certain that there is no single pathogenetic mechanism which applies to all cases of endometriosis. The aetiology of endometriosis, as distinct from the pathogenesis, is also uncertain but genetic, familial and immunological factors probably play important roles.

The pathology of endometriosis is, in essence, simple, for the only diagnostic criterion is the presence of histologically recognizable endometrial glands and stroma in an ectopic site (Fig. 6.11). Unfortunately, however, the situation is complicated by the tendency towards haemorrhage that is so characteristic a feature of endometriosis. Bleeding into the lesion itself can cause considerable tissue damage and a 'self-destruction' of the endometrial tissue, thus leaving the pathologists bereft of specific histological findings. Furthermore, haemorrhage into the surrounding tissues releases free iron which is intensely fibrogenic and promotes dense adhesions which tend to obscure the primary lesion.

The early stages of ovarian endometriosis appear to the naked eye as reddish-blue surface implants which may be raised or dimpled and which can measure from 1 mm to 5 mm across. It is usual for tiny cysts to appear and for these to enlarge progressively and grow into the ovarian tissue, usually reaching a size of 2–5 cm across but occasionally attaining a diameter of up to 10 cm (Fig. 6.12). The cysts have a smooth or granular brownish-yellow lining and their walls, originally thin, eventually become thick and fibrotic. Their content of old, semi-fluid or inspissated blood commonly has a dark brown or black appearance, a feature which has led to the use of the terms 'chocolate' or 'tarry' cyst. There is a marked tendency for blood to leak out from endometriotic cysts and this results in the formation of firm adhesions which bind the enlarged ovary down to the posterior surface of either the broad ligament or the uterus, any attempt at separating the ovary from these structures leading to an escape of brown or black cyst contents. Peritubal adhesions are frequently seen and the tubes are often kinked and distorted. However, the tubal ostia are usually patent and the tubal lumen is rarely obstructed.

The histological diagnosis of ovarian endometriosis is readily made if endometrial glands and stroma are still present in recognizable form in the lesion. However, it is by no means unusual for the endometrial lining of the cysts either to be so attenuated as to be unrecognizable as such or to be largely or completely lost. If the endometrial lining has been totally destroyed, the appearances will be those of a simple haemorrhagic cyst lined by granulation tissue and with a fibrous wall in which aggregates of iron-containing macrophages are usually present (Fig. 6.13). Under these circumstances it is justifiable to conclude that the appearances are 'compatible with a diagnosis of endometriosis' or even to make a diagnosis of 'presumptive endometriosis', but it would be unwise to venture beyond these rather tentative

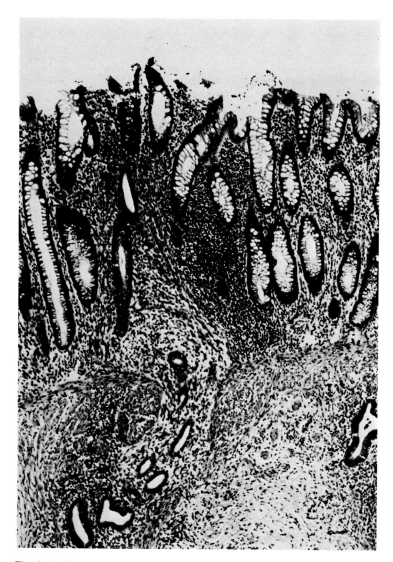

Fig. 6.11 The rectum of a woman, aged 35 years, in which there was a large pelvic mass due to endometriosis of the large bowel. Glands of endometrial type and endometrial stroma can be seen disrupting the submucosa and mucosa (H. & E. × 45).

conclusions. Any endometrial tissue that is present may show the full range of normal cyclical changes but is often inactive or shows only proliferative activity. Under the latter circumstance there may be progression to a simple or an atypical hyperplasia, changes which have to be distinguished from the reactive atypia which is not infrequent in endometrial epithelium.

Extraovarian pelvic endometriosis, e.g. in the uterosacral and round ligaments, pouch of Douglas, rectovaginal septum or on the surface of the uterus, is seen as multiple bluish-red nodules, patches or cysts, almost invariably with accompanying fibrous adhesions. The lesions are usually small but ligamentous foci may attain a size sufficient to be easily palpable, whilst endometriotic foci in the rectovaginal septum can not only lead to fixation of the rectum but can extend into the vaginal vault or the rectum to form small haemorrhagic nodules or polypi.

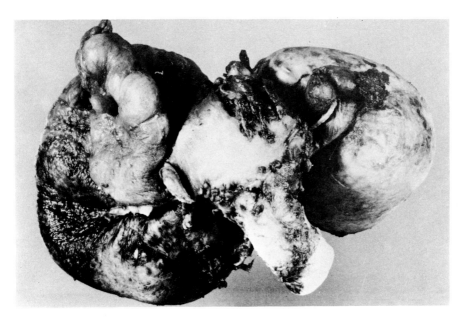

Fig. 6.12   Endometriosis of the ovaries and pelvic peritoneum. Dark deposits of endometriosis stud the uterine serosa and the ovaries are enormously enlarged by the presence of cystic endometriosis (chocolate cysts).

Women with endometriosis commonly complain of pelvic and back pain just before and during the menstrual period, deep pain on sexual intercourse and rectal discomfort or bleeding. Recurrent hormonally induced swelling of foci in the uterosacral ligaments is thought to account for the perimenstrual pain, whilst similar swelling and engorgement of lesions in the rectovaginal septum are considered to be responsible for dyspareunia and rectal symptoms. Infertility is common but, as discussed in Chapter 14, the reasons for this are incompletely understood; the reduced fertility does not appear to be due to tubal obstruction or to any other simple mechanistic factor. It is of interest that neither the incidence of infertility nor of the other symptoms of endometriosis is clearly related to the extent of the disease, since women with extensive endometriosis may be symptom free, whilst others with only minimal disease have striking symptoms.

Endometriosis can undergo neoplastic change and in ovarian foci this is often preceded by an atypical hyperplasia which, when sufficiently severe, can be regarded as either an adenocarcinoma *in situ* or as an endometrioid tumour of borderline malignancy. Any of the malignant tumours which can occur in the normally sited endometrium (see Chapter 10) can also arise in endometriotic foci but those encountered most commonly are endometrioid and clear cell adenocarcinomata. Very rarely will an endometrial stromal sarcoma of the ovary develop from the stromal component of the lesion. Only a minority of ovarian endometrioid adenocarcinomata arise in pre-existing foci of endometriosis but it is difficult to assess the magnitude of this minority, for it is unusual to be able to trace a direct continuity between an endometrioid adenocarcinoma and a focus of endometriosis. There is often only a presumption of such an origin based on the finding of endometriosis in the contralateral ovary or elsewhere in the pelvis. Extraovarian endometriosis can also undergo neoplastic change and give rise to an endometrioid adenocarcinoma in such sites as the uterine ligaments, pouch of Douglas, rectovaginal septum, bladder or large bowel. These occur uncommonly but are by no means of exceptional rarity.

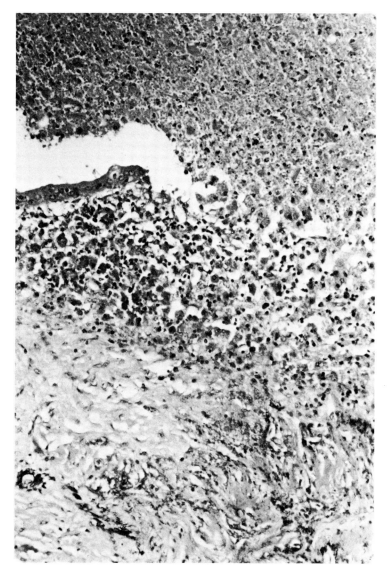

Fig. 6.13 Ovary: endometriotic cyst. The cyst lumen, at the top of the section, contains altered blood. The wall is formed by granular macrophages, non-specific granulation tissue and fibrous tissue. Note the remnant of the original endometrial-type epithelium to the left of the section (H. & E. × 108).

Tubal epithelium

Small cystic nodules lined by tubal-type epithelium and often containing psammoma bodies may be found scattered on the surface of the uterus, on the pelvic peritoneum and in the omentum. This condition of *endosalpingiosis* has been attributed to the displacement of tubal tissue but it is much more probable that it is due to multifocal tubal differentiation within the loose connective tissue immediately deep to the mesothelium. This tissue has a propensity for müllerian differentiation and is sometimes classed as the secondary müllerian system. The major significance of endosalpingiosis is that the lesions may be misinterpreted as metastases, or implants, from an ovarian serous adenocarcinoma or serous tumour of borderline malignancy. Atypical proliferation does occur within endosalpingiotic foci and gives a picture of borderline malignancy and whilst, occasionally, progression to an adenocarcinoma occurs, it is highly probable that this is the pathogenesis of primary papillary serous adenocarcinomata of the peritoneum.

Endocervical epithelium

Tiny cysts lined by endocervical-type epithelium may occur in the same sites as areas of endosalpingosis. These foci of *endocervicosis* probably arise as a result of endocervical differentiation within the secondary müllerian system and can, occasionally, give rise to an extraovarian mucinous tumour.

Mixed müllerian epithelia

A variety of different types of müllerian epithelia may occur ectopically in the vagina in the condition known as *vaginal adenosis*. This abnormality, which is usually asymptomatic but occasionally associated

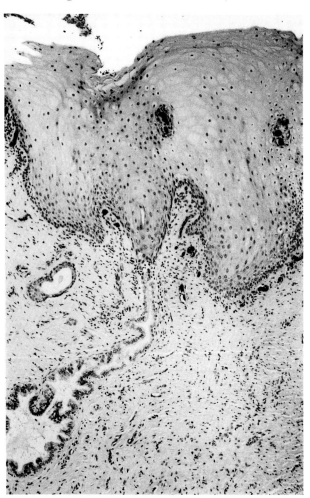

Fig. 6.14 Vaginal adenosis. The vagina is lined by a mature metaplastic squamous epithelium, beneath which there are glandular spaces lined by a columnar epithelium. The epithelium is of endometrial and cervical types (H. & E. × 93).

with a mucoid vaginal discharge, appears to the naked eye as a reddish roughening of the vaginal mucosa, most commonly on the anterior wall of the upper portion. Histologically, the condition is characterized by the presence of glandular structures in the lamina propria of the vagina (Fig. 6.14). These glands are, in the majority of cases, lined by a mucinous epithelium of endocervical type, but a minority of glands contain endometrial- or tubal-type epithelium. The glands can sometimes be seen to be opening into the vaginal lumen and their lining epithelium may extend on to the surface. The epithelium, whether it be in the glands or on the surface, has a marked tendency to undergo squamous metaplasia and the resultant multiple foci of squamous epithelium lying deep to the surface may give rise to a suspicion of invasive squamous cell carcinoma. However, even in cases where the glandular epithelium has been completely replaced it is usually possible to demonstrate small pools of mucus in the squamous foci.

Vaginal adenosis is thought to be due to sequestration of müllerian remnants during the upgrowth of the squamous epithelium of the urogenital sinus. It is unusually common in girls who have been exposed prenatally to diethylstilboestrol (DES), this lesion being found in about 70 per cent of those exposed to DES before the eighth week of gestation. Clear cell adenocarcinoma of the vagina in DES-exposed girls almost certainly arises from vaginal adenosis and is usually preceded by atypical changes within endometrial-type glands within the adenosis.

Adrenal tissue

Tiny nodules of ectopic adenocortical tissue are a quite common finding in the mesovarium; they are of no importance and do not give rise to neoplasms. Contrary to what is often thought, intraovarian ectopic adrenal tissue is of the greatest rarity.

Breast tissue

Ectopic breast tissue is sometimes found in the vulva, usually in the labia major. It tends to present as a painless lump during pregnancy and histological examination reveals morphologically normal breast tissue showing pregnancy changes. Rarely, a benign or malignant neoplasm may develop in ectopic breast tissue.

Key References

Baggish M S and Woodruff J D. (1967) The occurrence of squamous epithelium in the endometrium. *Obstetrical and Gynecological Survey* **22**, 69–115.

Buckley C H and Fox H. (1989) *Biopsy Pathology of the Endometrium.* Chapman and Hall, London.

Clement P B. (1987) Endometriosis, lesions of the secondary Müllerian system and pelvic mesothelial proliferations. In: *Blaustein's Pathology of the Female Genital Tract, 3rd edn.* pp. 516–59. Edited by R J Kurman, Springer-Verlag, New York.

Coleman D V and Evans D M D. (1988) *Biopsy Pathology and Cytology of the Cervix.* Chapman and Hall, London.

Czernobilsky B. (1987) Endometriosis. In: *Haines and Taylor, Obstetrical and Gynaecological Pathology, 3rd edn.* pp. 763–77. Edited by H Fox, Churchill Livingstone, Edinburgh.

Desmopoulos R J and Greco M A. (1983) Mucinous metaplasia of the endometrium: ultrastructural and histochemical characteristics. *International Journal of Gynecological Pathology* **1**, 383–90.

Emge L A. (1962) The elusive adenomyosis of the uterus. *American Journal of Obstetrics and Gynecology* **83**, 1541–63.

Ferenczy A and Winkler B. (1987) Anatomy and histology of the cervix. In: *Blaustein's Pathology of the Female Genital Tract, 3rd edn.* pp. 141–57. Edited by R J Kurman, Springer-Verlag, New York.

Fox H and Buckley C H. (1984) Current concepts of endometriosis. *Clinics in Obstetrics and Gynaecology* **11**, 279–87.

Fruin A H and Tighe J R. (1967) Tubal metaplasia of the endometrium. *Journal of Obstetrics and Gynaecology of the British Commonwealth* **74**, 93–7.

Fu Y S and Regan J W. (1989) *Pathology of the Uterine Cervix, Vagina and Vulva.* W B Saunders, Philadelphia.

Gugliotta P, Fibbi M, Fessia L, Canevini P and Bussolati G. (1983) Lactating supernumerary mammary gland tissue in the vulva. *Applied Pathology* **1**, 61–5.

Hendrickson M R and Kempson R L. (1980) Endometrial epithelial metaplasias: a study of 89 cases and proposed classification. *American Journal of Surgical Pathology* **4**, 525–42.

Hsu Y K, Parmley T H, Rosenshein N B, Ghaganan B S and Woodruff J D. (1980) Neoplastic and non-neoplastic proliferations in pelvic lymph nodes. *Obstetrics and Gynecology* **55**, 83–8.

Kurman R J and Scully R E. (1974) The incidence and histogenesis of vaginal adenosis. *Human Pathology* **5**, 265–76.

Molitor J J. (1971) Adenomyosis: a clinical and pathologic appraisal. *American Journal of Obstetrics and Gynecology* **110**, 275–82.

Shatia N N and Hoshika M G. (1982) Uterine osseous metaplasia. *Obstetrics and Gynecology* **60**, 256–9.

Singer A. (1987) Anatomy of the cervix and physiological changes of the epithelium. In: *Haines and Taylor, Obstetrical and Gynaecological Pathology, 3rd edn.* pp. 217–36. Edited by H Fox, Churchill Livingstone, Edinburgh.

Trowell J E. (1985) Intestinal metaplasia with argentaffin cells in the uterine cervix. *Histopathology* **9**, 551–9.

Tyagi S P, Saxena K, Rizvi R and Langley F A. (1979) Foetal remnants in the uterus and their relation to other uterine heterotopia. *Histopathology* **3**, 339–45.

Zinsser K R and Wheeler J E. (1982) Endosalpingiosis in the omentum: a study of autopsy and surgical material. *American Journal of Surgical Pathology* **6**, 109–17.

7

Non-neoplastic cysts

A wide variety of non-neoplastic cysts is found in the female genital tract, many arising from developmental remnants, others being due to blockage of gland ducts and yet others to epithelial or mesothelial inclusions. Endometriotic cysts are common but these are considered separately in Chapter 6.

Vulva

Sebaceous cysts, which are quite common, are so called because they result from the blockage of one of the numerous sebaceous glands of the vulval skin. The cysts are usually in the labia and, although mobile, they elevate and are fixed to, the overlying skin, which invariably shows a punctum at its summit. The cysts contain greasy or pultaceous yellow-white material and this is occasionally protruded through the punctum to form a scab-like crust. Histologically, the cysts are most commonly lined only by stratified squamous epithelium and only rarely does the epithelium show sebaceous differentiation. However, it is by no means uncommon for a sebaceous cyst to become infected and this may result in destruction of the lining epithelium and spillage of the cyst contents into the surrounding tissue, with production of a foreign body-type granulomatous reaction.

Many vulval cysts are of the *epidermoid* type. These are lined by regular squamous epithelium and their whitish, flaky or cheesy contents consist of laminated keratinous material. Epidermoid cysts may result from trauma but also arise at sites of fusion of epidermal structures during embryogenesis and they are found most commonly on the labia and around the clitoris.

Cysts may develop in the vulva from remnants of the mesonephric duct and these, also known as *Gartner's duct cysts*, are found on the lateral aspect of the vulva. They are thin walled, contain clear colourless fluid, are lined by low columnar or cuboidal cells and usually have a smooth muscle component in their wall.

Mucinous cysts, lined by a columnar epithelium similar to that of the endocervix (Fig. 7.1), occur in the vulva and were previously thought to arise from paramesonephric remnants. However, the paramesonephric (or müllerian) system plays no role in the development of the vulva and it is now established that tiny mucinous glands, almost certainly of urogenital sinus origin, are normally present in the vulva, the cysts arising as a result of obstruction to the neck of one of these glands. The rare *serous cysts* of the vulva, lined by a tubal-type epithelium, similarly develop from minute intravulval serous glands.

A *cyst of the canal of Nuck* develops from a peritoneal fragment or inclusion which is carried by the round ligament as it passes through the inguinal canal to insert into the labium major. Such a cyst, which is found in the upper part of the labia majora, is thus analogous to a hydrocele in the male.

A *Bartholin's duct cyst* develops as a consequence of obstruction to the main duct of Bartholin's gland and presents as a firm swelling in the inferior part of the labium major. These cysts can measure anything from 1 cm to 10 cm across and contain clear, sometimes slightly mucoid, fluid. They are lined by transitional epithelium which frequently shows focal squamous metaplasia. Compressed glandular acini

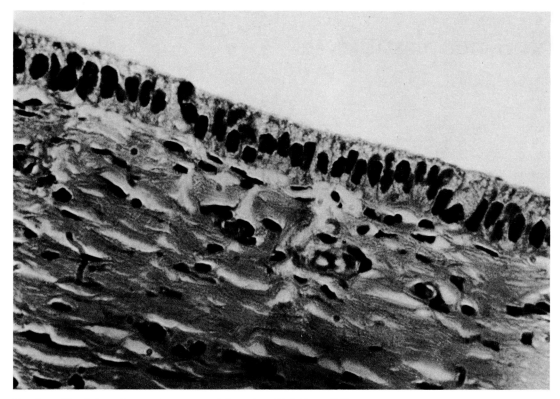

Fig. 7.1   The lining of a mucinous cyst of the vulva (H. & E. × 405).

are often present in the outer part of the wall (Fig. 7.2). A Bartholin's duct cyst is prone to infection and may therefore present as a localized abscess.

Vagina

Cysts of the vagina are uncommon, the type encountered most frequently being the *mesonephric (or Gartner's duct) cyst*, which is found on the anterolateral wall of the vagina and which, although usually small, may attain a size sufficient to present at the vulva. The histology of these cysts is identical to those of similar origin occurring in the vulva, i.e. a lining of cuboidal or low columnar epithelium and a wall containing smooth muscle (Fig. 7.3). These cysts are sometimes multiple and may form a chain along the vaginal wall. Removal of one of the cysts may, therefore, lead to the formation of a fistula from which serous fluid drains.

Epidermoid cysts are usually a result of trauma inflicted during parturition and, although most commonly found on the posterior wall, can occur at any site in the vagina; they are lined by squamous epithelium and contain keratinous material.

Cysts lined by endocervical-, tubal- or endometrial-type epithelium are sometimes encountered in the vagina and are often classed as *paramesonephric* or *müllerian cysts*; it being postulated that they derive from remnants of müllerian epithelium left behind as this is replaced during development by the squamous epithelium of the urogenital sinus. However, an origin from urogenital sinus cannot be specifically refuted

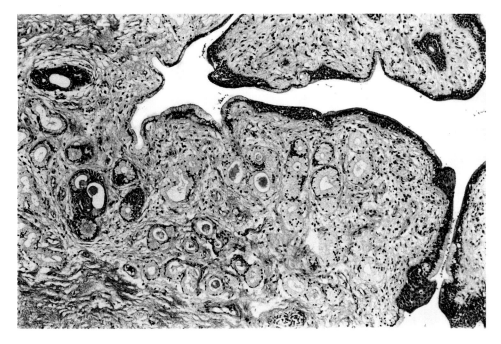

Fig. 7.2 A Bartholin's duct cyst. The cyst is partly lined by mucinous epithelium and partly by transitional epithelium which, in places, is replaced by metaplastic squamous epithelium. The gland acini and smaller ducts are present within the wall (H. & E. × 93).

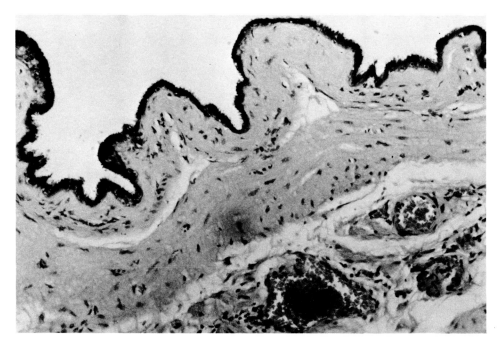

Fig. 7.3 The wall of a Gartner's duct cyst of the vagina. The cyst is lined by a columnar epithelium and the wall contains smooth muscle (H. & E. × 108).

and it is important to stress that these cysts do not appear to arise from or be associated with, vaginal adenosis (see Chapter 6).

Emphysematous cysts of the vagina are distinctly uncommon; they present as gas-filled blebs bulging through the mucosa and, whilst often producing no symptoms, are occasionally associated with a vaginal discharge or with complaints of a popping noise from the vagina as a cyst ruptures. Histological examination shows a cystic space deep to the epithelium which has no lining and is surrounded by lymphocytes, histiocytes and, very commonly, foreign body-type giant cells. The aetiology and pathogenesis of this condition are uncertain but it tends to be diagnosed particularly during pregnancy (probably fortuitously) and is not uncommonly associated with trichomonal infection.

Cervix

Ubiquitously found in the cervix are *retention cysts*, also known as *nabothian follicles*. These are seen as bulging, pearly grey protuberances in the vicinity of the external os and, although usually very small and multiple, may occasionally be as large as 2 cm in diameter, a single cyst of this size sometimes replacing one lip of the cervix. Retention cysts may form if the neck of an endocervical gland, or more exactly a crypt, is blocked with inspissated mucus. More commonly, the cystic change is secondary to obstruction of the neck by squamous metaplasia of the surface epithelium, the squamous epithelium growing over and obliterating the surface opening of the crypt. Histologically, the cysts are lined by flattened endocervical epithelium (Fig. 7.4).

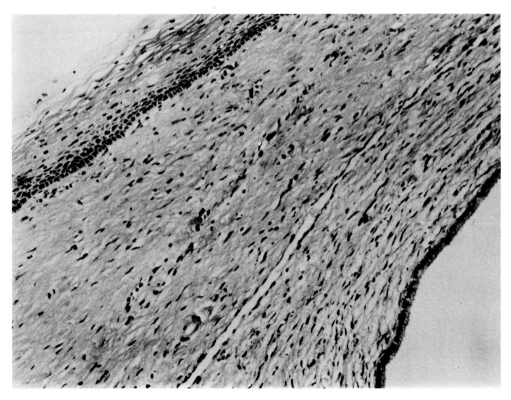

Fig. 7.4   A retention cyst (or nabothian follicle) of the cervix. The cervical squamous epithelium is above and to the left; the cyst is below and to the right (H. & E. × 108).

Mesonephric duct cysts, identical histologically to those of the vulva and vagina, are occasionally found in the lateral cervical wall, whilst the very uncommon *epidermoid cyst* of the cervix is usually a consequence of implantation of fragments of squamous epithelium into the deeper tissues by surgical or obstetric trauma.

Endometrium

Most apparent cysts of the endometrium are cystically dilated glands as found either in a florid simple hyperplasia or as encountered in the atrophic cystic endometrium of the postmenopausal woman. *Emphysematous cysts*, similar in type to those occurring in the vagina, have been recorded but are of exceptional rarity.

Myometrium

The most common cause of cyst formation in the uterine wall is cystic degeneration of a leiomyoma, but occasionally *mesonephric* or *paramesonephric cysts* are encountered, these having the same characteristics as those of similar origin occurring in the vagina. A curiosity is the exceptional development of a *hydatid cyst* of the myometrium, but *mesothelial cysts* of the peritoneal covering of the uterus are relatively common and are usually lined by a single layer of flattened cells.

Fallopian tube

Hydatid cysts of Morgagni are extremely common and are seen as pedunculated, translucent cysts dangling from the fimbrial end of the tube. They rarely measure more than 1 cm in diameter and contain clear colourless fluid. The stalk is formed of fibromuscular tissue whilst the thin delicate wall contains connective tissue fibrils. The cyst is lined by columnar or cuboidal cells of tubal type, these are often ciliated. These cysts are of paramesonephric origin and are nearly always asymptomatic, only very rarely undergoing torsion and thus producing abdominal pain.

Cystic Walthard's rests (Fig. 7.5) are found immediately below the tubal serosa, usually in the outer third of the tube, and are seen as tiny white nodules. Small *mesothelial inclusion cysts* are also occasionally encountered on the tubal surface; neither of these types of cyst is of any clinical significance.

Broad ligament

Paraovarian cysts are of two types; the majority are of paramesonephric (müllerian) origin and are often considered to develop from blind accessory tubal lumena. Such cysts are usually between 5 cm and 10 cm in diameter but can occasionally grow to massive proportions. They lie within the ligament with the tube stretched over their upper surface (Fig. 7.6) and, if very large, compressing and even flattening the ovary. The cysts are freely movable within the ligament and easily enucleated. They are unilocular,

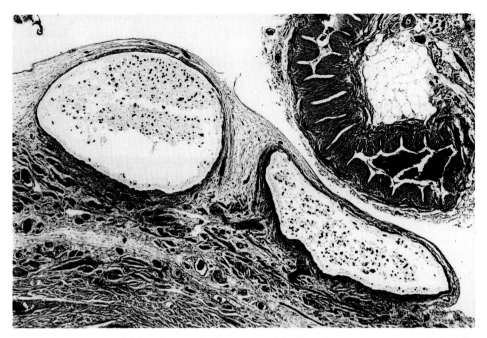

Fig. 7.5   Two cystic Walthard's rests, in the centre of the field, lie in the subserosa of the fallopian tube (H. & E. × 47).

contain clear fluid, have a wall formed by connective tissue and smooth muscle and are lined by epithelium of tubal type which may, if the cyst is large, be flattened (Fig. 7.7). The less common variety of paraovarian cyst is of mesonephric origin and, although grossly similar to that of paramesonephric derivation, is usually smaller and away from the tube, which is not stretched over its surface; it cannot be enucleated from the ligament. Histologically, this type of cyst has a rather thick fibromuscular wall and is lined by

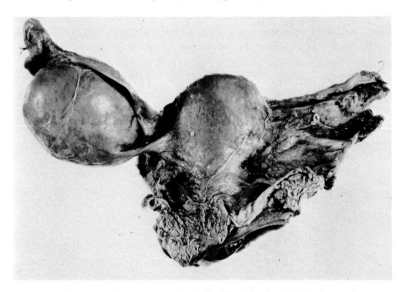

Fig. 7.6   A paraovarian cyst (on the left). The tube is stretched over the upper surface of the cyst and the ovary is flattened and lies behind the cyst.

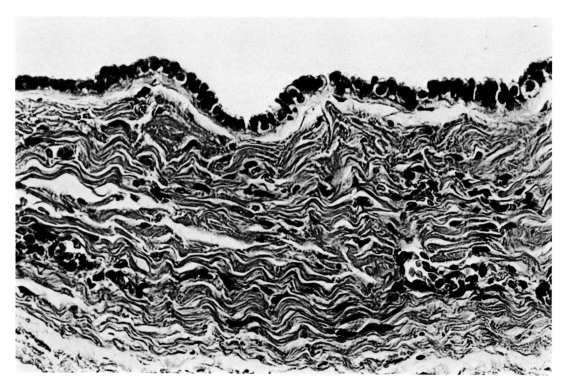

Fig. 7.7   The wall of a paraovarian cyst. The cyst is lined by darkly staining tubal-type epithelium and the wall contains smooth muscle (H. & E. × 270).

a single layer of non–ciliated cuboidal cells. Paraovarian cysts of either variety may undergo torsion, can rupture and sometimes become infected.

A *Kobelt's cyst* is similar macroscopically to a hydatid cyst of Morgagni but is of mesonephric origin and lies towards the lateral border of the broad ligament. Its thin wall is formed of delicate connective tissue and it is lined by a flattened or cuboidal epithelium.

Cysts of the *paroöphoron* develop from remnants of the tubules of the paroöphoron and are therefore of mesonephric origin. They are small (usually less than 1 cm in diameter) and lie between the ovary and the uterine cornu. The cysts contain clear fluid, are lined by low cuboidal cells and have a relatively thick fibromuscular wall; they are usually an incidental finding of no clinical significance.

Ovary

Non-neoplastic cysts of the ovary may develop from the surface epithelium (mesothelium) or from the follicles and are the most common cause of ovarian enlargement. Non-neoplastic cysts developing in foci of endometriosis or as a consequence of tubo–ovarian inflammation are described in Chapters 5 and 6.

Cysts of mesothelial origin

Simple inclusion cysts

These common, hormonally inactive, cysts develop at any age as invaginations of the surface epithelium into the ovarian cortex which gradually enlarge due to secretion of serous fluid by the epithelium. They may be single or, particularly when small, multiple, and occur most frequently after the menopause. They lie superficially or deep in the cortex and vary in size from a few millimetres to several centimetres. The distinction between simple inclusion cysts and benign serous cysts, which have the same histological features, is usually made arbitrarily on size, those lesions measuring less than 3 cm in diameter being designated simple inclusion cysts.

The cysts are thin-walled, their outer surface and lining are smooth and they are lined by cuboidal epithelium of tubal or, less commonly, endocervical or endometrial type. The contents are clear and serous but, if the cyst has undergone torsion, the fluid may be blood stained.

Cystic Walthard's rests

Cystic Walthard's rests
When the serosal lining of the inclusion cyst undergoes metaplasia to a transitional type, a cystic Walthard's rest, similar to that seen on the surface of the fallopian tube, results.

Cysts of follicular origin

Follicular cysts
Prior to the menopause, many follicles begin to mature at the beginning of each menstrual cycle, but at all stages of their development the majority become atretic. It is from follicles which have reached a partial degree of maturation and then undergone atresia that the majority of follicular cysts develop.

These cysts are extremely common, lie just below the surface of the ovary, are usually tiny and often multiple. They may very occasionally reach up to 10 cm in diameter and, exceptionally, very large follicular cysts may be encountered in pregnancy.

The cyst wall is thin, the surface and lining are smooth and the contents clear and watery. In a proportion of cases, haemorrhage occurs into the cyst lumen from a perifollicular haematoma, a feature which is of no pathological significance. The cyst is lined by stratified granulosa cells beneath which lies the theca interna (Fig. 7.8). In some cysts the granulosa cells are luteinized, this depending upon the maturity of the follicle when it became atretic and hence its capacity to respond to luteinizing hormone. As the cyst enlarges, the granulosa cells tend to reabsorb and the cyst becomes lined only by theca cells or fibrous tissue. Its appearance may then be entirely non-specific and the term 'simple' or 'indeterminate' cyst is applied.

Occasionally, the cyst develops not from an atretic follicle, but from one in which the granulosa cell layer, and sometimes the ovum, is well preserved; such cysts are lined by active granulosa and thecal cells and the cyst contents are high in oestrogen. Patients with such cysts, who are often anovulatory as a result of pituitary dysfunction, commonly have endometrial hyperplasia and irregular uterine bleeding.

Follicular cysts which regress spontaneously are a common finding in children with precocious pseudopuberty, whilst multiple follicular cysts are a feature of the polycystic ovary syndrome (which is discussed in Chapter 14).

In some women, the high levels of pituitary gonadotrophin which occur around, or just after, the time of the menopause are sufficient to stimulate a previously dormant follicular cyst into activity and may result in postmenopausal bleeding, as a consequence of inducing endometrial proliferation, or even in hyperplasia.

Large or giant luteinized follicular cysts of pregnancy and the puerperium
These rare cysts present as palpable abdominal swellings in pregnancy or the puerperium or may be found unexpectedly at caesarean section. The cysts range in size from 8 to 25 cm, have thin walls and

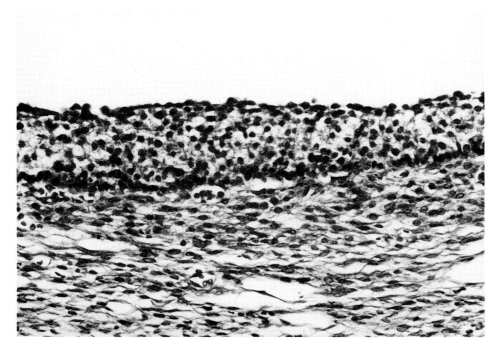

Fig. 7.8 A follicular cyst of the ovary. The cyst is lined by stratified granulosa cells (above). Beneath is the theca interna (H. & E. × 297).

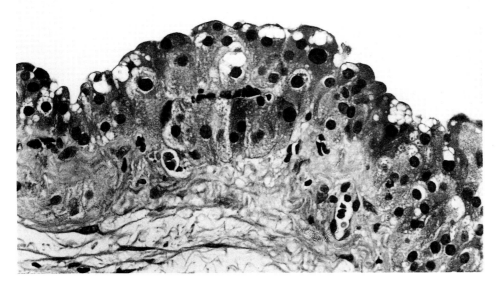

Fig. 7.9 Giant luteinized follicular cyst of pregnancy. The cyst is lined by several layers of heavily luteinized granulosa cells in which there is moderate nuclear pleomorphism and cytoplasmic vacuolation (H. & E. × 465).

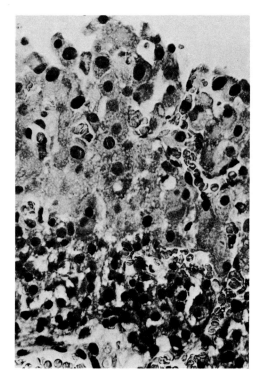

Fig. 7.10   A luteal cyst. The cyst is lined by lutenized granulosa cells (above) and deep to this are clusters of thecal cells (H. & E. × 320).

contain clear or blood stained serous fluid or, occasionally, mucoid material. They are lined by multiple layers of heavily luteinized granulosa cells, the cytoplasm of which may be densely eosinophilic or vacuolated. The nuclei may be small and regular but, not infrequently, are bizarre, pleomorphic and hyperchromatic (Fig. 7.9). Mitoses are not seen. With the fibrous tissue of the cyst wall there may be clusters of luteinized cells, similar to those lining the cyst but, unlike common follicular cysts, there is no differentiation into granulosa and thecal cell layers.

Corpus luteum cysts
Luteal cysts are usually single and an artificial distinction is sometimes made between a cystic corpus luteum and a corpus luteum cyst, a distinction which is without clinical value or pathological validity. A luteal cyst may result when the central cavity of the corpus luteum is unusually large, as may happen in a normal corpus or in pregnancy; it may occur when the central cavity undergoes organization rather slowly and a thin layer of fibrous tissue forms on its inner surface or, most commonly, it may be the sequel to a corpus luteum haematoma, a term applied to the condition in which the amount of blood extravasated into the corpus is excessive.

The cyst is lined by luteinized granulosa cells, deep to which small wedge-shaped clusters of luteinized thecal cells are usually visible (Fig. 7.10). Whilst the luteinized granulosa cells persist, progesterone secretion continues and delayed menstruation and continuous uterine bleeding may occur. As the luteal tissue becomes hyalinized, progesterone secretion falls and ultimately a hormonally inert *corpus albicans cyst* results. Occasionally, a luteal cyst may rupture into the pelvis, and blood loss, though usually slight, may sometimes be profuse.

Theca lutein cysts

These are follicular cysts with an intensely luteinized theca interna. The cysts may be quite small but occasionally, in a normal or twin pregnancy, in some patients receiving gonadotrophin therapy and in up to 50 per cent of patients with hydatidiform mole or choriocarcinoma, the ovaries may form multicystic nodular masses up to 20 cm in diameter — this condition is sometimes known as *ovarian overstimulation syndrome*.

The surface of the ovary is smooth and bosselated and its cut surface is multicystic with focal yellow nodules and haemorrhage in the cyst walls. The cyst fluid is usually clear and yellow but may be blood stained when there has been haemorrhage. The cyst lining is smooth and histological examination shows luteinized thecal cells. Granulosa cells are usually few but occasionally there is a well marked, or strikingly luteinized, granulosa cell layer.

Spontaneous regression is the rule after removal of the cause, which is excessive gonadotrophic stimulation, whether this be endogenous or exogenous. However, while the cysts are actively growing they may be complicated by haemorrhage, torsion or rupture.

Key references

Blaustein A, Kantius M, Kaganowicz A, Pervez N and Wells J. (1982) Inclusions in ovaries of females aged day 1–30 years. *International Journal of Gynecological Pathology* **1**, 145–53.

Caspi E, Schreyer P and Bukovsky J. (1973) Ovarian lutein cysts in pregnancy. *Obstetrics and Gynecology* **42**, 388–98.

Clement P B. (1987) Nonneoplastic lesions of the ovary. In: *Blaustein's Pathology of the Female Genital Tract, 3rd edn*, pp. 471–515. Edited by R J Kurman, Springer-Verlag, New York.

Clement P B and Scully R E. (1980) Large solitary luteinized follicle cyst of pregnancy and puerperium: a clinicopathological analysis of eight cases. *American Journal of Surgical Pathology* **4**, 431–8.

Fox H and Buckley C H. (1988) Tumour-like lesions and cysts of the vulva. In: *The Vulva*, pp. 228–34. Edited by C M Ridley, Churchill Livingstone, Edinburgh.

Gardner G H, Greene R R and Peckham B. (1949) Normal and cystic structures of broad ligament. *American Journal of Obstetrics and Gynecology* **55**, 917.

Pradhan S and Tobon H. (1986) Vaginal cysts: a clinicopathological study of 41 cases. *International Journal of Gynecological Pathology* **5**, 35–46.

Robboy S J, Ross J S, Prat J, Keh P C and Welch W R. (1978) Urogenital sinus origin of mucinous and ciliated cysts of the vulva. *Obstetrics and Gynecology* **51**, 347–51.

Schmidt W A. (1987) Pathology of the vagina. In: *Haines and Taylor, Obstetrical and Gynaecological Pathology, 3rd edn*, pp. 168–73. Edited by H Fox, Churchill Livingstone.

Strickler R C, Kelly R W and Askin F B. (1984) Postmenopausal ovarian follicle cyst: an unusual cause of estrogen excess. *International Journal of Gynecological Pathology* **3**, 318–22.

8

Benign neoplasms of the female genital tract

Most benign neoplasms of the female genital tract arise from the connective tissues rather than from the epithelial component. Certain tumours, such as leiomyomata or fibromata, can occur in any part of the genital tract and hence any systematic account of benign neoplasms is bound to be somewhat repetitive, saved from monotony only by the paradox that although most of these tumours are extremely rare, one, the uterine leiomyoma, is the most commonly occurring neoplasm to which the human body is prone. The reasons for this disparity are far from obvious and it is perhaps too simplistic to seek aetiological refuge in the sensitivity of the uterine musculature to oestrogenic stimulation and its constant process of hyperplasia and regression. It is also remarkable that benign epithelial neoplasms are so uncommon in the female genital tract, for in a comparable epithelial structure, the gastrointestinal tract, many malignant tumours develop in more frequently occurring benign lesions, such as adenomata.

Vulva

With the exception of condyloma acuminata, benign epithelial neoplasms of the vulva are rare; the type most commonly diagnosed being the squamous papilloma. Most, if not all, such tumours are in reality, fibroepithelial polypi (skin tags), viral warts, basal cell papillomata or condylomata acuminata. *Basal cell papillomata*, sometimes incorrectly known as 'seborrhoeic keratoses', are occasionally encountered in the vulval skin and are seen as flat, slightly warty, pigmented lesions with a curiously superficial 'stuck-on' appearance. Histologically they are characterized by multiple intraepithelial keratin cysts and sheets of immature epithelial cells; they are fully benign and lack malignant potential (Fig. 8.1).

Condylomata acuminata are contagious, sexually transmitted, benign epithelial neoplasms caused by the DNA-containing human papilloma virus (HPV). They occur particularly in patients with spontaneous or iatrogenic immune impairment, in those with poor perineal hygiene, in pregnancy (when they may grow very rapidly) and in patients with diabetes mellitus.

They occur typically along the edges and inner surfaces of the labia minora, between the labia minora and majora or around the introitus, sometimes extending onto the perineum and perianal area, and are seen as papillary or verrucous lesions which may be sessile or pedunculated (Fig. 8.2). The condylomata are usually multiple and sometimes confluent. Histologically, fibrovascular cores are covered by acanthotic squamous epithelium which shows parakeratosis and often hyperkeratosis (Fig. 8.3). Epithelial multinucleation, mild nuclear enlargement and pleomorphism and perinuclear haloes (koilocytic atypia) are characteristic features. There is usually a mild chronic inflammatory cell infiltrate of the underlying dermis. Although condylomata usually grow slowly, they occasionally enlarge quite rapidly to form the *giant condyloma of Buschke–Loewenstein*. However, many lesions thus designated are verrucous carcinomata that have been malignant *ab initio* and relatively few are true large condylomata. In fact, the development of a carcinoma in a true condyloma is extremely rare, although treatment with podophyllin causes increased cellularity, pleomorphism, increased mitotic activity and cellular enlargement, features which may lead to a mistaken impression of malignancy.

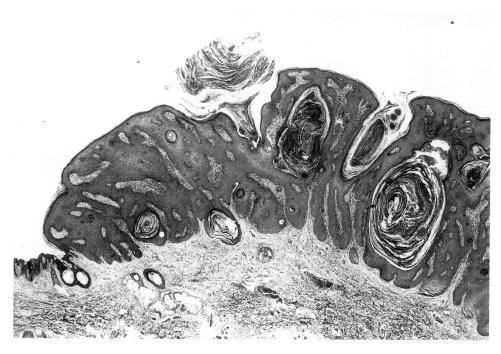

Fig. 8.1 Basal cell papilloma of the vulva. The exophytic, papillary lesion is composed of variably pigmented sheets of cells resembling the normal basal cells of the epidermis and enclosing cysts in which there is laminated keratin (H. & E. × 18.5).

True *naevi*, usually of the intradermal type, but occasionally of junctional or compound type, are found in the vulva, but more common are a variety of connective tissue neoplasms such as *leiomyomata, fibromata, lipomata, neurofibromata* and *neurilemmomata*. Some of these, particularly the fibromata and leiomyomata, may attain a considerable size and, because of the effects of gravity, tend to become pedunculated. Ulceration and secondary infection of such tumours is common, because of local moisture and warmth accentuated by the effects of tight clothing, and the macroscopic appearance of such an ulcerated neoplasm, often accompanied by enlargement of the regional lymph nodes, may give a false clinical impression of malignancy.

Tumours of sweat gland origin occur with modest frequency in the vulva, an organ rich in adnexal glands. The *papillary hidradenoma* is a neoplasm virtually confined to the anogenital region of middle-aged women and presents, usually on the labia majora or in the interlabial fold, as a firm, oval, painless subcutaneous swelling which rarely measures more than 2 cm in diameter. The overlying elevated skin is often reddened, because of frictional trauma, and may become ulcerated, the raspberry-red tumour tissue then protruding through the skin surface to present a misleadingly ominous naked-eye appearance. On histological examination, the neoplasm shows a complex tubular, acinar and papillary pattern with the epithelium covering the papillae and lining the acini and often, but not always, showing a characteristic double layer of large cuboidal or columnar cells, sometimes showing apocrine features, overlying a layer of small cuboidal or spindle-shaped myoepithelial cells (Fig. 8.4). The microscopic features of a papillary hidradenoma may at first sight be alarming and, indeed, a mistaken diagnosis of adenocarcinoma is sometimes made. However, the neoplasm is invariably benign. *Clear celled hidradenomata*, formed of solid tubules of large clear cells separated by delicate strands of connective tissue, can also occur in the vulva.

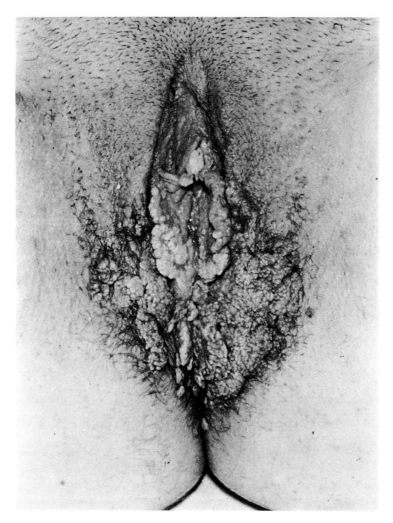

Fig. 8.2 Vulval condylomata. The labia minora, labia majora and introitus are studded by sessile, papillary and verrucous lesions.

A rare sweat gland tumour is the *syringoma*, which is seen as a small fleshy papule and consists histologically of multiple dilated ductal structures within the dermis.

Vascular neoplasms of the vulva, such as *haemangiomata*, are sometimes encountered, but not with unusual frequency. A particular variety of vascular neoplasm, the *angiokeratoma* is, however, virtually confined to the vulval skin and presents as a small purplish nodule which, on microscopy, consists of large dilated vascular channels separated from each other by strands and cords of squamous cells which grow down from the overlying hyperkeratotic epidermis (Fig. 8.5).

An uncommon neoplasm, but one which has a slight predilection for the vulva, is the *benign granular cell tumour*, which can occur at any age. This forms a well-circumscribed, non-tender swelling on the labium major. It elevates the overlying skin, which may be depigmented, and usually measures less than 4 cm in diameter. The nodule is commonly mobile but when it lies in the upper dermis it may be tethered to the overlying skin. It is greyish-brown on section and consists of sheets or nests of large cells with abundant acidophilic granular cytoplasm and indistinct cell boundaries. There has been considerable

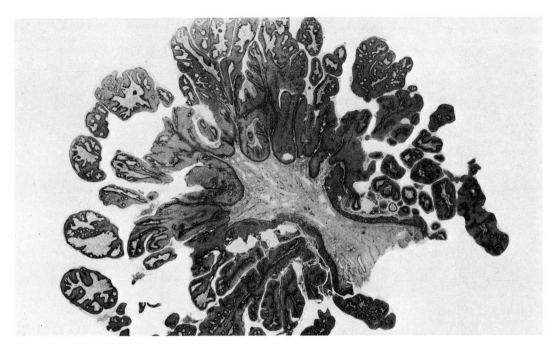

Fig. 8.3 Vulval condyloma. The papillary fibrovascular cores covered by acanthotic epithelium can be seen in this low magnification microphotograph (H. & E. × 7.2).

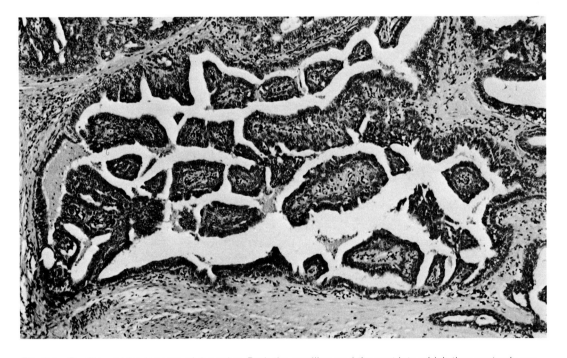

Fig. 8.4 Papillary hidradenoma of the vulva. Both the papillae and the cyst into which they protrude are covered by a double layer of epithelium. The inner layer is shallow columnar, the outer flattened cuboidal (H. & E. × 45).

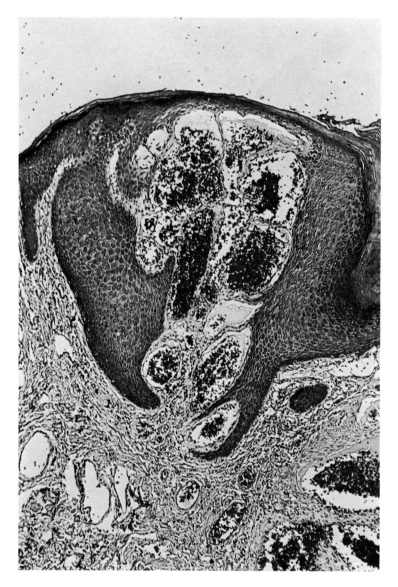

Fig. 8.5   Angiokeratoma of the vulva. A cluster of dilated, subepithelial vascular channels is surrounded by acanthotic squamous epithelium (H. & E. × 45).

controversy as to the nature of this tumour but, on the basis of morphological, ultrastructural and histochemical studies, it is now known to be derived from the Schwann cells of the nerve sheath.

Finally, three oncological curiosities are the development of a *fibroadenoma* or *duct papilloma* in ectopic breast tissue situated in the vulva, and the occurrence of an *adenoma* of Bartholin's gland.

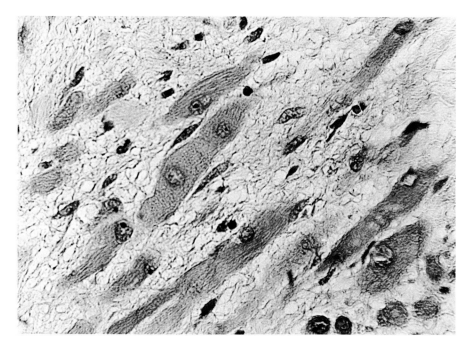

Fig. 8.6 Vaginal rhabdomyoma. Well-differentiated striated muscle fibres showing neither pleomorphism nor mitotic activity, which are characteristic of this benign neoplasm (H. & E. × 405).

Vagina

This is an uncommon site for benign tumours. *Squamous papillomata* are occasionally found, whilst *leiomyomata, fibromata, lipomata* and *granular cell tumours* all occur with extreme rarity. The most common benign vaginal neoplasm is the *condyloma acuminatum*, which is usually multiple and almost invariably associated with vulval and cervical lesions. The condylomata are usually small but may occasionally attain a size sufficient to obstruct the vagina.

A very uncommon tumour of the vagina is the *rhabdomyoma*. This presents as a well defined nodule which is seen to consist of regular striated muscle fibres showing no pleomorphism or mitotic activity (Fig. 8.6). This can occur at any age and care has to be taken to distinguish this fully benign tumour from a rhabdomyosarcoma or carcinosarcoma with heterologous elements. Another rare neoplasm is the *benign mixed tumour* in which islands of squamous epithelium are set in a fibrous stroma.

A curious lesion of the vagina, which is of unknown nature and probably not neoplastic, is the *benign vaginal nodule*. This is seen as a polypoid mass which histologically consists of rather non-specific connective tissue. It occurs at any age and has been described in neonates.

Cervix

Papillomata of the cervix are uncommon and should not be confused with a viral wart or a condyloma acuminatum. They consist of a focal papillary projection of thickened, regular squamous epithelium supported on a core of fibromuscular tissue. Malignant change has been described with some frequency in papillomata but there is a strong possibility that most such cases were misdiagnosed verrucous carcinomata that had been malignant from the start.

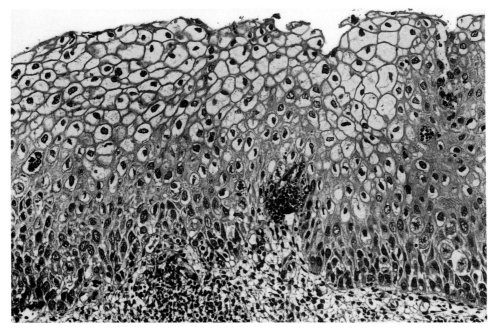

Fig. 8.7   A flat condyloma of the cervix (subclinical HPV infection). The superficial layers of the squamous epithelium are occupied by cells with vacuolated cytoplasm; some of these cells are multinucleated (H. & E. × 186).

Condylomata acuminata occur with some frequency on the cervix, often in association with vulval and vaginal condylomata, which they resemble histologically. They typically form pedunculated filiform lesions which may, rarely, be seen as large tumour-like masses but HPV infection may also occur without the development of exophytic lesions. These are the so-called flat condylomata (Fig. 8.7), also known as non-condylomatous wart virus infection (NCWVI) or sub-clinical HPV infection. These latter lesions are detectable only on colposcopy but their presence may be suspected when koilocytes are found in a cervical smear from an apparently normal cervix. Intraepithelial neoplasia is frequently found in association with condylomata, particularly the flat variety, and this has led to the suggestion that both may have a common aetiology. The topic is considered again in the section on intraepithelial neoplasia (page 112).

About 5–7 per cent of uterine leiomyomata are found in the cervix, where they arise from the muscle fibres of the cervical stroma. The tumour is usually confined to one side of the cervix and may impinge on, and distort, the endocervical canal. *Lipomata*, *fibromata*, *ganglioneuromata* and *haemangiomata* are uncommon, but documented, neoplasms of the cervix and in recent years there have been a number of reports of cervical *blue naevi*, lesions characterized by the presence of melanin-containing fusiform cells with dendritic cytoplasmic processes. The cells, which are possibly neurilemmal in origin, lie deep to the surface epithelium and there is no risk of malignancy.

The *benign mixed tumour* or *adenofibroma* of the cervix is a polypoid tumour with numerous branching clefts and papillary excrescences which are lined, usually, by cells of endocervical type. However, the epithelium is sometimes partially or totally of tubal, endometrial or squamous type. Glands and cysts lined by similar epithelia are also present. The stroma is formed of compact cellular fibrous tissue and there are no features to suggest malignancy in either the stromal or epithelial components of the tumour. This lesion is now considered to be a benign mixed neoplasm lying at one end of the spectrum which ranges through the adenosarcoma to the carcinosarcoma.

Endometrium

All benign endometrial neoplasms are rarities, the least uncommon being the *benign stromal nodule*. This is considered to be the benign equivalent of an endometrial stromal sarcoma and, although often very small, can form a quite large, fleshy, grey or tan-coloured mass. The tumour is composed of cells similar to those of the normal proliferating endometrium, has a pushing, rather than an infiltrating, edge and contains less than ten mitotic figures per ten high power microscopic fields. However, its diagnosis should be made only when its discrete and benign nature can be confirmed by examination of the whole uterus. *Adenofibromata* (benign mixed tumours), identical to their cervical counterparts, sometimes occur in the endometrium, whilst occasional intraendometrial *leiomyomata* are encountered.

A lesion which occupies the borderline between neoplasm and focal hyperplasia is the *atypical polypoid adenomyoma*, which forms, as its name suggests, an intrauterine polyp which may be sufficiently large to protrude through the external cervical os. It is composed of a fibromuscular tissue in which there are glands of irregular shape and architecture, which may be crowded or widely spaced, and which are lined by epithelium of endometrial type which, focally, may have undergone squamous metaplasia (Fig. 8.8). This is not a malignant lesion but will recur if not completely removed.

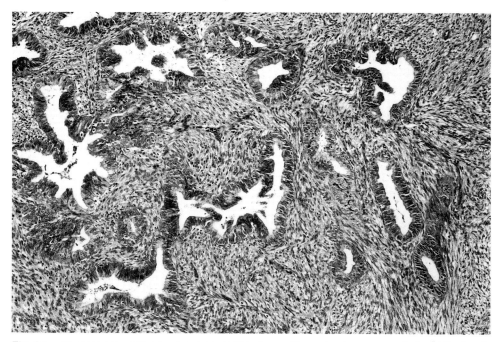

Fig. 8.8 Atypical polypoid adenomyoma of the uterus. The polyp is composed of architecturally atypical glands, lined by epithelium of endometrial type set in a fibromuscular stroma (H. & E. 93).

Myometrium

Leiomyomata originate from, and are tumours of, the smooth muscle cells of the myometrium. There is commonly an intermingling with fibrous tissue and these neoplasms are often, but inaccurately, known both in the lay and gynaecological vernacular as 'fibroids'. Myometrial leiomyomata are extremely common, being present in at least 20 per cent of women above the age of 35, and there is considerable

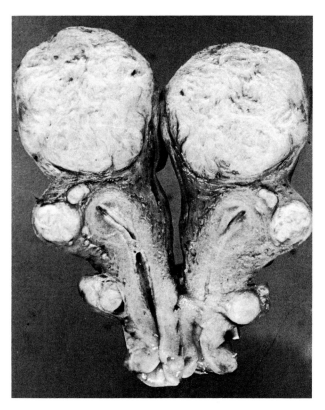

Fig. 8.9 Multiple leiomyomata of the uterus. Typical well-circumscribed whorled masses lie in the subserosa.

circumstantial, but by no means absolute, evidence that oestrogenic stimulation plays a role in their pathogenesis. Certainly, these tumours appear to be, at least partially, under hormonal control for they occur most frequently during the reproductive years, enlarge during pregnancy and may regress after the menopause. The tumours (Fig. 8.9) are usually multiple and vary in size from tiny seedlings only just visible to the naked eye, to huge masses which may fill the abdomen. Leiomyomata may be within the uterine wall, i.e. intramural, in a submucosal site immediately below the endometrium or lie just below the peritoneal covering of the uterus in a subserosal site. Submucosal leiomyomata bulge into and distort the uterine cavity, with thinning of the overlying endometrium, and sometimes become pedunculated to form a mass which not only fills the cavity but may extend through the endocervical canal into the vagina. Subserosal tumours grow out from the uterine surface and can extend into the broad ligament. Such a neoplasm may become pedunculated and can become attached to the omentum or pelvic peritoneum where, after shedding its peduncle, it derives a new blood supply and can flourish as a *parasitic leiomyoma*. Leiomyomata have a well defined regular outline and a surrounding pseudocapsule of compressed muscle fibres. On section, they tend to bulge out from the surrounding myometrium and to have a firm, white whorled or trabeculated surface. Histologically (Fig. 8.10) a leiomyoma consists of smooth muscle fibres arranged in bundles and whorls. The muscle fibres are elongated with spindle-shaped nuclei but bundles of fibres are often cut in cross-section and then appear as rounded cells with centrally placed round nuclei. Some tumours, known as *cellular leiomyomata*, contain densely packed spindle cells with elongated nuclei (Fig. 8.11). Occasionally, the smooth muscle cells are polygonal with a centrally placed nucleus and clear, slightly vacuolated cytoplasm (Fig. 8.12), tumours containing such cells are known as *epithelioid leiomyomata*, *clear cell leiomyomata* or *leiomyoblastomata*. Other variants on the

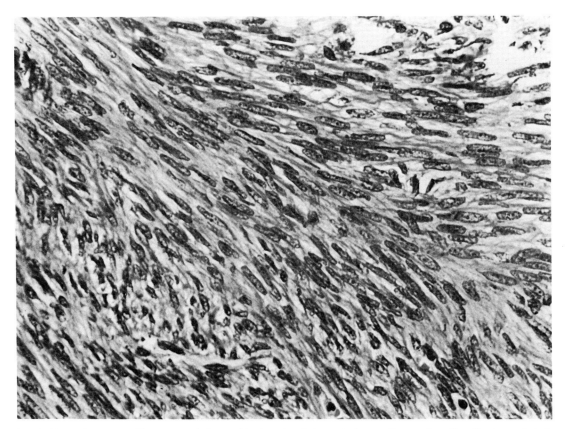

Fig. 8.10 Leiomyoma. The tumour is formed by bands of elongated smooth muscle cells with characteristic oblong nuclei (H. & E. × 270).

usual pattern are the *palisaded leiomyoma*, in which the nuclei show a palisading pattern very similar to that seen in a neurilemmoma; the *myxoid leiomyoma*, in which relatively few muscle cells are set in an abundant, loose myxoid stroma; the *leiomyoma with tubules*, in which an otherwise typical leiomyoma contains epithelial-like tubules; and the *lipoleiomyoma*, in which the neoplasm contains clusters of mature adipose cells (Fig. 8.13): all these various histological variants are fully benign.

In all except the smallest leiomyomata, fibrous tissue is intermixed with the smooth muscle fibres and the appearances are also commonly altered by a variety of degenerative changes which are due to the neoplasm outgrowing its blood supply. Thus, hyaline change, calcification, cystic change, myxoid degeneration, patchy necrosis and fatty change are common. A specific form of necrosis occurring particularly, but not only, during pregnancy is 'red degeneration' and this is characterized by a dull, beefy red appearance of the tumour (Fig. 8.14), which may also have a slightly fishy odour. This change can be accompanied by pain and fever and the presence of thrombosed vessels suggests that it represents haemorrhagic infarction of an extremely hyalinized neoplasm.

Cells near to an area of necrosis in a leiomyoma may contain large, bizarre, hyperchromatic nuclei and form multinucleated giant cells (Fig. 8.15). Similar changes are sometimes seen during pregnancy, or discovered incidentally during the routine histological examination of leiomyomata and this finding is not an indication of malignancy unless mitotic figures are also present. In fact, malignant change is rare in leiomyomata and the only histological feature indicative of such change is the presence of many mitotic figures. However, certain variants of leiomyomata, which histologically show no malign features, do

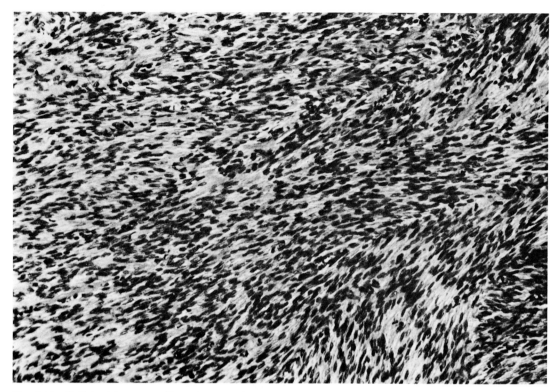

Fig. 8.11 Cellular leiomyoma. Densely packed cells form this neoplasm (H. & E. × 108).

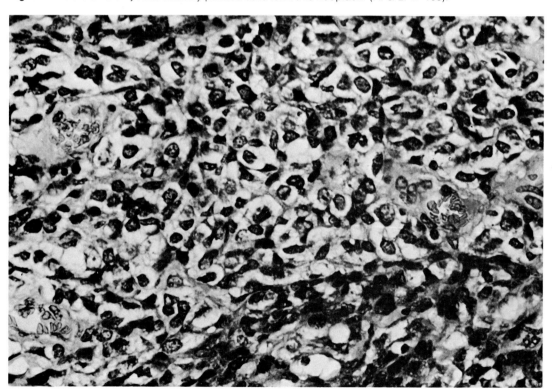

Fig. 8.12 Clear cell (epithelioid) leiomyoma. The smooth muscle cells have vacuolated clear cytoplasm and contain a central nucleus (H. & E. × 270).

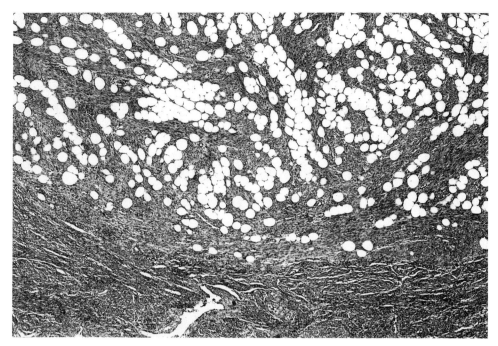

Fig. 8.13 Lipoleiomyoma of the myometrium. Clusters of mature adipose cells with clear cytoplasm lie between the bands of smooth muscle cells (H. & E. × 37).

appear to straddle the rather ill-defined border between benignity and malignancy. *Intravenous leiomyomatosis* is a condition in which cords of smooth muscle are found in uterine and parauterine veins (Fig. 8.16), usually in association with more conventional leiomyomata elsewhere in the myometrium. This rare lesion can sometimes be suspected macroscopically by recognizing prominent veins containing easily extruded worm-like masses, whilst histological examination shows plugs of smooth muscle within sinusoidally dilated vessels. Occasionally, plugs of tumour extend as far as the inferior vena cava and can even grow into the right atrium. It is not clear whether this condition is due to a special form of leiomyoma which, despite its benign nature, invades veins, or whether the tumours arise from the muscle of the vein wall. A condition possibly related to intravenous leiomyomatosis is benign *metastasizing leiomyoma*, in which apparently benign uterine tumours appear to give rise to metastases which show no histological evidence of malignancy. Some such cases probably represent the simultaneous development of uterine and pulmonary leiomyomata, whilst others may result from dissemination of a benign uterine leiomyoma by surgical trauma, e.g. curettage. In *disseminated peritoneal leiomyomatosis*, small leiomyomatous nodules are found scattered about the peritoneum and omentum in association with uterine leiomyomata. This condition occurs most commonly in pregnancy and the nodules are thought to arise *in situ* from the mesenchyme of the peritoneal mesothelium.

Fibromata, *lipomata* and *haemangiomata* can all occur in the myometrium but are extremely rare. *Lymphangiomata* have been described in the myometrium but it is probable that many of these have been misdiagnosed adenomatoid tumours. A variant of a lymphangioma is the *lymphangiocystic fibroma*, which consists of large lymphatic channels in a matrix of highly cellular fibrous tissue, which in some areas forms broad bands of collagen.

Adenomatoid tumours of the myometrium are, quite common if sought, probably occurring in 1 per cent of uteri. They are usually small, less well delineated than a leiomyoma and found on the posterior surface of the uterus near the cornua, just beneath the serosa. Histologically (Fig. 8.17), these tumours

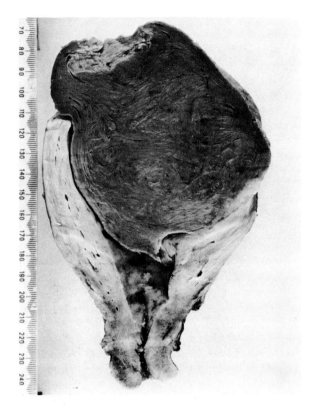

Fig. 8.14 Red degeneration of a leiomyoma. Even in a black and white print the dusky hue of the degenerate leiomyoma is apparent and contrasts with the usual appearance (*see* Fig. 8.9).

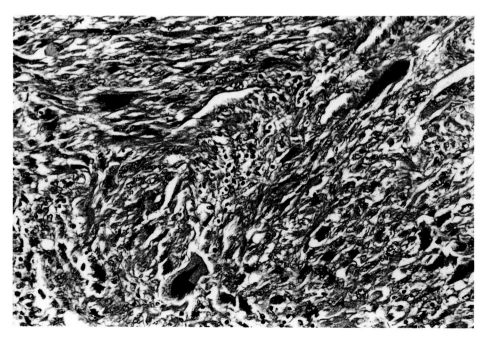

Fig. 8.15 Bizarre leiomyoma. There is no mitotic activity in this benign lesion, despite the cellular pleomorphism and cellular hyperchromatism (H. & E. × 232).

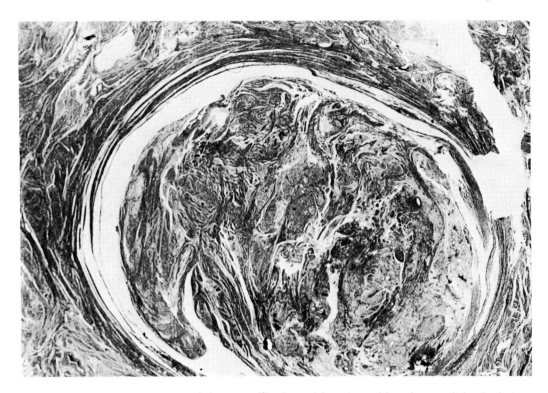

Fig. 8.16 Intravenous leiomyoma. At low magnification, a leiomyoma with a characteristic whorled pattern distends a small vein (H. & E. × 17.5).

usually consist of complex multiple gland-like spaces of various sizes which are lined by a flattened or low cuboidal epithelium and are separated from each other by strands of fibromuscular tissue. A plexiform arrangement of cuboidal cells is sometimes seen in these small neoplasms, which are almost invariably asymptomatic incidental findings and are thought to be benign mesotheliomata originating from the overlying mesothelial serosa. Indeed, in many cases serial sampling reveals a continuity with the overlying peritoneum.

A further rare, usually small and asymptomatic smooth muscle neoplasm is the *plexiform tumourlet*. This is often rather irregular and is less well defined than a typical leiomyoma. It is usually less than 1 cm in diameter and consists of nests and anastomosing strands of small cells set in an eosinophilic, collagenous richly vascularized, matrix (Fig. 8.18).

Fallopian tube

Benign tumours of the tube are all extremely rare and are commonly asymptomatic, being discovered incidentally during surgery, on pathological examination of resected specimens or at autopsy. The *adenomatoid tumour* is the least uncommon benign salpingeal neoplasm and is usually found in a subserosal site, compressing the muscularis into the tubal lumen. It is rarely more than 1–2 cm in diameter and is well circumscribed, firm and yellowish white. The histological appearances and nature of these tumours are identical with those of uterine adenomatoid tumours. *Leiomyomata* are probably the next most common benign tumour, although their rarity in the tube contrasts with their frequent occurrence in the

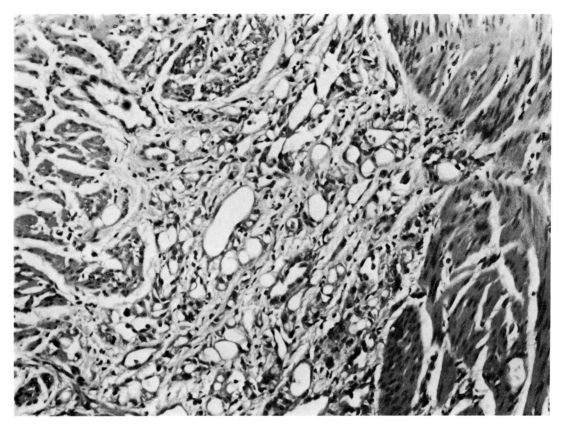

Fig. 8.17 Adenomatoid tumour of the myometrium. The tumour forms a complex of small acini lined by flattened cuboidal epithelium and, in some cases, careful serial sectioning will reveal its continuity with the covering serosa (H. & E. × 108).

uterus, a disparity due possibly to the myometrium having a greater sensitivity to oestrogens than the tubal musculature. Rare instances of *lipoma*, *fibroma*, *haemangioma* and *neurilemmoma* have also been recorded. These mesenchymal neoplasms do not usually produce symptoms but some, particularly the leiomyomata, occasionally attain a size sufficient to present as a pelvic mass or to cause pelvic pain. Torsion either of a pedunculated tumour or of a tube containing a large neoplasm may lead to presentation as an acute abdominal catastrophe, whilst intratubal bleeding can occur from a haemangioma.

Benign epithelial neoplasms of the tube are exceptionally rare and it is probable that most so-called *papillomata* are of an inflammatory rather than a neoplastic nature, whilst reported instances of *adenomata* have usually been either examples of adenomatoid hyperplasia provoked by infection or foci of endo-salpingeal endometriosis which develop secondary to tubal obstruction. Very rarely, however, true adenomata and papillomata do occur. The *metaplastic papillary tumour* of the tube resembles an ovarian papillary serous tumour of borderline malignancy, although the epithelial cells have abundant eosinophilic cytoplasm. These lesions involve only part of the circumference of the mucosa and have been incidental findings in pregnant women. The exact status of this lesion is uncertain and it is not established whether they are truly neoplastic or not. *Papillary adenofibromata* of the tube are very uncommon. They tend to form spongy multicystic masses, which may distend the tube and which consist histologically of papillae formed of fibrous tissue and covered by cuboidal or low columnar cells.

Mature cystic teratomata (dermoids) can occur in the tube and probably develop from germ cells

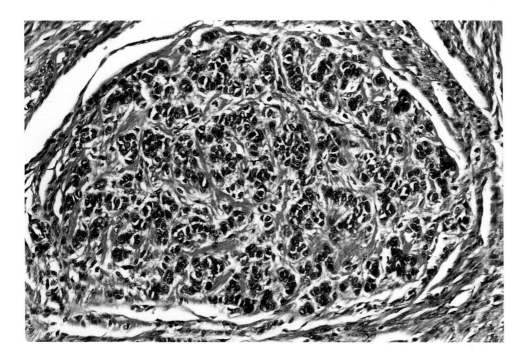

Fig. 8.18 A plexiform tumourlet of the myometrium. A well-demarcated lesion composed of cells with small, darkly staining nuclei lying in a collagenous vascular stroma (H. & E. × 232).

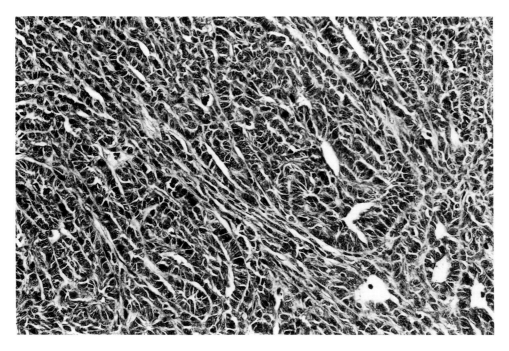

Fig. 8.19 Benign adnexal tumour of wolffian origin. The mixed tubular and trabecular pattern seen in this area is typical (H. & E. × 232).

that have become arrested during their passage through the salpingeal lumen. These tumours are morphologically identical to their commonly occurring ovarian counterparts and, although usually small and devoid of clinical significance, can be sufficiently large to be associated with abdominal or pelvic pain and do occasionally rupture either into the tubal lumen or through the wall of the tube into the peritoneal cavity.

Broad ligament

Leiomyomata, to be distinguished from subserous uterine leiomyomata pursuing an intraligamentary course, are the most common benign neoplasm of the broad ligament and arise from the sparse smooth muscle fibres found between the layers of the ligament. These neoplasms can attain a huge size and have been known to compress the ureter, producing a hydronephrosis, or the iliac vessels, with subsequent leg oedema. *Fibromata* can also develop in this site and may similarly reach large proportions. Rare neoplasms include *neurilemmomata, ganglioneuromata, lipomata, haemangiomata* and *adenomatoid tumours. Serous cystadenomata* and *cystadenofibromata*, identical to their ovarian counterparts, can occur in the ligament and in some cases clearly develop in paratubal cysts, others presumably arise from paramesonephric duct remnants. The *adnexal tumour of wolffian origin* is usually a moderate-sized mass which, histologically, consists of cellular cords, trabeculae, solid alveoli and tubules set in a scanty stroma (Fig. 8.19). Despite its name, the wolffian (or mesonephric) origin of this tumour is a mere assumption, based largely on its site of occurrence, there being nothing in either the light or electron microscopic appearances to suggest a mesonephric derivation. It is almost invariably benign, although there has been a well documented example of recurrence. There have been occasional well documented, but largely inexplicable, instances of *Brenner tumours* and *granulosa cell neoplasms* occurring in the broad ligament.

Key references

Altaras M, Jaffe R, Bernheim J and Ben-Adaret N. (1985) Granular cell myoblastoma of the vulva. *Gynecologic Oncology* **22**, 352–5.

Anders K H, Hall T L and Fu Y S. (1986) Epidemiologic and histopathologic studies of female genital warts. In: *Progress in Surgical Pathology, vol. 6*, pp. 33–47. Edited by C M Fenoglio, M W Woolf and F Rilke, Field and Wood, Philadelphia.

Barnes H M and Richardson P J. (1973) Benign metastasising fibroleiomyoma: a case report. *Journal of Obstetrics and Gynaecology of the British Commonwealth* **86**, 569–73.

Chabrel C M and Beilby J O W. (1980) Vaginal rhabdomyoma. *Histopathology* **4**, 645–52.

Fox H and Buckley C H. (1988) Non-epithelial and mixed tumours of the vulva. In: *The Vulva*, pp. 235–62. Edited by C M Ridley, Churchill Livingstone, Edinburgh.

Kaminski P F and Tavassoli F A. (1984) Plexiform tumorlet: a clinical and pathologic study of 15 cases with ultrastructural observations. *International Journal of Gynecological Pathology* **3**, 124–34.

Kluzak T R and Kraus F T. (1987) Condylomata, papillomas and verrucous carcinomas of the vulva and vagina. In: *Pathology of the Vulva and Vagina*, pp. 49–77. Edited by E J Wilkinson, Churchill Livingstone, New York.

Kurman R J and Norris H J. (1976) Mesenchymal tumors of the uterus VI. Epithelioid smooth muscle tumors including leiomyoblastoma and clear cell leiomyoma: a clinical and pathologic analysis of 26 cases. *Cancer* **37**, 1853–65.

Meisels A, Fortin R and Roy M. (1977) Condylomatous lesions of the cervix II. Cytologic, colposcopic and histopathologic study. *Acta Cytologica* **21**, 379–90.

Nogales F F, Navarro N, de Victoria J M M, Contreras F, Redondo C, Herraiz M A, Seco M A and

Velasco A. (1987) Uterine intravascular leiomyomatosis: an update and report of seven cases. *International Journal of Gynecological Pathology* **6**, 331–9.

Norris H J and Parmley T H. (1975) Mesenchymal tumors of the uterus V. Intravenous leiomyomatosis: a clinical and pathologic study of 14 cases. *Cancer* **36**, 2164–78.

Novick N L. (1985) Angiokeratoma vulvae. *Journal of the American Academy of Dermatology* **12**, 561–3.

Persaud V and Arjoon P D. (1970) Uterine leiomyoma: incidence of degenerative change and a correlation of associated symptoms. *Obstetrics and Gynecology* **35**, 432–6.

Saffos R O, Rhatigan R M and Scully R E. (1980) Metaplastic papillary tumor of the Fallopian tube — a distinctive lesion of pregnancy. *American Journal of Clinical Pathology* **74**, 232–6.

Sirota R L, Dickersin G R and Scully R E. (1981) Mixed tumors of the vagina: a clinicopathological analysis of eight cases. *American Journal of Surgical Pathology* **5**, 413–22.

Sivathondan Y, Salm R, Hughesdon P E and Faccini J M. (1979) Female adnexal tumour of probable Wolffian origin. *Journal of Clinical Pathology* **32**, 616–24.

Tavassoli F A and Norris H J. (1979) Smooth muscle tumors of the vulva. *Obstetrics and Gynecology* **53**, 213–7.

Tavassoli F A and Norris H J. (1982) Peritoneal leiomyomatosis (leiomyomatosis peritonealis disseminata): a clinicopathologic study of 20 cases with ultrastructural observations. *International Journal of Gynecological Pathology* **1**, 59–74.

Tiltman A J. (1980) Adenomatoid tumours of the uterus. *Histopathology* **4**, 437–43.

Vellios P, Ng A B P and Reagan J W. (1973). Papillary adenofibroma of the uterus — a benign mesodermal mixed tumor of Müllerian origin. *American Journal of Clinical Pathology* **60**, 543–51.

Woodworth H, Dockerty M B, Wilson R B and Pratt J H. (1971) Papillary hidradenoma of the vulva: a clinicopathologic study of 69 cases. *American Journal of Obstetrics and Gynecology* **110**, 501–8.

Young R H, Treger T and Scully R E. (1986) Atypical polypoid adenomyoma of the uterus: a report of 27 cases. *American Journal of Clinical Pathology* **86**, 139–45.

9

Epithelial abnormalities of the female genital tract and their malignant potential

The concept of morphological precursors of invasive epithelial neoplasms is now well established. A wide range of epithelial abnormalities of the female genital tract are regarded as possible precursors of invasive neoplasia and these fall into two broad groups. First, there are those abnormalities which are regarded as *premalignant*, i.e., whilst they are not in themselves neoplastic they are, in a proportion of cases, complicated in the long term by the development of a neoplasm. Second, there are abnormalities in which cells considered to be of a neoplastic nature are present in, and are confined to, the epithelium, i.e., they represent *preinvasive*, or *intraepithelial*, *neoplasms*. The diagnosis of both premalignant and preinvasive neoplastic epithelial lesions is usually based solely upon histopathological criteria and an understanding of their natural history has been determined by studying large numbers of patients over a period of years. In this chapter all epithelial abnormalities of the genital tract that predispose, even to the most limited degree, to the development of a carcinoma, or that represent forms of carcinoma that are either intraepithelial or fall short of being frankly invasive, are considered.

Vulva

The term *vulval dystrophy* was introduced in 1961 by Jeffcoate and Woodruff to encompass a wide variety of squamous epithelial abnormalities, some of which were preinvasive neoplasms, some of which seemed to be premalignant and yet others which would more correctly be classified as dermatological disorders. In 1976 the International Society for the Study of Vulvar Disease (ISSVD) modified the classification of the dystrophies, but there remained drawbacks to these modifications. First, the groups included both benign and neoplastic conditions of quite different prognosis. Second, they continued to draw an artificial distinction between a squamous epithelium in which there are cytologically atypical cells showing some differentiation (dystrophy with atypia) and an epithelium composed of cells showing little or no differentiation, involving the full thickness of the epithelium and termed carcinoma *in situ*. It is clearly inappropriate to consider such a disparate group of disorders as a single entity and hence the current classification for vulval epithelial abnormalities, recommended by the International Society of Gynaecological Pathologists, abandons the term 'dystrophy' and attempts to distinguish between, on the one hand, epithelial abnormalities that are not premalignant and in which there is no cytological atypia and, on the other hand, those that are intraepithelial neoplasias.

Clinical criteria alone are insufficiently discriminating to permit specific diagnosis of the various forms of epithelial abnormality. A wide variety of histopathological conditions with very different malignant potentials may present identical macroscopic appearances. Hence, imprecise clinical terms such as 'leukoplakia' or 'kraurosis' have no place in the modern classification of vulval epithelial abnormalities and no diagnosis is complete without histopathological confirmation of the condition.

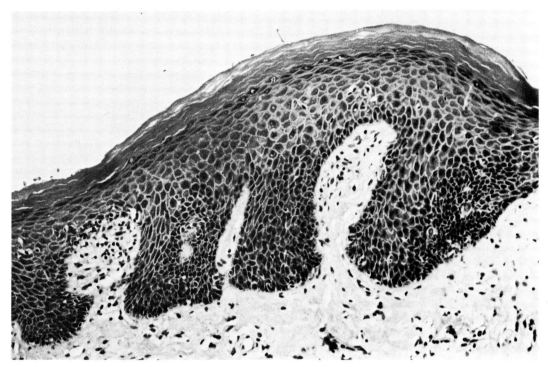

Fig. 9.1 Squamous epithelial hyperplasia of the vulva. There is acanthosis (hyperplasia), widening of the rete ridges and marked hyperkeratosis but no cytological atypia (H. & E. × 108).

Non-neoplastic epithelial disorders

Lichen sclerosus (et atrophicus)

Lichen sclerosus is described fully in Chapter 18 but is included here because, in approximately 3–4 per cent of cases the vulval lesions will be complicated by the development of a squamous cell carcinoma. It is important to recognize, however, that lichen sclerosus is not a preinvasive malignancy and that cytological atypia is not a feature of pure lichen sclerosus.

In about 10–15 per cent of cases the squamous epithelium becomes hyperplastic or develops the characteristics of vulvar intraepithelial neoplasia (see below).

Squamous epithelial hyperplasia and lichen simplex

The histological term 'squamous epithelial hyperplasia' is synonymous with the dermatological diagnosis of lichenification. It occurs in women with underlying dermatological disease as well as in women with pruritus vulvae but no dermatological disease. Most women with epithelial hyperplasia are less than 50 years old and any part of the vulva may be affected. The abnormal skin is thickened, slightly scaly, pale or earthy with accentuated markings and has ill-defined margins. In places, the epithelium may be markedly white, indicating hyperkeratosis, or it may be eczematoid; fissuring is not uncommon. The lesions vary in appearance from area to area and from time to time, because of variations in moisture, scratching and treatment. The appearances correspond histologically with changes in the squamous epithelium characterized by hyperkeratosis or parakeratosis, acanthosis (with irregular thickening of the Malpighian layer), elongation of the rete ridges and with a non-specific chronic inflammatory cell infiltrate in the dermis which may also be oedematous (Fig. 9.1). Cytological atypia is not a feature of the epithelium.

Those cases in which the hyperplasia cannot be attributed to any morphologically recognizable cause are described by the pathologist as squamous epithelial hyperplasia and by the dermatologist as lichenification. If there is associated chronic dermal inflammation, the condition is known as lichen simplex. Cases in which there is also evidence of lichen sclerosus, described previously as a mixed dystrophy, are regarded by the pathologist as showing squamous epithelial hyperplasia superimposed on the dermatosis.

In the absence of cytological atypia there is no risk of progression of epithelial hyperplasia to invasive carcinoma.

Neoplastic epithelial disorders

Vulvar intraepithelial neoplasia

The term vulvar intraepithelial neoplasia (VIN) is applied only to preinvasive malignancy of the squamous epithelium. Non-squamous forms (e.g. Paget's disease) are considered below.

Clinically, VIN may resemble squamous epithelial hyperplasia and is similarly very variable in appearance; a multicentric growth pattern is not unusual. Lesions may be discrete and sharply localized to the labia and/or perineum or may affect the whole vulva. Spread to the perianal area and anal canal occurs in between 14 and 35 per cent of cases, particularly when the vulval lesions lie posteriorly. The affected tissue often has a variegated appearance with granular dull red, or white, areas interspersed with 'warty' lesions. Intraepithelial or intradermal melanin often renders the lesions dark brown or black. Some of these pigmented lesions present a specific clinical picture of multiple, discoid, flat grey-brown or red-brown papular or verrucous lesions and are known as multicentric pigmented *Bowen's disease* or *Bowenoid papulosis*. Histologically, however, these lesions are indistinguishable from non-pigmented forms of VIN and their clinical behaviour is similar.

VIN may occur in hyperplastic skin, condylomata or skin in which there is no other disease process. Histologically, VIN is recognized by disturbances of epithelial stratification and maturation and by the presence of atypical mitoses. Two forms are recognized, that in which the epithelium is partly or completely replaced by non-stratified cells resembling those of the basal or parabasal cells of the normal epithelium (Fig. 9.2) and that which is characterized by the presence of individually keratinized cells, corps ronds and koilocytes (Fig. 9.3), so-called 'Bowenoid' VIN. The two forms frequently coexist. It has been customary to recognize three grades of VIN, according to the proportion of squamous epithelium lacking differentiation. VIN I representing well differentiated intraepithelial neoplasia, VIN II moderately differentiated intraepithelial neoplasia and VIN III poorly differentiated intraepithelial neoplasia. However, most lesions recognized as VIN affect the whole thickness of the epithelium and the majority are, in practice, VIN III.

'Bowenoid' VIN is often associated with HPV infection. It is increasing in incidence and many individuals with this lesion are quite young. In about 25 per cent of cases there is also cervical or vaginal intraepithelial or invasive neoplasia, though the conditions do not necessarily occur simultaneously, and this finding lends support to the concept of a field change within the lower female genital tract.

It is recognized that in up to 4 per cent of cases, particularly in the immunosuppressed or elderly, VIN may progress to invasive carcinoma. On the other hand, a small proportion of histologically proven cases of VIN spontaneously regress. Recognition of the low invasive potential of the condition has led to an increasing tendency to treat the disease as conservatively as possible. However, in planning treatment it is important to remember that VIN often extends into the skin appendages, is frequently multicentric and that when invasion does occur it too may be multifocal, making multiple biopsies mandatory.

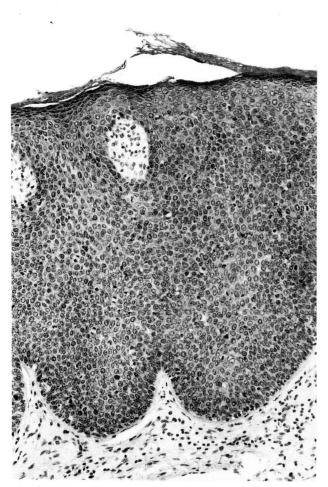

Fig. 9.2 Vulvar intraepithelial neoplasia. The epithelium is occupied by a fairly uniform population of cells which resemble those of the normal parabasal layer (H. & E. × 108).

Microinvasive carcinoma

This term was introduced as a counterpart to the well defined microinvasive carcinoma of the cervix (see later) but whilst the prognosis of the carefully defined and selected cervical lesion has been clearly demonstrated to be similar to that of intraepithelial neoplasia, no such certainty applies to even the most minimally invasive vulval lesion. It is agreed, therefore, that the term microinvasive carcinoma of the vulva is misleading and dangerous when applied to confluent invasive vulvar carcinoma, defined either in terms of volume or depth of invasion, and that such a designation may lead to inappropriate treatment. It is recommended that the designation 'stage 1a carcinoma of the vulva' should be used to describe solitary confluent lesions confined to a maximum of 2 cm diameter and up to 1 mm in depth (ISSVD, 1984). This recommendation is clearly justified but it does not mean that attempts to define a minimally invasive lesion which can be treated conservatively should be abandoned. Indeed, non-confluent invading foci, single or multiple, which arise from an epithelium with the features of VIN, are contained within the papillary dermis, do not extend into the stroma for more than 2 mm and are not associated with vascular space permeation, can probably be treated conservatively.

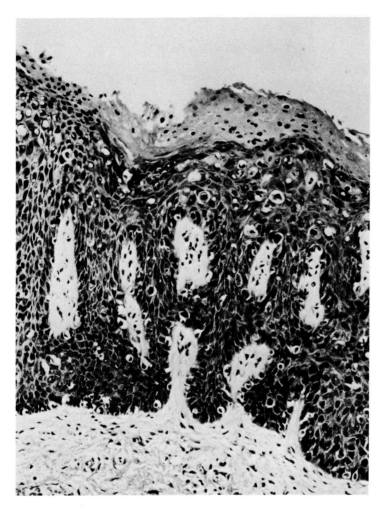

Fig. 9.3   Vulvar intraepithelial neoplasia ('Bowenoid' or HPV associated VIN). There is a lack of orderly maturation of the epithelium and vacuolated cells (koilocytes) are present: there is parakeratosis and mitoses are frequent (H. & E. × 108).

Paget's disease

Paget's disease of the vulva is rare and occurs most commonly in postmenopausal women in whom it presents as poorly demarcated, and often multifocal, erythematous, eczematoid weeping areas on the vulva. Histological examination (Fig. 9.4) shows large round or oval cells with pale cytoplasm lying singly or in nests within the epidermis. Microscopic disease often extends beyond the margins of the macroscopic lesion. The histogenesis of Paget's disease is not always clear but in up to 50 per cent of patients the condition is associated with intraepithelial or invasive neoplasia in the adjacent cutaneous adnexae, and it appears that in such cases the Paget cells are malignant cells that have migrated into the epidermis from the underlying structures. In other cases, however, there is no associated neoplasia and it is believed that in this situation the Paget cells develop *in situ* from undifferentiated or uncommitted cells in the germinative zone of the epithelium or, more probably, from the ductal portions of sweat glands. In such circumstances the Paget cells are thought to represent a form of primary intraepithelial neoplasia

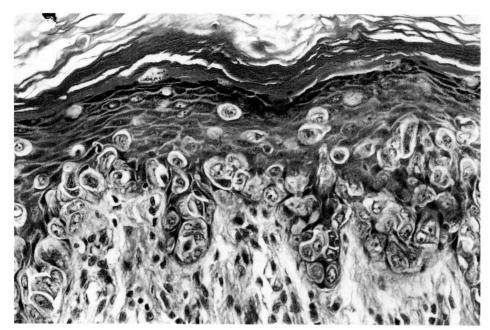

Fig. 9.4 Paget's disease of the vulva. Large pale cells which stain positively for mucin have infiltrated the epidermis (H. & E. × 370).

and, although very exceptional cases of invasion of the dermis by Paget cells have been recorded, it appears to be a slowly progressive, indolent and usually localized process.

The prognosis will obviously depend on the presence or otherwise of associated neoplasia and in patients with invasive adnexal tumours at the time of diagnosis, is poor. The outlook is better for patients with no associated neoplasia but the extension of the disease beyond the visible margins and its development *in situ* probably explain the fact that local recurrence occurs in nearly 40 per cent of cases. Recurrence may be delayed for many years and repeated resections are not uncommon; recurrence in grafted skin has been recorded.

Vagina

Intraepithelial neoplasia

Intraepithelial neoplasia in the vagina (VAIN) may appear as a poorly or sharply defined area of increased or abnormal vascularity, or as a whitish patch or verrucous lesion. Often, however, this lesion is not visible to the naked eye. Histologically, the appearances are similar to those seen in cervical intraepithelial neoplasia (see below) but the natural history of the vaginal lesion is less well understood, although it has been suggested that 20 per cent of cases of VAIN III will eventually progress to carcinoma.

In women with VAIN, there is frequently a history of preceding or simultaneous cervical intraepithelial or invasive neoplasia and it is not always clear whether the vaginal lesion is an extension of the cervical abnormality or a separate and independent focus of neoplastic change. What is clear, however, is that in some women, particularly those in whom there is HPV infection associated with the intraepithelial neoplasia, there is a field change affecting the entire lower genital tract and vulval neoplasia may also be present.

Vaginal adenosis

This heterotopic condition (discussed in Chapter 6) is considered to be a precursor of clear cell carcinoma of the vagina, although the incidence of neoplastic change is low and evidence of cellular atypia within foci of vaginal adenosis has very rarely been observed. In women using oral contraceptives, a microglandular hyperplasia, similar in all respects to that more commonly encountered in the cervix (see below), may develop in vaginal adenosis; such a lesion has no malignant potential.

Cervix

Squamous intraepithelial neoplasia

Preinvasive neoplastic squamous lesions of the cervix have been more extensively studied that those occurring elsewhere in the female genital tract, partly because of their frequency and partly because of the ease with which they can be identified by relatively easy, rapid, non-invasive techniques. They are entirely asymptomatic.

The term cervical intraepithelial neoplasia (CIN) is now well established and describes a single disease process. It begins at one end of the spectrum with well differentiated squamous intraepithelial neoplasia, or CIN I — previously known as mild dysplasia — and ends with invasive carcinoma. There are intermediate grades of moderately differentiated squamous intraepithelial neoplasia, CIN II, previously known as moderate dysplasia, and poorly differentiated squamous intraepithelial neoplasia, CIN III, encompassing those conditions known previously as severe dysplasia and carcinoma *in situ*. CIN is recognized histologically by abnormalities of cellular organization and maturation in the metaplastic squamous epithelium of the transformation zone, the cells showing nuclear and cytoplasmic characteristics of malignancy. Loss of polarity, an absence of stratification and increased mitotic activity are indicative of the abnormal pattern of growth, whilst an increased nucleocytoplasmic ratio, nuclear hyperchromatism, an irregular distribution of nuclear chromatin and the presence of abnormal mitotic figures, indicate the neoplastic nature of the cells.

CIN is graded according to the proportion of the squamous epithelium occupied by undifferentiated cells, although it should be recognized that this does not imply division into separate diagnostic categories and that the grade of the lesion should not be used as a basis for differing therapeutic strategies. The only truly critical decision, from a clinical point of view, is whether the neoplasm is intraepithelial or has progressed to invasion. In CIN I (Fig. 9.5), only the basal third, or less, of the epithelium is occupied by undifferentiated cells; the lesion is classed as CIN II (Fig. 9.6) if such cells occupy between one-third and two-thirds of the thickness of the epithelium. A diagnosis of CIN III is made (Figs. 9.7 and 9.8) if more than two-thirds of the epithelial thickness is occupied by undifferentiated cells. The cells which are shed from the surface of the abnormal epithelium closely reflect the abnormality in the underlying epithelium and their examination is the basis of the cervical smear test. The differentiation of CIN is rarely uniform throughout the affected transformation zone, the outer, ectocervical, part being generally better differentiated whilst that adjacent to the endocervical columnar epithelium is more poorly differentiated. It should be appreciated that inadequate sampling from the endocervical canal, particularly in the older woman in whom the transformation zone has withdrawn to within the endocervical canal, is most likely to miss the least well differentiated component of the CIN.

CIN III is usually assumed to be a squamous intraepithelial neoplasm but can be closely mimicked by poorly differentiated adenocarcinoma *in situ*, which can be recognized only by the use of mucin stains.

Features of HPV infection (the presence of koilocytes, epithelial multinucleation and individual cell keratinization) are present in many cases of CIN. These abnormalities are most evident in CIN I and II

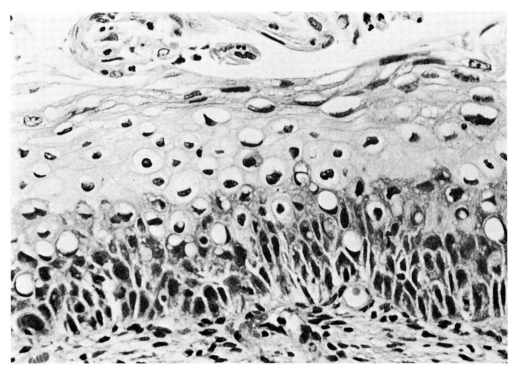

Fig. 9.5 CIN I. The basal third of the epithelium is occupied by atypical cells and while some cytoplasmic maturation occurs as the cells become more superficial, nuclear atypia persists. The cells with clear perinuclear haloes and abnormally-shaped nuclei in the superficial layers of the epithelium (koilocytes) are indicative of HPV infection (H. & E. × 255).

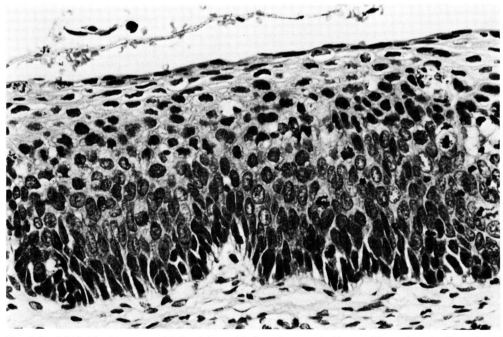

Fig. 9.6 CIN II. The lower two-thirds of the epithelium is occupied by undifferentiated cells and, while the upper third of the epithelium shows cytoplasmic maturation, abnormal nuclei persist to the surface (H. & E. × 255).

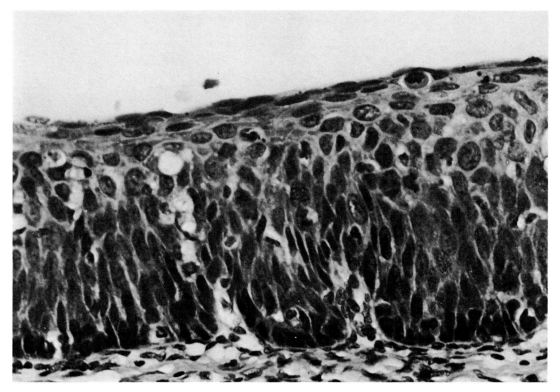

Fig. 9.7 CIN III (previously severe dysplasia). More than two-thirds of the epithelial depth is occupied by neoplastic cells with a high nucleocytoplasmic ratio. The minor degree of cytoplasmic maturation shown by the superficial layers of cells does not alter the grade of this lesion (H. & E. × 270).

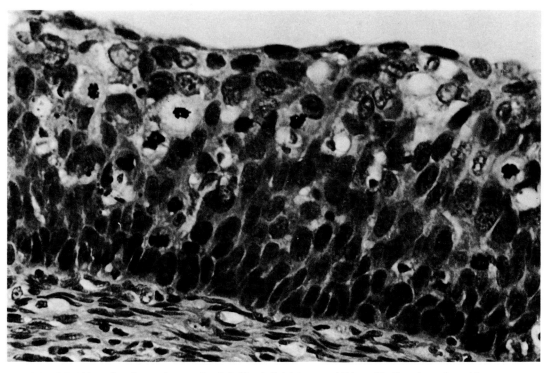

Fig. 9.8 CIN III (previously carcinoma *in situ*). The full thickness of this epithelium is replaced by undifferentiated neoplastic cells. Mitoses can be seen in the superficial third (H. & E. × 270).

and are less apparent in CIN III, in which integration of the viral genome into the DNA of the epithelial cell nucleus has become complete.

The fact that a lesion is neoplastic in nature does not necessarily imply that it will inevitably progress and the frequency of progression and the rate of change from one stage to another cannot be predicted with certainty for cases of CIN; the natural history of this lesion can be markedly modified not only by treatment but also by diagnostic procedures. However, it has been estimated that, within 20 years of diagnosis, between 35 and 40 per cent of cases of CIN III will progress to invasive cancer, whilst an unknown number of lesions will apparently regress following diagnostic procedures. The long term risk of invasion in cases of CIN I and II is less well defined but progression to CIN III is not necessary before invasion occurs, there being well documented examples of invasion from lesser grades of CIN. Hence, all cases of CIN, irrespective of grade, must be treated in the same manner; it is not the grade of CIN but rather its extent which is of importance to the individual patient.

The CIN probably arises from malignant change in a single cell situated in the transformation zone. The malignant clone originates most commonly on the anterior lip of the cervix and then spreads horizontally, to involve the whole of the transformation zone, stopping abruptly at the junction with the original ectocervical squamous epithelium. The abnormal epithelium is seen not only on the surface but also within the underlying crypts and extensive crypt involvement is sometimes mistaken for invasion.

The aetiological factors involved in the development of CIN are similar to those for invasive cervical squamous carcinoma, which are discussed in Chapter 10: the peak incidence of CIN was in women aged 30 years to 40 years but in recent years there has been a sharp increase in incidence in women under the age of 30 years, this now being the most commonly affected group.

Microinvasive squamous cell carcinoma

This condition should, by rights, be considered in Chapter 10 because it is a form of invasive neoplasm and not one which is still confined within the limits of the epithelium. However, the term 'microinvasive' is applied to a neoplasm which, although minimally invasive, can for all practical purposes be treated as if it were purely intraepithelial, since it is not associated with any risk of nodal metastases.

Invasion is first recognized by an increase in the amount of cytoplasm and eosinophilia of the cytoplasm of one or more cells in the basal layer of an epithelium which shows the features of CIN and which covers the surface of the cervix or lines one of the crypts. Subsequently, the deep margin of the epithelium becomes irregular and jagged as tongues of infiltrating cells penetrate the underlying stroma (Fig. 9.9) where there is usually a lymphocytic infiltrate and reactive fibrosis. Invasion may be multifocal or limited to a single focus; it may be confluent or form discrete, non-confluent tongues of tumour.

Non-confluent lesions which consist only of small tongues of invading cells are described as 'early stromal invasion' (Stage Ia1 cervical carcinoma). Confluent, microinvasive carcinoma (Stage Ia2 cervical carcinoma) is less than 500 mm^3 in volume, must not exceed 1.0 cm in its greatest horizontal axis and must not penetrate the stroma for more than 0.5 cm. A minor degree of lymphatic permeation in the immediate vicinity of the neoplasm in those lesions under 200 mm^3 does not exclude the lesion from this category. The term 'microinvasive carcinoma' should not be used unless there has been complete excision of both the invasive component and the associated CIN, affording complete assessment of the lesion.

Adenocarcinoma *in situ*

An intraepithelial, non-invasive stage of endocervical adenocarcinoma is now well recognized, although the relative rarity of this lesion has limited knowledge of its natural history.

Adenocarcinoma *in situ* may occur in any part of the cervix where columnar cells are to be found, i.e. on an ectopy, within the surface epithelium of the endocervical canal or within the endocervical crypts. It is characterized by cytological atypia within the columnar cells, cellular stratification, increase in the

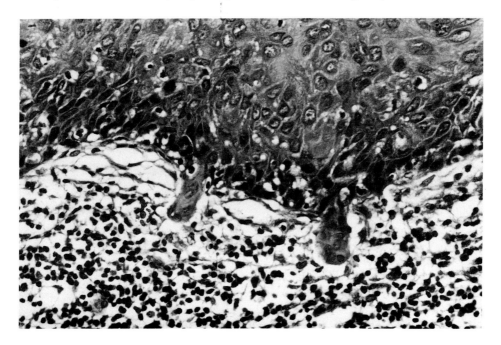

Fig. 9.9 Microinvasive squamous cell carcinoma of the cervix (early stromal invasion). Two infiltrating tongues of atypical squamous cells arise from the base of an epithelium with the features of CIN. Note the lymphocytic response at the site of invasion (H. & E. × 370).

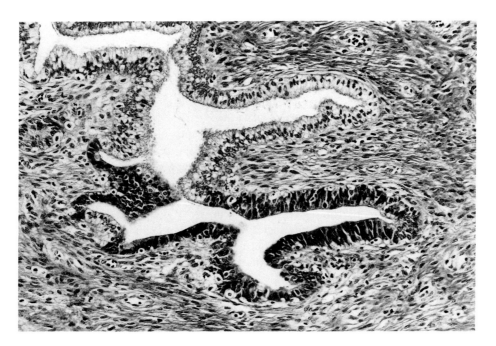

Fig. 9.10 Cervical adenocarcinoma *in situ*. The endocervical crypt is lined in its upper part by normal, pale-staining, mucus-secreting columnar cells and in its lower part by stratified cells with larger, darkly-staining nuclei and scanty cytoplasm. The latter is typical of adenocarcinoma *in situ* (H. & E. × 186).

nucleocytoplasmic ratio, loss of mucin secretion, loss of nuclear polarity, nuclear hyperchromasia and many mitotic figures, some of which may be atypical (Fig. 9.10). There is also often an alteration in the configuration of the affected endocervical crypts — outpouchings, budding and close packing of glandular acini being typical. It is not unusual to find associated intraepithelial neoplasia of the adjacent squamous epithelium. The latter should be distinguished from poorly differentiated adenocarcinoma *in situ*, with which it is easily confused unless mucin stains are performed.

Lesser degrees of cytological atypia than those described as adenocarcinoma *in situ* have been reported but their recognition is more difficult and the criteria for their diagnosis less well established. They and adenocarcinoma *in situ* are known collectively as cervical glandular intraepithelial neoplasia (CGIN).

Microglandular hyperplasia

This is a benign lesion of the endocervical epithelium which occurs in women using oral steroid contraceptives and during pregnancy. It is thought to be progesterone induced but may persist for some time after the original progestational stimulus has been withdrawn. Commonly, microglandular hyperplasia is a symptomless condition, apparent only on histological examination but, in a proportion of cases, the lesion may assume a polypoid form and be responsible for postcoital bleeding or spotting. Histologically, there are tightly packed glandular acini lined by flattened or cuboidal cells. Squamous metaplasia is a common feature (Fig. 9.11) and occasionally a sheet-like proliferation is seen. There may be a modest amount of nuclear pleomorphism and hyperchromasia but mitotic figures are rarely seen and the lesion is always fully benign.

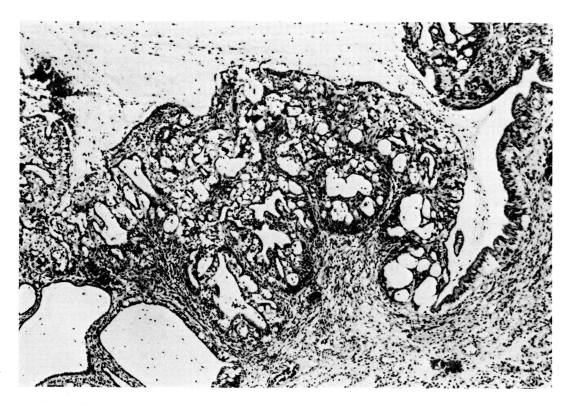

Fig. 9.11 Microglandular hyperplasia of the cervix. The closely packed, small acini lined by flattened cubocolumnar cells and focal squamous metaplasia are typical of this lesion (H. & E. × 45).

Endometrium

Simple hyperplasia

This is a true hyperplasia of the uterus, which is usually slightly or moderately enlarged. The endometrium is thickened, bulky and, not uncommonly, polypoid. Curettage yields abundant soft, red, sometimes velvety, material in which tiny cysts may be apparent on naked-eye examination (Fig. 9.12(a) and (b)).

The entire endometrium, including both glands and stroma, is involved and the normal distinction between basal and functional zones tends to be lost (Fig. 9.13). The endometrial glands show a proliferative pattern but vary markedly in calibre, some being unusually large, others being of normal size and yet others being unduly small. The glands usually have a smooth rounded contour, although some degree of budding into the stroma is not uncommon. They are lined by regular, tall cuboidal or columnar cells which have strongly basophilic cytoplasm and round, basally or centrally sited nuclei. There is commonly a degree of multilayering but intraluminal tufting, loss of polarity and cytological atypia are not seen. Tubal or squamous metaplasia is common.

In simple hyperplasia the stroma shares in the hyperplastic process and hence the gland-to-stroma ratio is normal, there being no glandular crowding. The stroma is usually hypercellular and resembles that of a normal proliferative endometrium. Focal areas of stromal necrosis and haemorrhage are not uncommon.

Mitotic figures, both in the glands and in the stroma, may be abundant or sparse but are invariably of normal form.

A simple hyperplasia is due to prolonged, unopposed oestrogenic stimulation of the endometrium and may thus complicate the administration of exogenous oestrogens, oestrogenic ovarian tumours or the polycystic ovary syndrome. However, the most common cause is a sequence of anovulatory cycles and hence simple hyperplasia tends to occur predominantly at the menarche or in the perimenopausal years, when such cycles occur with greatest frequency. Patients with this form of hyperplasia tend to suffer episodic bleeding which is often heavy and prolonged. It is assumed, perhaps rather simplistically, that this is due either to intermittent waning of oestrogen levels or to the endometrium attaining a bulk that surpasses the supportive capacity of the oestrogens.

If ovulation occurs in a patient having anovulatory cycles, or if a progestagen is administered, a simple hyperplasia will regress and the endometrium return to normal. It is of considerable importance to stress that a simple hyperplasia is not associated with any increased risk of the development of endometrial adenocarcinoma and that this form of hyperplasia is not a precursor of, and does not evolve into, an atypical hyperplasia.

Complex hyperplasia

This endometrial abnormality may occur under the same conditions as a simple hyperplasia but can also develop in normally cycling or atrophic endometria. A complex hyperplasia is restricted to the glandular component of the endometrium and is usually focal, or multifocal, rather than generalized. The hyperplastic glands are variable in size but are often larger and more numerous than normal with consequent crowding and a reduction in the amount of intervening stroma. The glands grow in an abnormal fashion with outpouchings, or budding, of the glandular epithelium into the surrounding stroma to produce a 'fingers-in-glove' pattern. Papillary projections of cells, with connective tissue cores, into the glandular lumens are not uncommon (Fig. 9.14). The glandular epithelium is regular and formed of tall cuboidal or low columnar cells with nuclei which can be ovoid or round and basally sited or central. Nucleoli are inconspicuous, multilayering is minimal, nuclear polarity is not lost and there is no cytological atypia. The stroma between the hyperplastic glands is compressed but not hypercellular. Mitotic figures can be fairly numerous in the glandular epithelium and are of normal form.

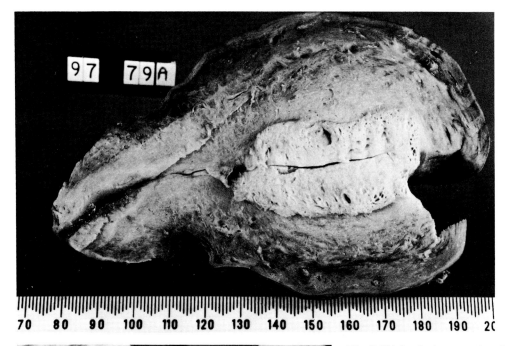

Fig. 9.12(a)   A uterus cut longitudinally to show the increased thickness of the endometrium and the finely cystic pattern of simple hyperplasia of the endometrium.

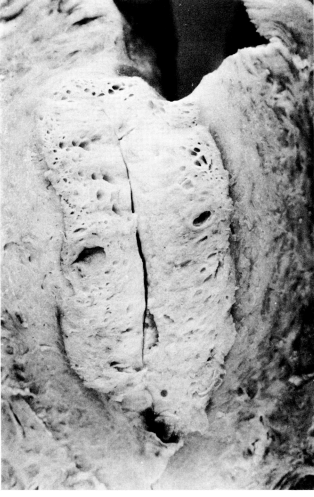

Fig. 9.12(b)   A higher magnification of Fig. 9.12(a), which emphasizes the widespread nature of the changes.

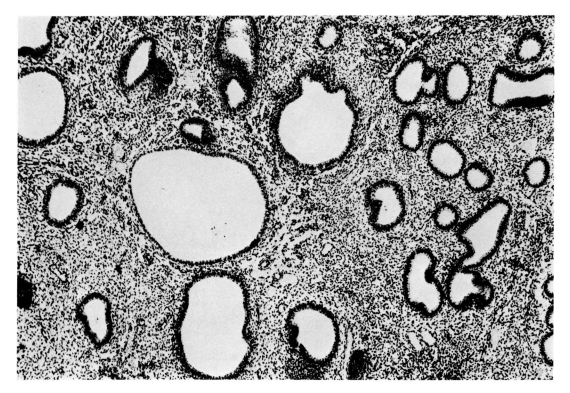

Fig. 9.13 Simple hyperplasia of the endometrium. There is an increase in the bulk of the stroma and many of the glands, which vary considerably in size, are cystically dilated (H. & E. × 45).

A complex hyperplasia may evolve into an atypical hyperplasia (see below) but in the absence of any superimposed cytological atypia a complex hyperplasia is not associated with any increased risk of development of a carcinoma.

Atypical hyperplasia

This form of hyperplasia is restricted to the endometrial glands and is always focal or multifocal, often quite sharply so. In the hyperplastic areas there is crowding of the glands with reduction in the amount of intervening stroma and, in severe cases, the glands may show a 'back-to-back' pattern, with the interglandular stroma being reduced to a thin wisp or completely obliterated. The glands are usually markedly irregular and their lining cells show varying degrees of atypia and pleomorphism (Fig. 9.15). In the milder forms of atypical hyperplasia the nuclei are ovoid, the nucleo-cytoplasmic ratio only slightly increased, the nucleoli are not enlarged and the nuclear chromatin is not clumped. In more severe cases the nucleo-cytoplasmic ratio is markedly increased, the nuclei are rounded, the nucleoli are enlarged and the nuclear chromatin clumped. There is a variable degree of loss of nuclear polarity, of multilayering and of intralumenal tufting and budding, the tufts sometimes fusing to give a cribriform pattern within the glands. The cytoplasm of the atypical cells may be relatively sparse but can also be unduly abundant. With increasing degrees of atypia greater numbers of mitotic figures are seen, these usually being of normal form.

An atypical hyperplasia of the endometrium may develop in some women whose endometria are

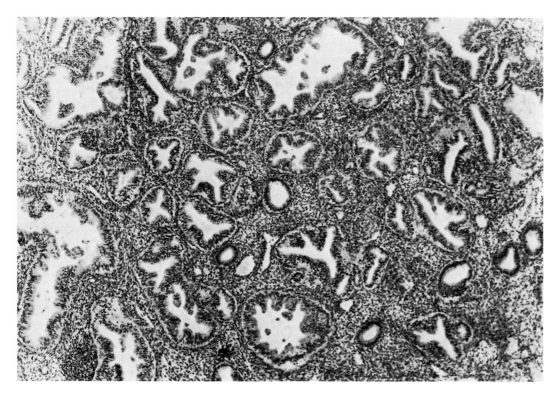

Fig. 9.14 Complex hyperplasia of the endometrium. A focus of rather crowded glands showing irregularity of outline due to abnormal branching and infolding (H. & E. × 108).

subjected to prolonged unopposed oestrogenic stimulation. It can also occur in women whose endometrium is otherwise atrophic or shows normal cyclical changes. This is the only form of endometrial hyperplasia which is associated with a risk of evolution into an adenocarcinoma, the magnitude of this risk being about 30–50 per cent in cases with severe atypia. However, exact assessment of the risk of development of an adenocarcinoma is made extremely difficult by the fact that the distinction between a severe atypical hyperplasia and an intraendometrial adenocarcinoma (see below) is often both subjective and arbitrary. There are, in fact, good grounds for believing that atypical hyperplasia of the endometrium is a neoplastic rather than a hyperplastic process, that attempts to draw a sharp distinction between severe atypical hyperplasia and an intraendometrial adenocarcinoma are unjustified and that both lesions should be considered together under the single heading of 'endometrial intraepithelial neoplasia' (EIN).

Intraendometrial adenocarcinoma

The term 'adenocarcinoma *in situ* of the endometrium' has been used in several different ways in accounts of endometrial pathology. Some have equated adenocarcinoma *in situ* with severe atypical hyperplasia whilst others, although drawing a distinction between these two conditions, have not always specified whether an *in situ* adenocarcinoma is one which is not invading the endometrial stroma or one which is not invading the myometrium. An adenocarcinoma *in situ* is, by presumed definition, a non-invasive lesion and therefore a true adenocarcinoma *in situ* of the endometrium is one in which the glands have

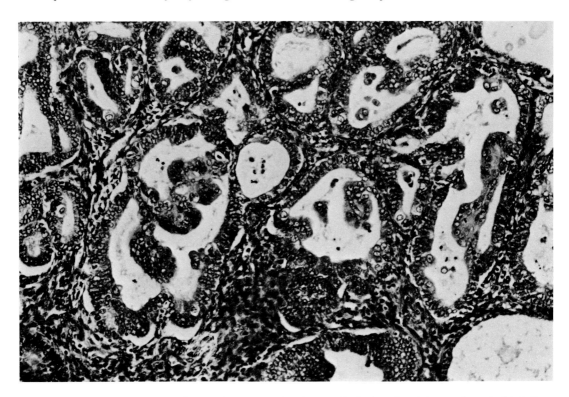

Fig. 9.15 Atypical hyperplasia of the endometrium showing cytological and architectural atypia (H. & E. × 108).

undergone neoplastic change but in which there is no invasion of the endometrial stroma. It is doubtful whether an adenocarcinoma of this type exists, or if it could be recognized even if it did. Hence, a term has to be found to describe a lesion which, although invasive, is confined to the endometrium and is not invading the myometrium. Of the various forms of nomenclature that have been proposed the name 'intraendometrial adenocarcinoma' seems to be the most appropriate.

An intraendometrial adenocarcinoma can be distinguished from a severe atypical hyperplasia if there is evidence of stromal invasion, i.e. stromal fibrosis, stromal necrosis or stromal polymorphonuclear leucocytic infiltration. However, in most cases these features are absent and, as already remarked, no differentiation between these two conditions can be made on objective grounds.

Fallopian tube

Premalignant abnormalities of the tubal epithelium are poorly documented and it has not yet been possible to define, with any degree of confidence, the criteria for the diagnosis of tubal intraepithelial neoplasia. Proliferative epithelial lesions, often with atypical features such as nuclear crowding, some loss of nuclear polarity, the presence of mitotic figures and a minor degree of nuclear stratification, are seen with some frequency in the tube. Such changes are often found in association with tubal inflammation and are seen most markedly in some cases of tubal tuberculosis where, indeed, they may be sufficiently marked as to be mistakenly interpreted as a carcinoma. There is no evidence that relatively minor proliferative lesions of this type, often known as *adenomatoid hyperplasia* (Fig. 9.16), progress to a carcinoma,

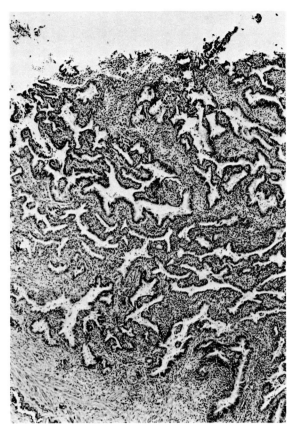

Fig. 9.16   Adenomatoid hyperplasia of the fallopian tube. The normal plical structure is replaced by a solid mass of branching papillary processes which may, on first examination, appear to be neoplastic (H. & E. × 34).

but an accepted morphological precursor of carcinoma is sometimes recognized. This is characterized by epithelium budding or a florid papillary pattern associated with nuclear enlargement, pleomorphism and hyperchromasia, prominent nucleoli, loss of cellular polarity and mitotic activity. How often such a lesion progresses to overt adenocarcinoma is, however, currently unknown.

Key references

Anderson M C. (1987) Premalignant and malignant disease of the cervix. In: *Haines and Taylor, Obstetrical and Gynaecological Pathology, 3rd edn*, pp. 255–301. Edited by H Fox, Churchill Livingstone, Edinburgh.

Buckley C H, Butler E B and Fox H. (1982) Cervical intraepithelial neoplasia. *Journal of Clinical Pathology* **35**, 1–13.

Buckley C H, Butler E B and Fox H. (1984) Vulvar intraepithelial neoplasia and microinvasive carcinoma of the vulva. *Journal of Clinical Pathology* **37**, 1201–11.

Buckley C H and Fox H. (1989) *Biopsy Pathology of the Endometrium*. Chapman and Hall, London.

Coleman D V and Evans D M D. (1988) *Biopsy Pathology and Cytology of the Cervix*. Chapman and Hall, London.

Crum C P. (1987) Vulvar intraepithelial neoplasia and associated viral changes. In: *Pathology of the Vulva and Vagina*, pp. 79–101. Edited by E J Wilkinson, Churchill Livingstone, New York.

Ferenczy A and Bergerson C. (1989) Endometrial hyperplasia and neoplasia. In: *The Biology of the Uterus*, pp. 333–53. Edited by R M Wynn and W P Jolly, Plenum, New York.

Ferenczy A and Winkler B. (1987) Cervical intraepithelial neoplasia and condyloma. In: *Blaustein's Pathology of the Female Genital Tract, 3rd edn*, pp. 117–217. Edited by R J Kurman, Springer-Verlag, New York.

Fox H and Buckley C H. (1982) The endometrial hyperplasias and their relationship to endometrial neoplasia. *Histopathology* **6**, 493–510.

Fu Y S and Reagan J W. (1989) *Pathology of the Uterine Cervix, Vagina and Vulva*. W B Saunders, Philadelphia.

Hilborne L H and Fu Y S. (1987) Intraepithelial, invasive and metastatic neoplasia of the vagina. In: *Pathology of the Vulva and Vagina*, pp. 181–207. Edited by E J Wilkinson, Churchill Livingstone, New York.

Lee S C, Roth L M, Ehrlich C and Hall J A. (1977) Extramammary Paget's disease of the vulva: a clinicopathologic study of 13 cases. *Cancer* **39**, 2540–9.

Moore S W and Enterline H T. (1975) Significance of proliferative epithelial lesions of the uterine tube. *Obstetrics and Gynecology* **45**, 385–90.

Norris H J, Connor M P and Kurman R J. (1986) Preinvasive lesions of the endometrium. *Clinics in Obstetrics and Gynaecology* **13**, 725–38.

Roth L M, Lee S C and Ehrlich C E. (1977) Paget's disease of the vulva: a histogenetic study of five cases including ultrastructural observations and review of the literature. *American Journal of Surgical Pathology* **1**, 193–206.

Silverberg S G. (1988) Hyperplasia and carcinoma of the endometrium. *Seminars in Diagnostic Pathology* **5**, 135–53.

Twiggs L B, Okagaki T, Clark B, Fukushima M, Ostrow R and Faras A. (1988) A clinical, histopathologic, and molecular biologic investigation of vulvar intraepithelial neoplasia. *International Journal of Gynecological Pathology* **7**, 48–55.

Wells M and Brown L J R. (1986) Glandular lesions of the uterine cervix: the present state of our knowledge. *Histopathology* **10**, 777–97.

10

Malignant neoplasms of the female genital tract

In this chapter consideration is given only to those neoplasms of the genital tract which are frankly invasive and overtly malignant.

Vulva

Squamous cell carcinoma

Ninety per cent of malignant vulval neoplasms are of squamous type and such tumours account for 4 to 5 per cent of cases of female genital tract cancer.

Aetiology
Most squamous cell carcinomata of the vulva develop against a background of chronic vulval irritation or intraepithelial neoplasia, although it is clear that some arise in previously healthy skin. Chronic granulomatous diseases of the vulva, such as syphilis, granuloma inguinale and lymphogranuloma venereum, appear to predispose to squamous cell carcinoma and vulval carcinoma occurs with greater frequency and at an unusually early age in countries where such diseases are common. The incidence of nulliparity is high amongst women with this neoplasm but the belief in an association with obesity, hypertension and diabetes mellitus is one that has not been upheld in controlled studies. There is a general, although partially anecdotal, belief that women of low socioeconomic status and who practise poor vulval hygiene are particularly prone to develop vulval carcinoma. A statistical association has been proved between vulval neoplasia and cigarette smoking, this apparently bizarre correlation being attributed to contamination of the vulva by urine containing a carcinogen derived from cigarette smoke.

Although the reproductive background of women with vulval carcinoma is, in general, different from that of patients with cervical carcinoma, it is by no means rare for women with vulval carcinoma to have cervical intraepithelial or invasive neoplasia and a variable, but significant proportion of women, particularly the younger patient in whom there is evidence of HPV infection, have a field change affecting the entire lower genital tract. Women with this pattern of disease are at particular risk of developing carcinoma should they be immunosuppressed, e.g. following renal transplantation.

Clinical findings
Squamous cell carcinoma is a disease of relatively elderly women, the peak incidence being at about 63 to 65 and one-third of patients being aged over 70. The usual symptoms are of pruritus, the finding of a

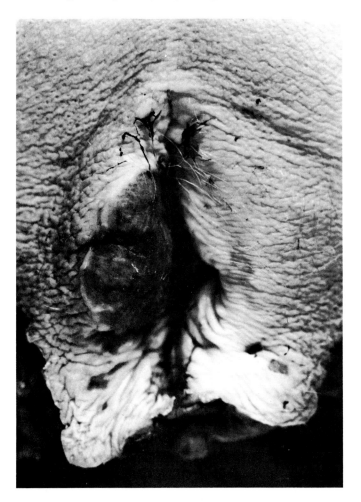

Fig. 10.1   A vulvectomy specimen showing a plaque of infiltrating squamous carcinoma invading the inner surface of the right labium major. White hyperkeratotic areas around the tumour and on the left labium major indicate the site of squamous, intraepithelial neoplasia

vulval ulcer or nodule, bleeding or pain, although in women with chronic vulval irritation, or VIN, the onset of an overtly malignant tumour may be very insidious.

Pathological findings
Seventy per cent of squamous cell carcinomata develop on the labia, most commonly in the anterior part; the clitoris is the next most common site, whilst tumours involving the mons or the urethral meatus are rather infrequent. The naked-eye appearances are usually of an indurated ulcer with raised, rolled edges but there may be a plaque or a papillary nodule (Fig. 10.1). The tumour is usually well differentiated with tongues and cords of squamous cells (Fig. 10.2) extending down into the dermis and subcutaneous tissue and forming well marked and abundant keratinizing epithelial pearls. The relatively uncommon tumours, which are poorly differentiated tend to grow in solid sheets. Rare histological variants include the *spindle cell type* of squamous cell tumour, the *pseudoglandular (adenoid squamous) carcinoma* which, is characterized by the presence of gland-like spaces formed as a result of extensive acantholysis. Very

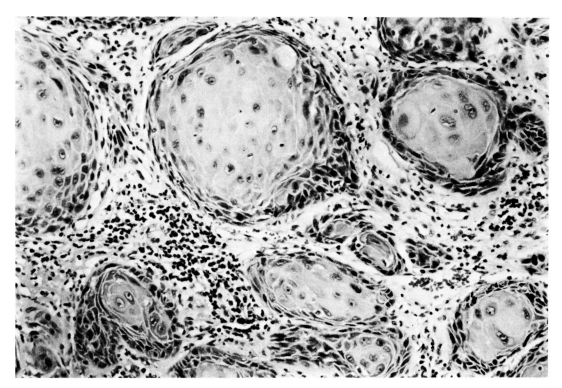

Fig. 10.2 Well-differentiated, invasive squamous cell carcinoma of the vulva forming epithelial pearls (H. & E. × 108).

exceptionally, a true *adenosquamous carcinoma*, containing an admixture of malignant squamous and glandular cells, is encountered in the vulva. The latter are believed to develop from cloacal remnants or skin appendages rather than directly from the epidermis.

Spread and prognosis
The carcinoma may spread directly to involve much of the vulva and can extend to the urethra, vagina, perineum and anal margin. Metastasis to lymph nodes is common and often occurs early in the course of the disease, large or poorly differentiated tumours being more likely to have metastasized via the lymphatics than small tumours or those which are well differentiated. Lymphatic spread occurs to the inguinal nodes initially and, because of anastomoses, the nodes on the contralateral side to that of the tumour are often also involved. From the inguinal nodes the tumour spreads to the node of Cloquet and thence to the deep pelvic nodes, the only exception to the general rule that if inguinal nodes are uninvolved the pelvic nodes will be free of metastases being in the case of clitoral and Bartholin's gland carcinoma, where there may be direct spread to Cloquet's node. Blood borne spread occurs late and principally to the liver, lungs and bones.

The clinical staging of vulval carcinoma takes into account both the size of the tumour and the extent of spread. However, clinical staging is intrinsically inaccurate, most commonly underestimating the presence of inguinal nodal metastases; on average there is an error of 25 per cent when a comparison is made between clinical and histologically confirmed stages. This error should be remembered when evaluating survival data.

Stage I. Lesion is less than 2 cm in diameter and no palpable groin nodes.

Stage II. Lesion is greater than 2 cm in diameter and no palpable groin nodes.

Stage III. Lesion extends beyond vulva without palable groin nodes *or* lesion of any size with unilateral regional node metastasis.

Stage IV. Bilateral node metastasis regardless of the extent of the primary tumour *or* lesion extends beyond the vulva to involve the mucosa of the bladder or rectum *or* there is evidence of metastatic disease anywhere.

The overall five-year survival rate (corrected) for women with a vulval squamous carcinoma is now in the region of 70 to 80 per cent. When the inguinal lymph nodes contain metastases an overall three-year survival rate of only 46 per cent is obtained. Survival for women with clinical stage I disease is between 90 and 100 per cent, falling to 80 per cent for stage II disease, 50 to 70 per cent for stage III disease and up to 20 per cent for stage IV disease. Recurrences, which may develop up to twelve years after treatment, occur in between a quarter and one-third of patients; they are usually vulval.

In general, the smaller the primary neoplasm and the less its depth of invasion, the lower the risk of nodal metastases and hence the better the prognosis. Indicators of poor prognosis, in terms of survival and/or recurrence, in addition to large tumour size, include deeply invasive tumours, poor tumour differentiation and vascular permeation around the primary neoplasm.

Verrucous carcinoma

This is a rare but distinctive variant of the squamous cell carcinoma. The tumour presents, usually in the postmenopausal years, as a bulky, fungating, cauliflower-like mass which is slowly growing but shows a progressive invasion of contiguous structures. Histologically, these macroscopically striking neoplasms have a remarkably bland appearance (Fig. 10.3). A superficial layer of hyperkeratotic or parakeratotic epithelium covers papillary fronds of well-differentiated squamous epithelium which shows little or no evidence of cellular atypia or mitotic activity. The base of the tumour is well circumscribed with broad, bulbous rete ridges which appear to be pushing against or compressing, rather than invading the stroma. Deep to the rete ridges there is usually a chronic inflammatory cell infiltrate.

These tumours rarely metastasize to lymph nodes but tend to show a relentless local invasiveness and commonly recur after excision. This is often surprising to the pathologist faced with a neoplasm that appears histologically benign, and the true diagnosis is often not made until the size and invasiveness of the tumour, and its tendency to recur, are seen to contrast sharply with the apparently innocuous microscopic appearances.

Surgery is the treatment of choice for verrucous carcinomata they are generally regarded as being radioresistant and, in some cases, radiotherapy has induced an anaplastic transformation with acceleration of growth and the development of metastases. Lymph node metastases are so uncommon that inguinal nodal dissection is not usually regarded as necessary. About 30 per cent of verrucous carcinomata recur locally but this is often the result of a failure to recognize the malignant nature of the neoplasm and hence carry out a sufficiently wide local excision.

Basal cell carcinoma

This is a slowly growing tumour of the vulva which usually occurs in postmenopausal women and which metastasizes with extreme rarity. It is uncommon and accounts for only 2 to 3 per cent of vulval neoplasms, its rarity being explicable on the basis of the infrequent exposure of the vulva to the only known aetiological agent, which is sunlight. The neoplasm usually arises on the labia majora and is seen as a slightly raised ulcerated nodule with rolled pearly margins. Histologically (Fig. 10.4), solid

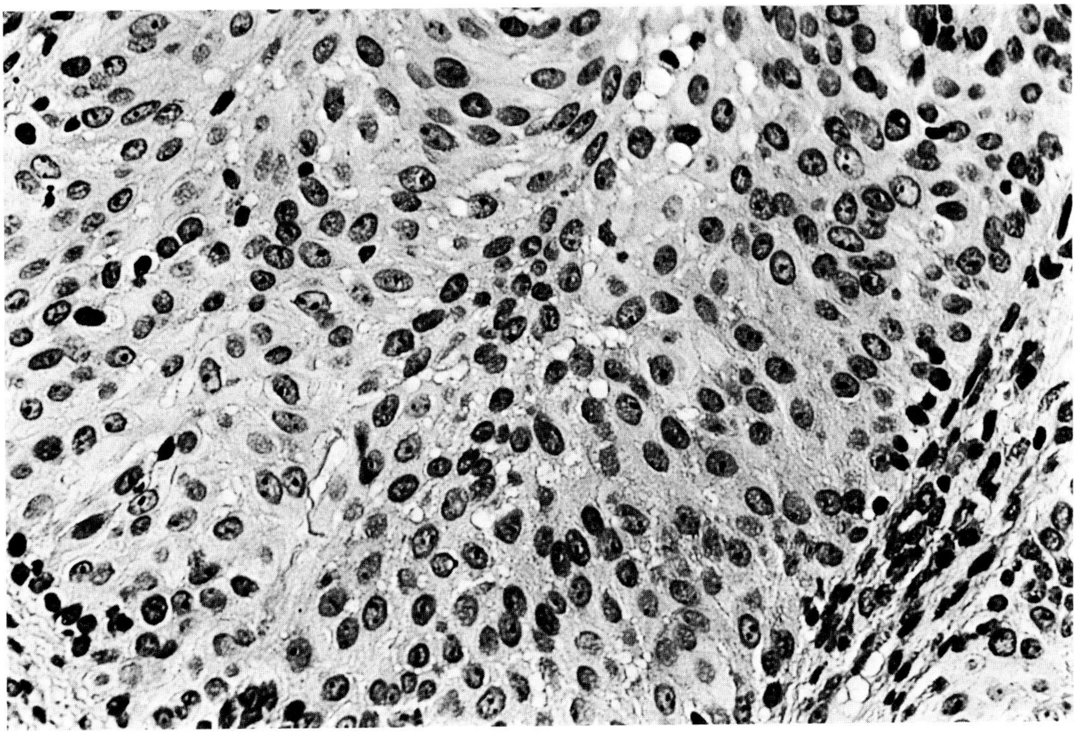

Fig. 10.3 A vulval varrucous carcinoma in which the papillary fronds are covered by very well-differentiated squamous epithelium showing an irregular pattern of growth but minimal cellular atypia and no mitoses (H. & E. × 270).

downgrowths of cells from the basal layer of the epidermis are apparent, these having rounded or angulated margins. A variety of patterns may be seen, such as cribriform or cystic, often in differing areas of the same tumour and it is not uncommon to find foci of squamous differentiation, a finding that does not alter the diagnosis. Mitotic figures are common.

These tumours are locally invasive and recur after removal in 20 per cent of cases. For practical purposes they can be regarded as non-metastasizing and no case of death resulting from a vulval basal cell carcinoma has ever been recorded.

Malignant melanoma

About 4 to 6 per cent of malignant melanomata occur on the vulva, arising either from a preexistent naevus or from previously normal skin. Melanomata account for approximately 3 per cent of malignant vulval neoplasms. The tumour occurs most commonly in women in their sixth, seventh or eighth decades. The site of predilection is the labia majora; melanomata of the labia minora are less common and 10–15 per cent of cases originate in the clitoris. The neoplasm presents as a raised smooth swelling which eventually ulcerates through the skin to present as a fungating tumour mass usually, but not invariably, bluish-black or dark brown in colour. Histologically (Fig. 10.5), most vulval melanomata are of either the superficial spreading type (in which large malignant melanocytes are seen in, and are largely confined to, the epidermis) or the nodular type (in which the rounded, polyhedral or spindle-shaped cells grow in clusters, pseudoalveoli or sheets and invade both dermis and epidermis). Pleomorphism is usually marked

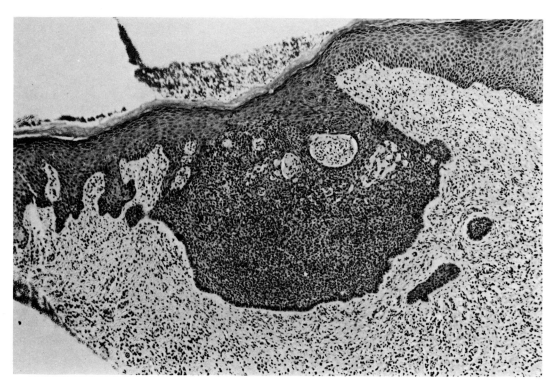

Fig. 10.4 Basal cell carcinoma of the vulva showing a solid angular mass of neoplastic cells arising from the basal layer of the epithelium (H. & E. × 45).

and mitotic figures abound. Melanin pigment may be a conspicuous feature but is often scanty and is absent from the rare *amelanotic melanoma*.

The over-all five-year and ten-year survival rates, adjusted for age, for women with a malignant melanoma are 30 to 35 per cent and 20 to 25 per cent respectively. The tumour tends to spread early to the inguinal lymph nodes and to be widely disseminated via the bloodstream. The most significant prognostic feature for cutaneous melanoma is the level of invasion into the dermis, the various defined levels, as measured from the granular layer of the epidermis, being:

Level 1. Confined to the epidermis.
Level 2. Extending for 1 mm or less into the dermis.
Level 3. Extending 1–2 mm into the dermis.
Level 4. Extending more than 2 mm into the dermis.
Level 5. Invading the subcutaneous fat.

Patients whose tumours are at levels 1 and 2 usually survive, but the five-year survival rate for levels 3 and 4 is only 40 per cent, whilst for level 5 it is 20 per cent. In practice, the majority of women with malignant melanomata have deeply penetrating tumours (more than 4 mm) at the time of presentation and as a consequence the over-all prognosis is poor. Other indicators of poor prognosis are ulceration of the neoplasm, epithelioid cell type, high mitotic rate and advanced patient age.

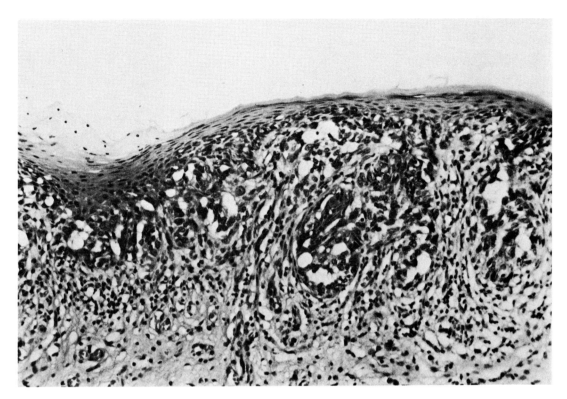

Fig. 10.5 Superficial spreading malignant melanoma of the vulva, showing clusters of malignant cells at the dermoepidermal junction and in the papillary dermis (H. & E. × 108).

Rare vulval tumours

All malignant mesenchymal tumours of the vulva are extremely rare, the most common being the *leiomyosarcoma*. *Malignant fibrous histiocytoma, fibrosarcoma, angiosarcoma, liposarcoma, haemangiopericytoma, aggressive angiomyxoma, Kaposi's sarcoma, malignant granular cell tumour, malignant Schwannoma, epithelioid sarcoma* and *alveolar soft part sarcoma* have all been encountered in the vulva. The majority of these rare neoplasms develop in the labia majora and there are no specific or diagnostic gross features. Haematogenous spread is a common feature but spread to the local lymph nodes is very variable. Vulval sarcomata tend to infiltrate locally and recur after excision.

Other rare neoplasms which have been reported in the vulva include *endodermal sinus tumour, non-Hodgkin's lymphoma, malignant mixed tumour* and *Merkel cell tumour*.

The *aggressive angiomyxoma*, which occurs more commonly as a tumour of the pelvis, may present as a vulval neoplasm and the bland histological appearances contrast sharply with its tendency to repetitive recurrence.

Primary adenocarcinoma of the vulva is rare and those that have been described are very variable in appearance and behaviour. They develop from the sweat glands, Bartholin's gland (see below), other similar, unnamed mucus-secreting glands in the vestibule, mesonephric (wolffian or Gartner's) duct remnants, cloacal remnants and breast tissue. The management is similar to that laid down for squamous carcinoma. *Cloacogenic carcinoma (basaloid carcinoma)* is believed to develop either from epithelial rests, remnants of the urogenital sinus or cloaca or from the transitional epithelium of the anal canal or excretory duct of Bartholin's gland. It lies deep in the labium major and is, in effect, a poorly differentiated adenosquamous cell carcinoma, the constituent cells resembling those of the basal cells of squamous epithelium; the prognosis is poor.

Metastatic tumours

The vulva is an uncommon site for metastases but deposits from squamous cell carcinoma of the cervix, adenocarcinoma of the endometrium and renal adenocarcinoma collectively account for approximately 8 per cent of vulval neoplasms.

Metastases are found most commonly in the dermis or subcutaneous tissue of the labia majora or around the clitoris. An expansile growth pattern, multiple lesions and an absence of an intraepithelial component all favour a diagnosis of metastatic rather than primary disease.

Bartholin's gland

Carcinomata of Bartholin's gland are rare. The mean age of presentation varies from 50 to 62 years, a proportion occurring in premenopausal women. The tumour usually presents as a nodule deep in the posterior part of the labium major, or with perineal pain. The presenting complaint in about a quarter of patients is of a Bartholin's gland abscess which fails to resolve following treatment and the failure to suspect a neoplasm often leads to delay in diagnosis of the carcinoma. The neoplasm is well circumscribed but not encapsulated, yellowish or grey-white and, although generally solid, may show areas of cystic change, necrosis or haemorrhage.

Histologically, the tumour may be an *adenocarcinoma*, a *squamous carcinoma*, an *adenoid cystic carcinoma*, a *mixed carcinoma* or a *transitional cell carcinoma*, whilst a small number are *undifferentiated neoplasms*. The adenocarcinomata may be mucin-secreting and have a papillary, tubular or cribriform pattern. They develop from either ductal or acinar cells. The squamous carcinomata probably arise from foci of metaplastic squamous epithelium within the ducts whilst the transitional cell carcinomata arise from the ductal epithelium which is normally of transitional type. Adenoid cystic carcinoma is a slowly growing and locally aggressive tumour which tends to recur locally, sometimes many years after its removal. However, metastases occur less commonly than with the other forms of carcinoma. The mixed tumours include adenosquamous carcinomata and mixed adenoid cystic/squamous cell carcinomata as well as adenocarcinomata in which there are foci of squamous metaplasia.

The adenocarcinomata and squamous cell carcinomata tend to avail themselves of the rich lymphatic drainage of Bartholin's gland and 35 to 50 per cent of patients already have inguinal nodal metastases at the time of diagnosis. Of these, 18 per cent already have metastases in the pelvic lymph nodes whilst occasionally pelvic nodal metastases are found in the absence of inguinal nodal metastases. The five-year survival rate is approximately 35 per cent.

Vagina

Malignant tumours of the vagina are uncommon and, indeed, a neoplastic lesion in the vagina is more likely to be a metastasis than a primary tumour. Squamous cell carcinomata account for the vast majority of primary vaginal neoplasms, although in recent years there has been, for reasons discussed below, a dramatic increase in the incidence of adenocarcinoma.

Squamous cell carcinoma

This accounts for between 1 and 1.5 per cent of female genital tract cancer and for 95 per cent of primary vaginal malignancies. However, the true incidence is not easy to determine for there is often doubt as to whether a neoplasm is truly arising in the vagina, it being a general clinical rule that a tumour in the vagina extending to the external os of the cervix should be considered as a carcinoma of the cervix, and that one involving the vulva should be regarded as a vulval carcinoma. The position is still further complicated by the fact that a proportion of women who appear to have been successfully treated for cervical carcinoma will later develop an apparently independent primary vaginal squamous cell carcinoma. Some such cases are, of course, really a recurrence of the cervical carcinoma but many are without doubt true independent neoplasms.

Aetiology

This is unknown and although it has been suggested that long standing procidentia and the wearing of a pessary possibly contribute to the development of a squamous cell carcinoma, these factors play little role in modern gynaecological practice. The fact that vaginal carcinoma probably evolves, in most cases, from previous intraepithelial neoplasia (see Chapter 9) and that vaginal and cervical lesions often develop in the same patient, may suggest a common carcinogenic stimulus acting on the lower genital tract, and the possibility of an oncogenic virus has been widely entertained. The role of HPV infection in the development of vaginal squamous carcinoma is, however, undetermined.

Clinical features

Squamous cell carcinoma of the vagina occurs principally in women aged 55–70, the peak incidence being about 63–65. Symptoms are usually consequent upon ulceration of the tumour and include vaginal bleeding or discharge and dyspareunia.

Pathological features

A squamous cell carcinoma develops most frequently in the upper third of the vagina and more commonly in the posterior than the anterior wall. It forms a small, soft tumour which is easily missed on palpation. The tumour may appear to the naked eye as a nodulopapillary exophytic growth or as an ulcerated endophytic lesion. Histologically the neoplasm is most commonly only moderately differentiated and it is unusual for there to be well-formed keratin pearls.

Spread and prognosis

The neoplasm tends to infiltrate locally, directly invading the paravaginal and parametrial tissues, the rectovaginal septum and either the bladder or the rectum. Rectovaginal or vesicovaginal fistulae may develop at a late stage in the disease. Lymphatic spread from tumours in the upper third of the vagina is to the pelvic nodes, whilst neoplasms in the middle and lower thirds also metastasize to the inguinal nodes. Blood borne spread, principally to bones and lungs, occurs late.

The tumour is staged according to the following criteria:

Stage I. The tumour is limited to the vaginal wall.
Stage II. The tumour has involved the subvaginal tissue but has not extended to the pelvic wall.
Stage III. The tumour has extended to the pelvic wall.
Stage IV. The tumour has extended beyond the true pelvis or has involved the mucosa of the bladder or rectum.

The five-year survival rate for patients with a Stage I carcinoma is in the region of 70 per cent, this figure

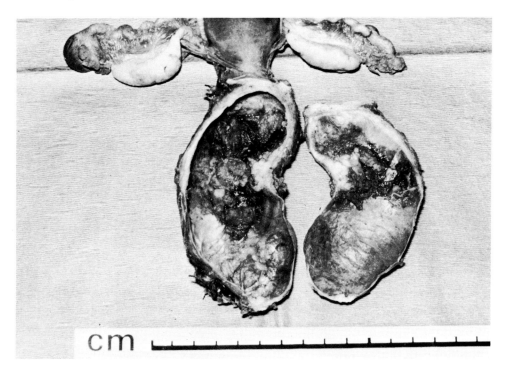

Fig. 10.6   Uterus, both adnexae and vagina from a 17-year-old girl whose mother had been given DES when she was pregnant. The vagina is studded with fungating nodules of haemorrhagic, clear cell carcinoma.

declining to 30–60 per cent for those with Stage II neoplasms, and to 24–35 per cent for patients in Stage III; it is unusual for patients with Stage IV carcinoma to survive for five years.

Adenocarcinoma

Vaginal adenocarcinoma was, until 20 years ago, one of the rarest tumours of the female genital tract and, indeed, it still is in Great Britain. However, some years ago it became apparent that in certain parts of the United States, there was a significant increase in the incidence of clear cell adenocarcinomata of the vagina, this increase being entirely in young girls who had been exposed prenatally to diethyl-stilboestrol (DES). This association has now been fully confirmed and a considerable number of cases has accumulated; the factor common to all being the administration to the mother of a synthetic oestrogen, usually DES, before the eighteenth week of pregnancy. Approximately 1 in 1000 young women exposed to this drug prenatally will develop a clear celled adenocarcinoma, the tumour usually becoming apparent between the ages of 14 and 23 years, most commonly in girls aged 17–19 years. The neoplasm develops from pre-existing vaginal adenosis (see Chapter 6) and is therefore of müllerian origin.

A clear cell adenocarcinoma usually develops in the upper third of the vagina, most commonly on the anterior wall. However, by the time of diagnosis, it may form a bulky mass which fills the entire length of the vagina. The neoplasm is seen as a polypoid, nodular or papillary mass (Fig. 10.6), although it is occasionally flat and sometimes ulcerated. Histologically (Figs. 10.7 and 10.8), there is a complex mixture of solid, papillary, tubular and cystic patterns, the solid areas being formed of sheets of cells with clear cytoplasm and the tubules being lined by 'hobnail' cells characterized by their scanty cytoplasm and large nuclei which protrude into the lumen. The cystic spaces tend to be lined by rather nondescript flattened cells.

The tumour spreads by local extension, by the lymphatics and by the bloodstream and, although the pelvic nodes are commonly the site of metastases, there is a surprisingly high incidence of spread to the supraclavicular nodes; blood borne spread is principally to the lungs. The five-year survival rate of Stage I cases is approximately 80 per cent, but this figure falls precipitously to 17 per cent for patients with a Stage II neoplasm and there are few or no five-year survivors amongst girls with Stage III or IV tumours.

Although a clear cell adenocarcinoma of the vagina probably always develops from vaginal adenosis, it has to be borne in mind that not all cases of vaginal adenosis are due to prenatal DES exposure and that, therefore, very exceptional instances of clear cell vaginal adenocarcinoma will be encountered in women not exposed to this substance. However, such patients tend to develop carcinoma at a rather later age than those whose tumours are related to transplacental carcinogenesis.

Rare vaginal tumours

A few *verrucous carcinomata* and *malignant melanomata* of the vagina have been recorded, the pathological features of these neoplasms being identical to their vulval counterparts. The malignant melanomata arise from the scattered melanoblasts normally present in the vagina and form pigmented nodules. The prognosis of these lesions is, if possible, even more gloomy than that for melanomata of the vulva. *Leiomyosarcoma* and *fibrosarcoma* of the vagina are extremely rare, the least uncommon sarcomatous vaginal neoplasm being the *sarcoma botryoides*, which arises during the first five years of life and forms a grape-like polypoid mass of greyish-red haemorrhagic tissue which may fill, and protrude from, the vagina. The tumour has a very oedematous myxoid stroma with a relatively small content of widely dispersed cells, appearances which may induce a falsely optimistic view of the nature of the lesion (Fig. 10.9). However, the scattered spindle-shaped or round cells are pleomorphic and show mitotic activity and, whilst many are of an immature mesenchymal nature, some will show differentiation into rhabdomyoblasts or striated muscle cells. The epithelial covering of the tumour is bland and the neoplastic cells tend to be condensed below this to form a 'cambium' layer. A sarcoma botryoides probably arises from primitive stroma in the area of the müllerian tubercle and is better considered as a form of embryonal rhabdomyosarcoma rather than as a variant of the mixed tumour. The neoplasm tends to invade locally and removal is usually followed by local recurrence. Blood borne spread occurs late and death, which is currently the rule, is due principally to the effects of pelvic infiltration.

A rare neoplasm, which macroscopically may resemble a sarcoma botryoides and also occurs in young children, is the *yolk sac tumour* of the vagina. These yolk sac tumours have the same histological features as those occurring more commonly in the ovary and are presumed to be derived from germ cells which have gone astray during their transit, in early embryonic life, from the gut to the developing gonad.

A few *synovial sarcoma-like tumours* of the vagina have been described. The true nature of these neoplasms is currently obscure.

Metastatic tumours of the vagina

A tumour in the vagina is more likely to be due to infiltration from a neoplasm in a neighbouring organ or to a metastasis than to a primary lesion. Spread to the vagina occurs principally from the cervix, endometrium, bladder, rectum (Fig. 10.10) and ovary, although metastatic nodules from renal adenocarcinoma also occur with some frequency. The vagina is a notoriously common site for metastatic deposits of choriocarcinoma.

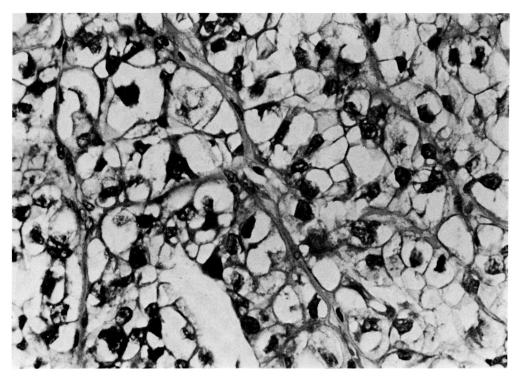

Fig. 10.7 Clear cell carcinoma of the vagina. Solid pattern, composed of pleomorphic cells with large hyperchromatic nuclei and clear vacuolated cytoplasm (H. & E. × 383).

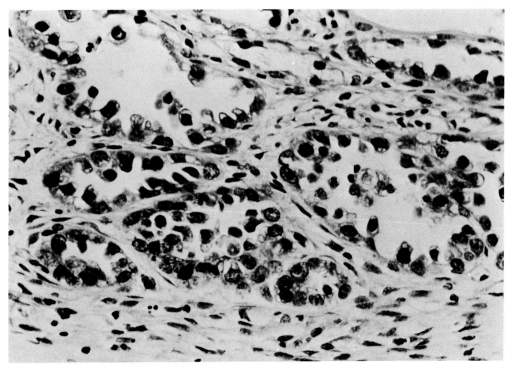

Fig. 10.8 A second pattern of clear cell carcinoma in which large pleomorphic cells with prominent nuclei (hobnail nuclei) and clear vacuolated cytoplasm line acini of variable size (H. & E. × 255).

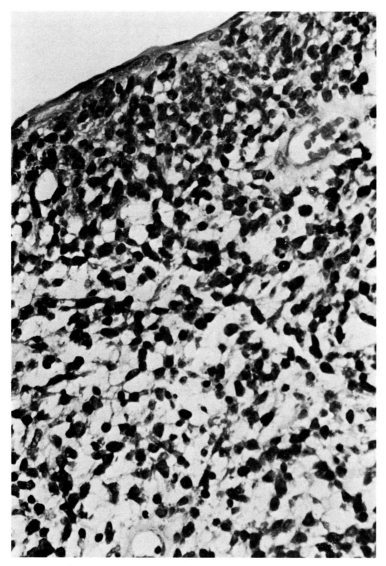

Fig. 10.9 Sarcoma botryoides arising in the lower vagina and showing undifferentiated immature cells, in a myxoid stroma, condensed beneath the covering layer of epithelium to form a 'cambium' layer (H. & E. × 270).

Cervix

Squamous cell carcinoma

In the last few years it has been recognized that, whilst squamous carcinoma remains the most common malignant neoplasm developing in the cervix, it constitutes only approximately 70 per cent of the total, the remainder being mainly adenocarcinomata and adenosquamous carcinomata.

In the last two decades the incidence of invasive carcinoma has declined sharply in the 4th and 5th decades of life, largely because cytological screening programmes have allowed for the detection, and

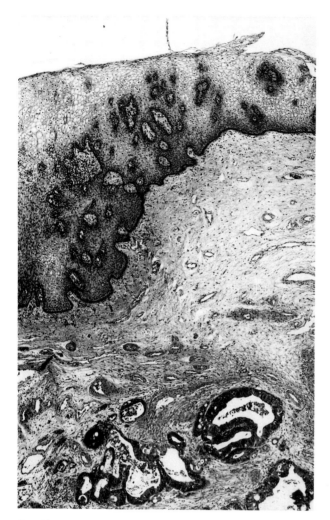

Fig. 10.10   Metastatic carcinoma in the vagina. Deep in the vagina wall (in the lower part of the tissue) there are foci of metastatic, well-differentiated adenocarcinoma which originated in the large intestine (H. & E. × 47).

eradication, of many cases which are still in the preinvasive stage. However, there has been a four- to five-fold increase in the incidence of carcinoma in women under the age of 35 years.

Aetiology and pathogenesis

It is, of course, now widely recognized that the vast majority of cervical squamous cell carcinomata do not arise abruptly from previously normal squamous epithelium but evolve over ten to fifteen years from an epithelium which shows cervical intraepithelial neoplasia. It is possible that a small proportion of cervical squamous cell carcinomata arise 'explosively' from a previously normal epithelium, but this is currently unproven.

There is an epidemiological association between squamous cell carcinoma of the cervix and early marriage, early pregnancy, a high number of pregnancies, sexual promiscuity, divorce, prostitution and low socioeconomic status. These findings clearly suggest a correlation with a particular lifestyle but it is

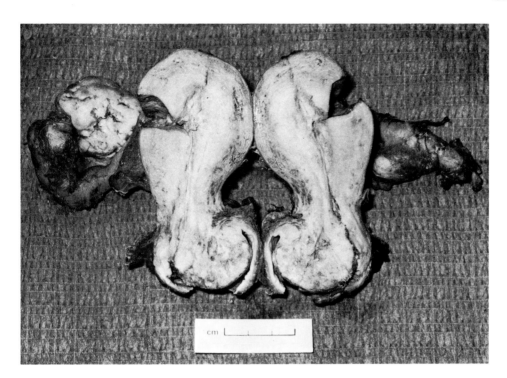

Fig. 10.11 A nodular squamous carcinoma occupies the posterior lip of the cervix in this bisected hysterectomy specimen.

virtually certain that the one common factor linking these disparate findings is early coitus, it being believed that a carcinogen is transmitted sexually by the male at a time when the epithelium is in an unstable state, i.e. when the transformation zone is undergoing squamous metaplasia during late adolescence (see Chapter 6). The nature of this carcinogenic agent is unknown but suspicion has fallen at different times on herpes virus type II and human papilloma virus (HPV) types 16 and 18. However, it is becoming increasingly clear that HPV is found so frequently in women with histologically normal cervices that its role as a carcinogen must be questioned. Present evidence, therefore, indicates that neither of these two viruses alone is the main aetiological agent but that, in the presence of additional factors, they may play a role. It has been known for some time, for example, that only a proportion of women with CIN develop an invasive neoplasm and that progression from CIN to carcinoma is most likely to occur when there is local immunosuppression produced by exposure to seminal plasma and metabolites of cigarette smoke, or when there is systemic immunosuppression. Cigarette smoking may also have a direct carcinogenic effect. Whatever the nature of the carcinogenic agent, or agents, that there is a sexually transmitted agent is further substantiated by evidence that barrier methods of contraception appear to confer some degree of protection against cervical squamous cell carcinoma and by the finding that the female partners of sexually promiscuous men have an increased risk of developing this neoplasm, even though they may well have confined themselves to a single partner. The previously held belief that male circumcision protects the female against the development of cervical carcinoma is no longer held to be valid, the relative lack of this neoplasm in the partners of circumcised men being more a reflection of the sexual mores of those ethnic groups which practise ritual circumcision rather than being attributable to any direct effect of the removal of the foreskin.

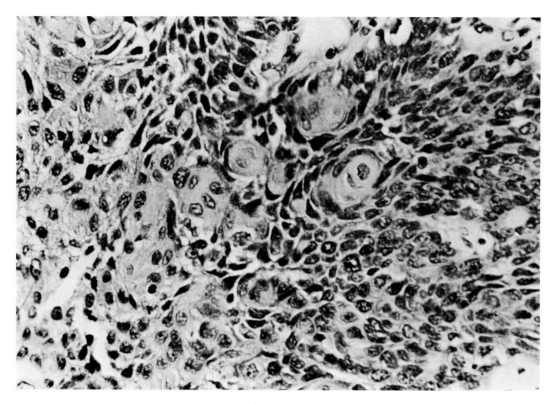

Fig. 10.12   A well-differentiated squamous cell carcinoma of the cervix. To the right the constituent cells are hyperchromatic and closely packed, whilst to the centre and left they are forming small keratinized pearls (H. & E. × 270).

Clinical features

Squamous cell carcinoma can occur at any age but reaches its peak incidence in women between the ages of 50 and 65; it is less common in the 40 to 50 year age group than it was 20 years ago. A second, smaller peak has developed in women under the age of 35 years. The common complaints are of abnormal, often postcoital vaginal bleeding, serosanguineous vaginal discharge and, in advanced cases, deep pelvic pain. Small carcinomata are often entirely asymptomatic and identifiable only by examination of cervical smears, colposcopy and biopsy.

Pathological findings

Squamous carcinomata develop either on the ectocervix, where they tend to grow in a predominantly exophytic manner to form a papillary or polypoidal mass, or in the endocervical canal where they commonly expand the cervix to form a hard barrel-shaped mass. The site of development is determined by the position of the abnormal transformation zone, and hence by the age of the patient, tumours in younger women developing more commonly on the ectocervix and those in older women being more likely to arise within the endocervical canal. Neoplasms that develop on the ectocervix may appear initially as a roughened, reddish, slightly raised area which bleeds easily to the touch, as a focal induration or as a shallow ulcer. More advanced tumours (Fig. 10.11) may form a bulky, friable mass, which may expand the upper vagina, or an excavating ulcer with indurated, raised margins.

Histologically, squamous cell carcinomata infiltrate the cervical stroma as a network of anastomosing

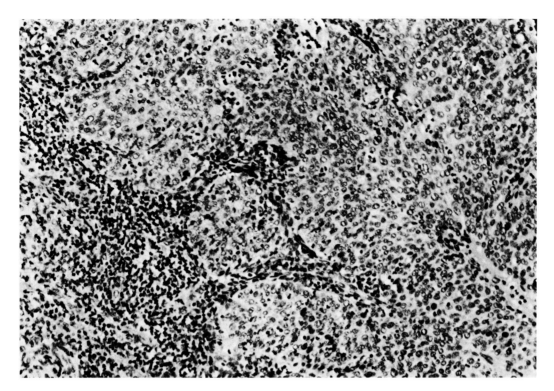

Fig. 10.13 A small cell, non-keratinizing squamous cell carcinoma of the cervix. A dense lymphocytic infiltrate can be seen (left) at the tumour margin (H. & E. × 108).

bands which appear on transection as irregular islands with spiky or angular edges. About 20 per cent of the tumours are of the well differentiated type (these also being known as 'large cell keratinizing tumours') and are formed of large, tightly packed cells with hyperchromatic nuclei (Fig. 10.12). Intercellular bridges are readily apparent and a striking feature is the formation of concentric whorls of keratin in the centre of the neoplastic cell islands ('keratin pearls'). Moderately differentiated tumours ('large cell focally keratinizing type') constitute about 60 per cent of the total and are formed of cells which are recognizably squamous but have larger and more irregular nuclei than the well differentiated type; intercellular bridges can rarely be recognized and keratin pearls are not seen. The remaining 20 per cent of cervical squamous cell carcinomata are poorly differentiated ('large cell non-keratinizing' or 'small cell non-keratinizing tumours') and consist of sheets of uniform large cells with pale cytoplasm and round or mildly irregular nuclei, or uniform cells with rather hyperchromatic nuclei (Fig. 10.13). Occasional foci of abortive squamous differentiation are sometimes apparent. In all cases, a diagnosis of squamous carcinoma should be made only when the absence of mucin has been confirmed by the use of special stains.

Two distinctive, and sometimes confusing, histological variants of cervical squamous cell carcinoma merit mention. In some tumours, usually of the well differentiated type, the squamous cells contain abundant glycogen and thus appear as 'clear' cells, whilst occasionally the poorly differentiated tumours assume a spindle-shaped cell form and thus superficially resemble a sarcoma.

The stroma of a squamous cell carcinoma is almost invariably infiltrated by lymphocytes and plasma cells and, occasionally, a heavy stromal infiltration by eosinophils is seen. Sarcoid-like granulomata are sometimes encountered in the stroma which may, on occasion, show a desmoplastic, or scirrhous, reaction to the neoplasm.

Spread and prognosis

Squamous cell carcinoma of the cervix spreads principally by direct local invasion of adjacent tissues and by the lymphatics; spread by the bloodstream is less common. The tumour spreads locally through tissue planes and in the perineural and perivascular spaces, upwards into the uterine body, downwards into the vagina, laterally into the parametrium, posterolaterally into the sacrouterine ligaments and anteriorly and posteriorly to the bladder and rectum. Eventually, neoplastic tissue may reach the pelvic wall and surround or compress the ureters as they cross the paracervical region. Lymphatic spread occurs first to the external iliac, hypogastric and obturator nodes; spread to sacral, aortic and inguinal nodes occurs later and less commonly. Blood borne metastases occur late in the course of the disease and usually not until there is very extensive pelvic infiltration and lymph node involvement. Haematogenous dissemination is principally to the lungs, liver and bone. In recent years, eradication of the primary tumour has become relatively more successful and death from cervical carcinoma is more commonly due to systemic dissemination of the neoplasm, i.e. carcinomatosis, than was previously the case.

The prognosis is linked to the stage of the disease at the time of initial diagnosis and for this purpose the FIGO staging system is widely used.

Stage I. Invasive carcinoma confined to the cervix.
Stage II. Invasive carcinoma which extends beyond the cervix but has not reached either pelvic wall; involvement of the vagina is limited to the upper two-thirds.
Stage III. Invasive carcinoma which extends to either lateral pelvic wall and/or the lower third of the vagina.
Stage IV. Invasive carcinoma which involves the urinary bladder and/or rectum or extends beyond the true pelvis.

It should be noted that Stage I is subdivided into Stages Ia and Ib, the former comprising microinvasive carcinoma and the latter comprising all other Stage I carcinomata, including those previously termed *occult invasive lesions*. It is also usual in Stage I and II tumours to differentiate between those that have spread to involve the endometrium and those that have not done so; such spread adversely affects the prognosis.

The overall five-year survival rate is in the region of 55 per cent. However, patients with a Stage I carcinoma have a five-year survival rate of 85–90 per cent, this figure falling to 70–75 per cent for Stage II cases, to 30–35 per cent for women with a Stage III carcinoma and to only 10 per cent for those with a tumour in Stage IV. Histological grading of the tumour bears little relationship to prognosis but there is some evidence that those cases in which there is a heavy lymphocytic infiltration of the stroma have a better outlook than those with only a sparse cellular response to the neoplasm.

Verrucous carcinoma

Tumours of this type occasionally occur in the cervix; their pathological characteristics are identical to those previously described for similar tumours in the vulva.

Adenocarcinoma

Adenocarcinomata constitute 12–16 per cent of malignant cervical tumours. They appear to fall into three distinct groups. First, those found in younger women and which have aetiological factors similar to those for squamous carcinoma. Second, those that develop in the older, nulliparous woman or the woman with low parity and a history of infertility or dysfunctional hormonal problems and who tends, on the whole, to be older than the woman with squamous carcinoma. Third, the clear cell carcinoma that develops in a young woman who may have been exposed, *in utero*, to diethylstilboestrol.

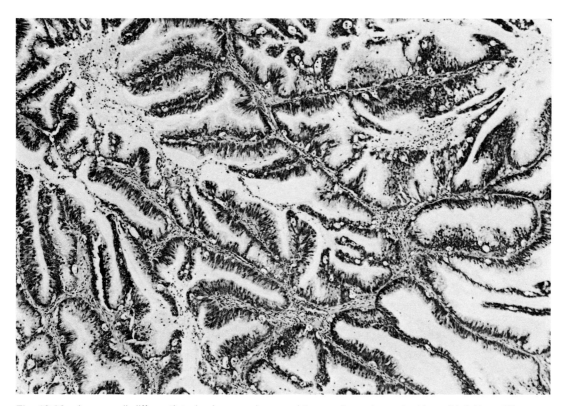

Fig. 10.14 A very well-differentiated adenocarcinoma of the cervix, endocervical type (H. & E. × 45).

Pathological features

Adenocarcinomata may adopt an exophytic, nodular, polypoid or ulceroinfiltrative form. There may rarely be a diffuse infiltration and enlargement of the cervix; it is not uncommon for the cervix to appear normal to the naked eye, the presence of a deep-seated intracryptal tumour being revealed only by endocervical curettage.

Histologically there are a number of differing types of adenocarcinoma and these are classified by cell type.

(a) *Endocervical type*. This is the most common form and accounts for about 75 per cent of cases. In many instances there is an associated adenocarcinoma *in situ*, situated on a cervical ectopy or in the lower endocervical canal, from which the tumour appears to arise. The most well differentiated form of this neoplasm is the rare minimal deviation adenocarcinoma. In tumours of this type there is little or no cytological atypia, the constituent cells closely resembling those of the normal endocervical epithelium. However, there is an increased complexity of the constituent glands, which are often sharply angulated and extend into the stroma to a greater depth than do their normal counterparts. Histological diagnosis of this neoplasm can be difficult.

The more typical well differentiated endocervical adenocarcinomata are formed of tall columnar cells which, although showing atypia and mitotic activity, bear some resemblance to those of the normal endocervical epithelium (Fig. 10.14). Well defined glandular acini are usually present and there may be a papillary or arborescent appearance. The less well differentiated forms of the tumour may take the form of glandular acini lined by very poorly differentiated cells or they may assume a solid pattern. Recognition of these poorly differentiated forms of endocervical adenocarcinoma is dependent upon finding mucus

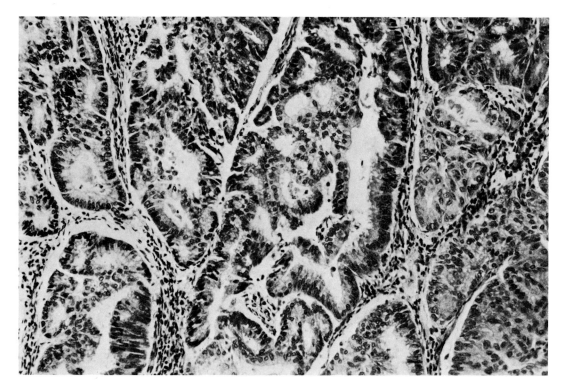

Fig. 10.15 Well-formed acini of cubocolumnar cells characterize this endometrioid adenocarcinoma of the cervix (H. & E. × 108).

within the tumour cells. Failure to carry out this simple investigation has led, in the past, to the considerable overestimation of the number of squamous cell carcinomata in the cervix, because the solid, poorly differentiated adenocarcinoma bears a striking morphological resemblance to a non-keratinizing squamous cell carcinoma. Sometimes the formation of mucus is excessive, with the development of pools of mucus which disrupt the acini and spill over into the stroma to produce the picture of a 'mucoid' or 'colloid' carcinoma. In other cases the poorly differentiated neoplasm is composed partly or completely of signet ring cells and care must be taken to distinguish this from a metastatic carcinoma. The endocervical-type adenocarcinoma is almost certainly derived from endocervical reserve cells.

(b) *Endometrioid type.* Neoplasms of this type are histologically identical to an endometrial adeno-carcinoma (Fig. 10.15). A proportion of these tumours probably arise from a focus of cervical endo-metriosis but most are thought to be derived from endocervical reserve cells which, being of müllerian origin, retain a potentiality for differentiating along endometrial rather than endocervical lines.

(c) *Serous adenocarcinoma.* Any adenocarcinoma of the cervix may grow in a papillary fashion but, occasionally, a papillary adenocarcinoma which mimics a tubal adenocarcinoma is encountered: such neoplasms probably indicate yet again the ability of the endocervical reserve cells to differentiate along a variety of müllerian pathways, these taking the tubal route. The tumour is distinct from the *villoglandular endocervical adenocarcinoma* of the cervix which has a more favourable prognosis.

(d) *Clear cell adenocarcinoma.* Some adenocarcinomata are formed, either wholly or in part, of cells with clear cytoplasm. These used to be regarded as of mesonephric origin but it is now clear that, with the exception of the extremely rare, deeply situated, more laterally placed neoplasm arising from Gartner's duct, they are of müllerian (paramesonephric) origin. The müllerian clear cell adenocarcinomata usually,

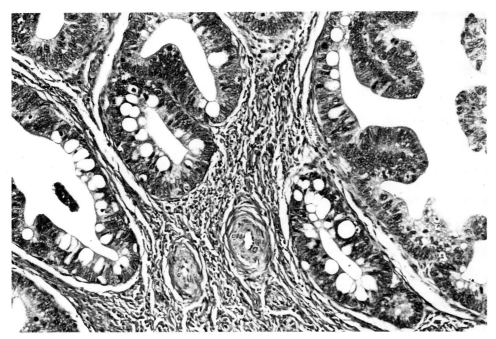

Fig. 10.16 Adenocarcinoma of the cervix of intestinal type. The tumour acini are lined by a stratified columnar epithelium in which there are goblet cells (H. & E. × 186).

although not invariably, occur in young girls with a prenatal history of DES exposure and their pathological characteristics are identical to those previously described for vaginal tumours of this type.

(e) *Intestinal type*. Less rarely than was previously supposed, a cervical adenocarcinoma may be histologically similar to an intestinal adenocarcinoma (Fig. 10.16), tumours of this type presumably arising from foci of cervical intestinal metaplasia. It is also not unusual to find small areas of intestinal metaplasia in otherwise typical carcinomas of endocervical type.

Spread and prognosis
Adenocarcinoma of the cervix spreads in a similar manner to that of squamous cell carcinomata but both local and lymph node extension tend to occur relatively early and the overall prognosis is considerably worse than is that for squamous cell carcinoma.

Mixed carcinomata

Four types of cervical neoplasm are included in this category. These all represent variations around a common theme and it is by no means certain that the distinction between each represents anything more than a variation of growth pattern and degree of differentiation.

(a) *Adenosquamous carcinoma* also known as 'mucoepidermoid carcinoma', tumours of this type contain both squamous carcinoma and adenocarcinoma and constitute up to 20 per cent of all cervical carcinomata. They probably develop from pluripotential cells and often arise from an epithelium with the features of CIN III. In the majority of cases they appear to have the same aetiological factors as squamous carcinomata and occur in the same age groups. Histologically, they range in appearance from the well differentiated, with a clearly identifiable keratinizing squamous component and well formed glandular acini to the poorly differentiated, so-called, *glassy cell carcinoma*. At presentation, adenosquamous carcinomata are

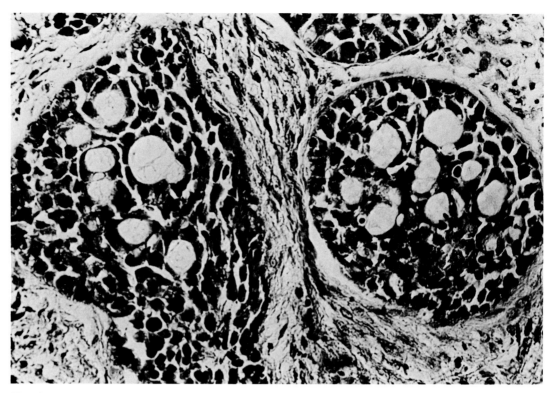

Fig. 10.17   Adenoid cystic carcinoma of the cervix. Nests of darkly staining basaloid cells with a cribriform pattern (H. & E. × 270).

found to have metastasized more frequently than squamous carcinomata and the poorly differentiated forms have a gloomy prognosis.

(b) *Adenoid cystic carcinoma.* Tumours of this type are rare in the cervix. They develop at a relatively late age, commonly in the seventh or eighth decade, and present as either a bulky ulcerated nodular mass or as a friable pedunculated polyp. Histologically (Fig. 10.17), they are formed of small, uniform basaloid cells with scanty cytoplasm and densely staining nuclei. The cells are arranged in sheets, solid masses or anastomosing cords and the solid masses have a cribriform pattern which is produced by the presence of rounded spaces containing hyaline or mucoid material.

In at least 75 per cent of cases of adenoid cystic carcinoma, the tumour is either admixed with a squamous cell carcinoma or an adenocarcinoma or is associated with CIN. This has led some to suggest that the adenoid cystic pattern is a non-specific one which may be adopted, either wholly or in part, by a squamous or glandular carcinoma. Others regard this tumour as one of pluripotential cells, which can partially differentiate into either squamous cell carcinoma or adenocarcinoma.

These neoplasms are locally aggressive and often associated with lymph node metastases; blood borne spread, although not uncommon, occurs late.

Small cell tumours

Small cell tumours of the cervix constitute a heterogenous group of neoplasms. Some are *endocrine cell* (*carcinoid* or *oat cell*) *tumours*, others are *basaloid carcinomata* and others are *small cell non-keratinizing squamous carcinomata.*

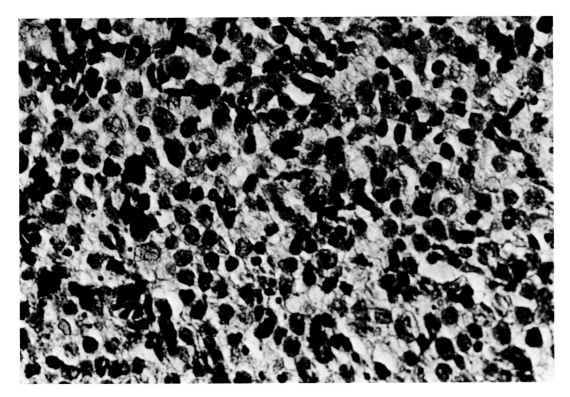

Fig. 10.18 Poorly-differentiated carcinoid tumour of the cervix. The constituent cells are hyperchromatic and pleomorphic, with scanty cytoplasm. The tumour thus appears highly cellular and closely resembles the oat cell carcinoma of the bronchus (H. & E. × 270).

(a) *Endocrine cell tumours* of the uterine cervix are rare and have a wide histological spectrum ranging from well differentiated types, which resemble a carcinoid tumour of the gastrointestinal tract, to the anaplastic forms which mimic an oat cell carcinoma of the bronchus (Fig. 10.18). A proportion of the cells are argyrophilic, as demonstrated by Grimelius stains, and a proportion contain electron dense neurosecretory granules. Some tumours secrete peptide substances and a paraendocrine syndrome may result (see Chapter 18). The endocervical epithelium contains a proportion of neuroendocrine cells and it is possible that endocrine cell tumours develop from the specific precursors of these cells. However, neuroendocrine tumours are frequently admixed with an intraepithelial or invasive squamous carcinoma or adenocarcinoma, findings which suggest that these neoplasms develop from the same pluripotential cells as the other cervical carcinomata. The tumours have a rather poor prognosis, particularly the poorly differentiated forms.

(b) *Adenoid basal carcinoma.* Tumours of this type are composed of small cells resembling those of the basal layer of squamous epithelium. They are frequently associated with CIN III or invasive squamous carcinoma.

(c) *Subcolumnar reserve cell carcinoma.* These rare neoplasms are composed of small, darkly staining cells which extend deeply into the stroma and form sharply defined nests. They are regarded as having a poor prognosis.

Malignant melanoma

Primary malignant melanoma of the cervix is extremely rare and may arise either in a focus of epidermal metaplasia or from the stromal melanocytes that are present in a small proportion of normal cervices. The neoplasm usually presents as a brown, black or bluish nodule or plaque on the cervical lip. The histological characteristics are identical to those already described for melanomata of the vulva.

Sarcomata

All sarcomata of the cervix are notably uncommon. Examples of *leiomyosarcomata* and *endocervical stromal cell sarcomata* have been described, whilst the *sarcoma botryoides* (embryonal rhabdomyosarcoma) of childhood sometimes develops in the cervix rather than in the vagina. The various forms of *carcinosarcoma* (mixed müllerian tumour) and *adenosarcomata* can also, on occasion, arise in the cervix and the pathology of these neoplasms is described in the section on endometrial neoplasms.

Metastatic tumours

Metastases in the cervix are most commonly from an endometrial adenocarcinoma. Choriocarcinoma also has a tendency to metastasize to the cervix, whilst secondary deposits from carcinomata of the breast or stomach are sometimes encountered.

Endometrium

Endometrioid adenocarcinoma

The vast majority of endometrial neoplasms are adenocarcinomata and most of these are of the endometrioid type, i.e. they show some degree of endometrial differentiation and bear a resemblance, albeit an anarchic one, to normal proliferative endometrium. The endometrioid adenocarcinoma is 'the usual type of endometrial adenocarcinoma' and when the term 'endometrial adenocarcinoma' is used without any qualification it should be taken as referring to the endometrioid form.

Aetiology and pathogenesis
It is widely believed that women who develop endometrial adenocarcinoma have a high incidence of associated obesity, hypertension and diabetes mellitus, that they are frequently unmarried, commonly nulliparous and often have a late menopause. The association with nulliparity and late menopause has withstood the test of controlled studies but there is considerable doubt as to whether there is any true association with either hypertension or diabetes mellitus. It is becoming increasingly accepted, however, that there is a very high incidence of obesity in women with endometrial adenocarcinoma, a finding the significance of which is discussed later.

The role of oestrogens in the aetiology of endometrial adenocarcinoma has given rise to much debate but it is now clearly established that the administration of exogenous oestrogens, either as postmenopausal replacement therapy or as a therapeutic measure for individuals with ovarian agenesis, is accompanied by a markedly increased risk (in the nature of × 10) of developing an endometrial adenocarcinoma. It is therefore established that oestrogens *can* cause endometrial adenocarcinoma but it remains uncertain as to whether that vast majority of women who develop an adenocarcinoma of the endometrium without being exposed to exogenous oestrogens do so because of an overproduction of endogenous oestrogens.

It is certainly the case that women with oestrogenic ovarian tumours, e.g. granulosa cell tumours, do have a notably high incidence of endometrial adenocarcinoma, but such cases account for only a tiny minority. A significant finding has been that women with endometrial neoplasia have an increased ability to convert androstenedione, produced by the adrenal gland, to oestrone, this conversion taking place in fat cells. It thus appears that the association between obesity and endometrial adenocarcinoma may well be explicable on the basis of the ability of obese patients, with their excess of body fat, to produce elevated levels of oestrone, it being proposed that the subsequent oestrogen excess could then induce endometrial neoplasia. A similar result would, of course, occur as a consequence of a primary overproduction of androstenedione and it is therefore of particular interest that endometrial adenocarcinoma, particularly in women aged less than 40, does show an association with the polycystic ovary syndrome, a condition in which there is an excess ovarian production of androstenedione, which is later converted to oestrone in extraglandular sites.

If excessive endogenous production of oestrogens is a significant factor in the aetiology of endometrial adenocarcinoma, it would be expected that endometrial hyperplasia would be an inevitable precursor of neoplasia in this site. However, simple hyperplasia of the endometrium is not associated with any significantly increased risk of adenocarcinoma, despite the fact that this abnormality is oestrogen dependent. On the other hand, atypical hyperplasia is a definite precursor of frank neoplasia (see Chapter 9). It nevertheless remains true that many endometrial adenocarcinomata arise from an atrophic endometrium, a finding that is not fully in accord with the results of endocrinological studies in women with endometrial adenocarcinoma.

In summary, therefore, exogenous oestrogens can cause endometrial adenocarcinoma and there is suggestive evidence that many women with this neoplasm produce an excess of endogenous oestrogens. Nevertheless, the oestrogenically induced simple hyperplasia of the endometrium is rarely complicated by the development of neoplasia and many carcinomata arise in an atrophic endometrium. Clearly, the question of the aetiology of endometrial adenocarcinoma is still far from fully understood.

Clinical features

Endometrial adenocarcinomata occur most commonly during the sixth decade, most patients being in the early postmenopausal years. About 5 per cent of cases are in women aged less than 40 years. The neoplasm presents as abnormal vaginal bleeding.

Gross pathology

The uterus containing an endometrial adenocarcinoma may be small, of normal size or enlarged. A carcinoma may be confined to a focal area of the endometrium and thus appear as a localized plaque, nodule or polyp. Lesions of this type, which are occasionally multiple, tend to develop in the upper part of the uterus, either on the posterior wall or near the cornua, and may be completely removed by diagnostic curettage. More commonly, the tumour diffusely involves the endometrium and no focal point of origin can be recognized (Fig. 10.19). In such cases, the neoplasm may appear as a generalized, irregular, nodular or polypoidal thickening of the endometrium or as a bulky, friable polypoid mass which fills, and distends, the uterine cavity and which shows areas of necrosis, haemorrhage or ulceration. Extension of tumour into the myometrium may not be apparent to the naked eye but is often seen as irregular areas of pale whitish tissue within the muscle coat. An unusual variant of this gross pattern is that in which the endometrium appears only a little nodular but in which the myometrium is diffusely thickened by an infiltration of carcinomatous cells.

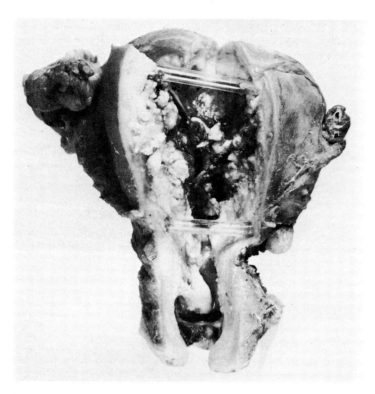

Fig. 10.19   A uterus which has been opened along its anterior surface to reveal a polypoidal mass of partly necrotic adenocarcinoma filling and distending the uterine cavity and extending into the cervix.

Histological features

All neoplasms in this category show, by definition, some degree of endometrial differentiation. The majority are well differentiated (Fig. 10.20) and consist of irregular, closely packed, complex glandular acini, which are lined by a cuboidal or low columnar epithelium of recognizable endometrial nature and which show a variable degree of pleomorphism, nuclear hyperchromatism and mitotic activity. The lining epithelium of the acini is often single-layered but foci of multilayering and intraluminal tufting are common. Intraglandular epithelial bridges, lacking any stromal support, are a characteristic feature and will, if widespread, impart a cribriform appearance to the neoplasm. The stroma is scanty and areas of haemorrhage, necrosis and polymorphonuclear leucocytic infiltration are common. The stroma may contain a number of foamy histocytes.

A minority of endometrioid adenocarcinomata are less well differentiated and have a partly acinar and partly solid growth pattern, whilst some have a predominantly solid appearance.

The pattern of growth is used to grade endometrioid adenocarcinomata:

Grade I. 5 per cent, or less, of the tumour shows a solid growth pattern.
Grade II. Between 5 and 50 per cent of the tumour is growing in a solid fashion.
Grade III. More than 50 per cent of the tumour shows a solid growth pattern.

This grading system requires modification to take into account not only the architectural features of the neoplasm but also the degree of cytological and nuclear atypia. Thus, if there is marked atypia those tumours falling into either Grade I or II are raised a grade.

A number of histological variants of an endometrioid adenocarcinoma merit attention. Many, indeed

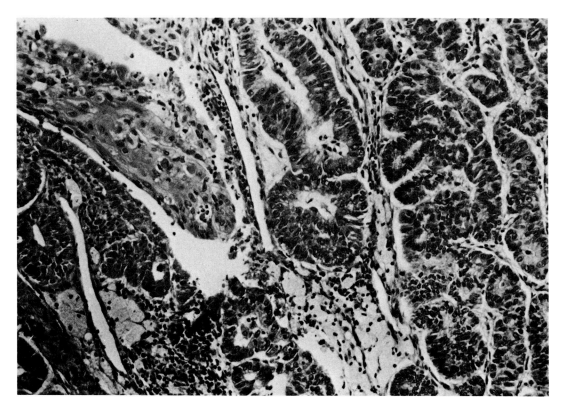

Fig. 10.20 A well-differentiated adenocarcinoma of the endometrium. Clusters of foamy macrophages can be seen in the stroma in the lower left of the field and, in the upper left, a tongue of tumour has a rather squamoid appearance (H. & E. × 108).

most, endometrioid adenocarcinomata contain areas of squamous metaplasia (Fig. 10.21), which occur as foci of bland, well differentiated squamous 'morules'. It has been suggested that those endometrioid adenocarcinomata in which squamous metaplasia is a prominent feature should be put into a separate category of *adenoacanthomata*. However, the frequency with which squamous metaplasia occurs in these tumours, the subjective criteria for the extent of such metaplasia to justify this diagnosis and the fact that squamous metaplasia, even if extensive, does not alter the prognosis for any given tumour have, or should have, led to the abandoning of the adenoacanthoma as a separate diagnostic category.

Many endometrioid adenocarcinomata show a papillary pattern in some areas. In a few, the *papillary endometrioid adenocarcinomata*, also known as *villoglandular endometrioid adenocarcinoma*, this pattern predominates.

Well differentiated endometrioid adenocarcinomata may undergo superimposed secretory changes, either because of the normal cyclical secretion of progesterone or because of therapy with a progestagen. However, there is no justification for considering 'secretory adenocarcinoma' as a distinct entity.

Spread and prognosis

Endometrioid adenocarcinomata are often slowly growing neoplasms, tending to spread initially by direct invasion of the myometrium and cervix. Later, the tumour may penetrate the uterine serosa and seed into the pouch of Douglas and onto the pelvic peritoneum. Cornual neoplasms often spread to the fallopian tube and malignant cells may pass out through the abdominal ostia of the tubes to be deposited on

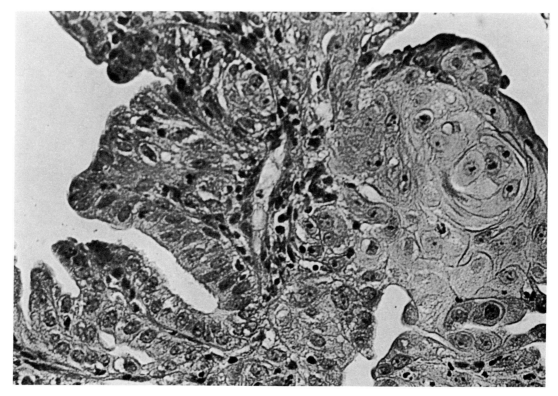

Fig. 10.21 Focal squamous metaplasia in a very well-differentiated endometrial adenocarcinoma (H. & E. × 270).

the ovaries or pelvic peritoneum. Local spread may also involve the broad ligament and the parametrium. Lymphatic spread is principally to the pelvic and para-aortic nodes, whilst haematogenous dissemination occurs late with the lungs, adrenals, liver and bones being the most common sites of distant metastases.

Endometrioid adenocarcinomata are usually staged as follows:

Stage I. The tumour is confined to the corpus.
Stage II. The carcinoma has spread to involve the cervix.
Stage III. The tumour has extended beyond the uterus but not outside the true pelvis.
Stage IV. The carcinoma has extended outside the true pelvis or has involved the mucosa of the bladder or rectum.

There is some controversy as to whether Stage I cases should be subdivided on the basis of the length of the uterine cavity but no dispute about the subdivision of neoplasms in this stage by histological grade. It should be noted that there must be true invasion of the cervical tissues for a tumour to be in Stage II, the mere extension of tumour into the endocervical canal not being of any prognostic significance. A further note of caution has to be sounded about grading tumours with apparent ovarian metastases as Grade III. In most instances the occurrence of an endometrioid adenocarcinoma in both uterine corpus and ovary is due to the occurrence of two independent primary neoplasms.

The prognosis for women with an endometrioid adenocarcinoma depends largely upon the stage and histological grade, although factors such as depth of myometrial invasion and the presence or absence of vascular space invasion are also of prognostic import. The overall five-year survival rate is in the region

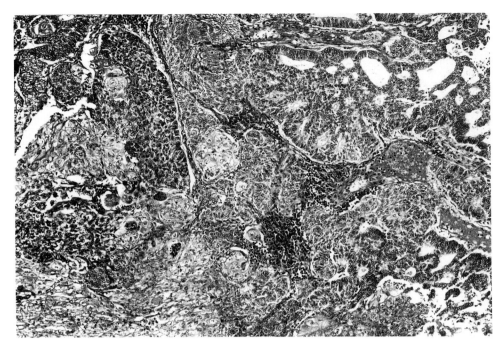

Fig. 10.22 Adenosquamous carcinoma of the endometrium. In the lower part of the section, to the left, there is infiltrating squamous carcinoma and, above, and to the right, there is well-differentiated infiltrating adenocarcinoma (H. & E. × 93).

of 66 per cent. For women with Stage I disease the survival rate is 75–80 per cent but this drops to 55–60 per cent for Stage II cases, to 30 per cent for women with Stage III tumours and to 10 per cent for those with Stage IV disease.

Adenosquamous carcinoma

This is a tumour containing an admixture of both adenocarcinoma and invasive squamous cell carcinoma (Fig. 10.22). The glandular element is usually an endometrioid adenocarcinoma. Adenosquamous carcinomata tend to develop at a relatively late age, the mean age at presentation being about 65 years, and they pursue an aggressive course, with a five-year survival rate of less than 40 per cent. About 5 per cent of all endometrial epithelial neoplasms are of this type and their incidence does not appear to be increasing.

The tumour described as a 'glassy cell carcinoma' of the endometrium is now recognized to be a poorly differentiated adenosquamous carcinoma.

Serous papillary carcinoma

These neoplasms are histologically identical with a papillary serous adenocarcinoma of the ovary (Fig. 10.23). Such tumours arise from foci of tubal metaplasia within the endometrium or from uncommitted cells which pursue an alternative route of müllerian differentiation along tubal lines. Serous papillary carcinomata tend to permeate, in a very extensive fashion, the uterine and adnexal lymphatic and vascular

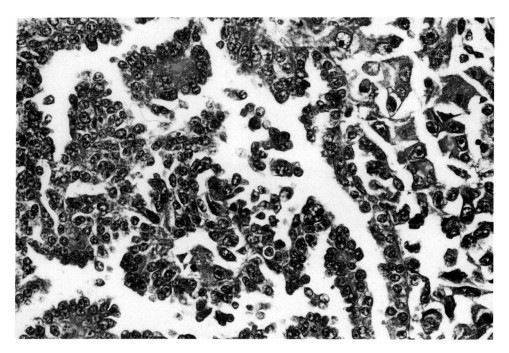

Fig. 10.23 Serous papillary carcinoma of the endometrium. Note the severe cytological atypia in the cells to the right of the figure (H. & E. × 370).

channels and, unlike the papillary form of endometrioid adenocarcinoma, are associated with a very gloomy prognosis.

Clear cell carcinoma

Endometrial neoplasms of this type are histologically identical to clear cell carcinomata of the ovary and vagina and behave in the same fashion as papillary serous carcinomata, sharing with these latter neoplasms a very poor prognosis.

Mucinous adenocarcinoma

A small proportion of endometrial adenocarcinomata are identical to mucinous adenocarcinomata of the ovary (Fig. 10.24). The prognosis for these tumours is similar to that for endometrioid adenocarcinomata of the same histological grade.

Squamous cell carcinoma

The endometrium is an extremely rare site for this type of neoplasm and the belief, propagated in older reports, that they tend to develop in elderly women with either a chronic pyometra or an ichthyosis uteri, seems less valid today. It should be noted that both condylomatous lesions of the cervix and cervical intraepithelial neoplasia can extend up into the uterine cavity and may here give rise to a squamous cell carcinoma.

The prognosis for a squamous cell carcinoma of the endometrium is usually poor.

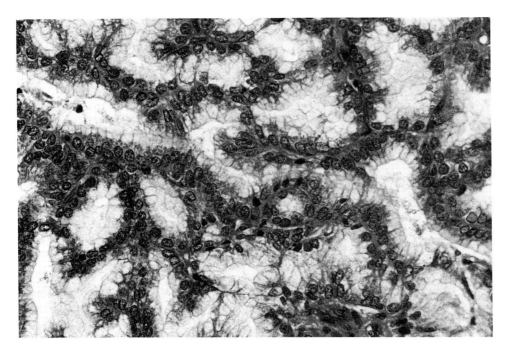

Fig. 10.24 Well differentiated mucinous carcinoma of the endometrium (H. & E. × 370).

Endometrial stromal sarcoma

Two forms of endometrial stromal sarcoma are now recognized, the *low grade stromal sarcoma* (previously known as 'stromal endometriosis' or 'endolymphatic stromal myosis') and the *high grade stromal sarcoma*. The low grade stromal sarcoma tends to produce a symmetrical enlargement of the uterus although a localized mass with ill-defined margins is sometimes seen. Because the neoplasm usually infiltrates the vascular and lymphatic channels of the myometrium, cords of tumour tissue may protrude from the cut surface of the uterus thus giving it a 'comedo' or 'rough towel' appearance. The tumour tissue is characteristically yellowish-grey and tends to stand out sharply from the surrounding myometrium. Histologically, the neoplasm is formed of irregular compact sheets or masses of spindle-shaped cells which usually resemble endometrial stromal cells of the non-secretory phase. The tumour infiltrates into the myometrium and has a particular tendency to grow into vascular or lymphatic spaces within the muscular wall of the uterus (Fig. 10.25). In some cases the tumour appears to lie entirely within such spaces with little or no infiltration of the adjacent myometrium. Occasionally, the infiltrating masses of tumour cells have a richly vascular pattern and may closely resemble a haemangiopericytoma. Mitotic figures are present but it is a defining feature of a low grade endometrial stromal sarcoma that there are fewer than ten mitotic figures per ten high power microscopic fields. The sarcoma with this degree of mitotic activity runs an indolently malignant course but tends to spread into the parametrium and often recurs locally, sometimes as long as twenty years after removal of the primary tumour. Distant spread can occur, principally to the lungs, but is rather unusual. Approximately 20 per cent of patients with this neoplasm will eventually succumb, often after an extremely protracted course.

High grade stromal sarcomata of the endometrium are less commonly associated with diffuse uterine enlargement and tend to present as soft, fleshy, white, fungating masses protruding into the uterine cavity. Myometrial invasion may or may not be macroscopically apparent but it is relatively unusual for a high grade stromal sarcoma to invade the myometrial vascular and lymphatic channels and thus present a

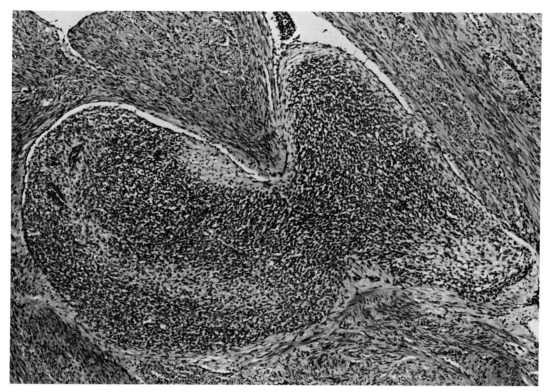

Fig. 10.25 Stromal sarcoma showing its typical growth pattern, in which it infiltrates the uterine vasculature (H. & E. × 45).

comedo appearance. Histologically, the tumour is highly cellular and grows as sheets and cords of endometrial stromal-like cells that extensively permeate the myometrium. The tumour cells show a greater degree of nuclear pleomorphism than is apparent in the low grade stromal sarcomata and invariably, and by definition, contain more than ten mitotic figures per ten high power microscopic fields. The five-year survival rate for women with this neoplasm is only between 15 per cent and 25 per cent, the tumour spreading rapidly to the parametrium and the mesentery. Pulmonary and vaginal metastases are common.

Mixed tumours

This group of neoplasms is considered here although it is not certain that all such tumours originate in the endometrium; it is possible that some arise primarily in the myometrium. Neoplasms of this type can also develop, albeit uncommonly, in the cervix.

Mixed tumours arise from müllerian stem cells which can differentiate along both epithelial and mesenchymal lines. If both epithelial and mesenchymal elements are benign the neoplasm is an *adenofibroma*, whilst if both components are malignant the tumour is a *carcinosarcoma*. In between these two extremes are neoplasms of low grade malignancy. Those with a benign epithelial element and a malignant stromal component are *adenosarcomata*, whilst the extremely rare tumours in which the epithelial component is benign and the stromal component malignant are classed as *carcinofibromata*.

The epithelial component of a mixed tumour is of a type normally found in the uterus whilst the stromal element usually shows either endometrial, stromal or smooth muscle differentiation but may also differentiate into tissues not normally present in the uterus, such as cartilage, striated muscle or bone. Thus any form of tumour may contain heterologous elements.

Despite the complexity of the nomenclature of these tumours, the malignant mixed tumours present in an almost stereotyped fashion. They occur principally in older women, the peak incidence being at nearly 70 years of age; patients usually present with vaginal bleeding. Pelvic pain and vaginal discharge are quite common complaints, whilst sometimes fragments of necrotic tumour are passed *per vaginum*. A significant proportion of women with this neoplasm have had prior uterine irradiation but the importance of this historical factor is not yet established. The uterus is almost invariably enlarged by a bulky, soft, fleshy, polypoid tumour mass which tends to fill the uterine cavity and to extend into the endocervical canal, sometimes protruding through the external os to present in the vagina. Foci of haemorrhage and necrosis are common. Histologically (Figs. 10.26 and 10.27), there is a mixture of carcinomatous and sarcomatous elements, the carcinomatous tissue usually being identical with an endometrial adenocarcinoma but sometimes resembling a tubal or endocervical carcinoma. Occasionally it may take the form of a squamous cell carcinoma. The sarcomatous component may be largely undifferentiated or resemble an endometrial stromal sarcoma and, if no heterologous stromal components are present, the neoplasm is classed as a *carcinosarcoma*. If heterologous sarcomatous elements are present, those most commonly noted are malignant striated muscle, cartilage or bone. Striated muscle fibres or rhabdomyoblasts containing striations are often seen, whilst large eosinophilic cells with granular cytoplasm, but lacking cross-striations, are frequently present, it being disputed as to whether these are rhabdomyoblasts or not. It is usual to find a mixture of heterologous components but sometimes the rhabdomyosarcomatous tissue predominates and, indeed, occasionally is the sole sarcomatous tissue present.

The pattern of spread of malignant mixed tumours is similar to that of endometrial adenocarcinoma, although the rate of advance is very much faster, this being a highly aggressive neoplasm. It is common for the tumour to have spread outside the uterus at the time of initial diagnosis and to be involving the pelvic peritoneum and lymph nodes. Metastases occur frequently to the lungs, liver and bone and these may be formed solely of sarcomatous tissue, purely of carcinomatous tissue or contain an admixture of carcinomatous and sarcomatous elements. The histological characteristics of a malignant mixed tumour are of little prognostic value and the best guide to the eventual outlook is the extent of tumour spread. Death is almost invariable and is rapid if the neoplasm has spread outside the uterus. Death remains the rule if the tumour, even though still confined to the uterus, has invaded the myometrium to an extent greater than 50 per cent of its thickness.

The adenosarcoma is a much less malignant neoplasm and, although often developing in the same age group as the malignant mixed tumour, tends to occur with greater frequency in younger women than does its more malign counterpart. However, the clinical features and macroscopic appearance of the adenosarcoma are often very similar to those of a malignant mixed müllerian tumour, although foci of haemorrhage and necrosis are less common and the tumour tends to have a more papillary appearance and to contain multiple small cysts on section. Histologically, the adenosarcoma has a benign epithelial component, comprising covering surface epithelium, glands and cysts, together with a sarcomatous stromal component (Fig. 10.28a and b). The epithelium of the glands and surface epithelium may be of endometrial, endocervical, tubal or squamous type, there commonly being a mixture of differing forms of epithelia, whilst the cystic spaces are usually lined by a flat or low cuboidal epithelium of rather nondescript type. The epithelial component may show a minor degree of atypia but otherwise appears fully benign. The stroma is of variable cellularity but is characteristically condensed around the glands and below the surface epithelium. A general appearance similar to that of an endometrial stromal sarcoma is the usual finding but heterologous elements such as striated muscle or cartilage may be present. The adenosarcoma is of relatively low grade malignancy and whilst pelvic or vaginal recurrence occurs in about half of patients after hysterectomy, distant metastases are distinctly uncommon. Even those patients with local recurrence tend to survive for prolonged periods.

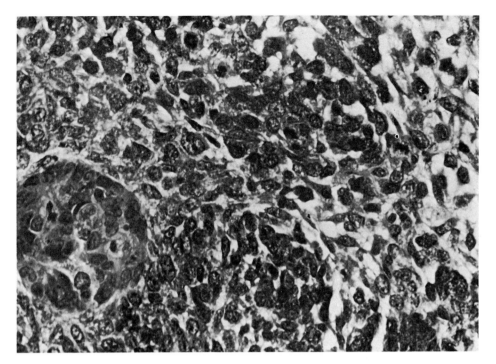

Fig. 10.26 A carcinosarcoma of the endometrium (malignant mixed tumour of homologous type). An acinus of poorly differentiated carcinoma is seen in the left of the field, whilst the remaining tissue resembles a stromal sarcoma (H. & E. × 240).

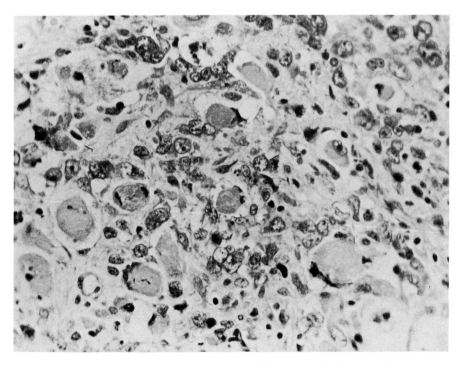

Fig. 10.27 A mixed tumour of heterologous type. The stroma in this example contains large cells with excentric nuclei and copious eosinophilic cytoplasm, these are rhabdomyoblasts (H. & E. × 240).

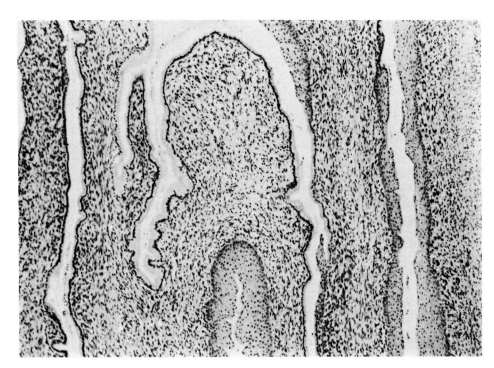

Fig.10.28(a) A uterine adenosarcoma at low magnification. The tissue clefts in this rather papillary tumour are lined by a mixture of benign squamous epithelium and columnar epithelium of endocervical type (H. & E. × 40).

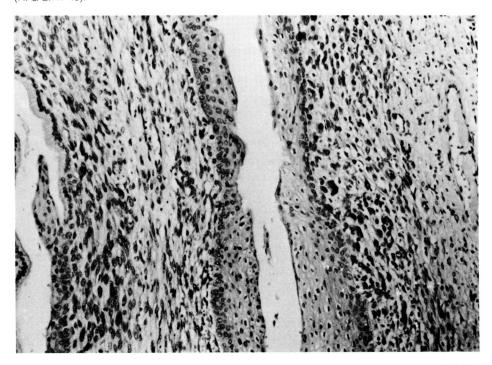

Fig. 10.28(b) A detail of the lower right corner of Fig. 10.28(a), showing the benign epithelium and pleomorphic sarcomatous stroma (H. & E. × 96).

Sex cord-like tumours

Very occasionally, neoplasms are encountered which appear to arise in the endometrium and to infiltrate the myometrium as cords, trabeculae or nests to produce a histological picture which mimics that of a sex cord tumour of the ovary. It appears that most such neoplasms are endometrial stromal sarcomata that are adopting an unusual pattern of growth although, exceptionally, adenosarcomata also grow, at least partly, in this fashion.

Rare endometrial neoplasms

Tumours which have been recorded as occurring in the endometrium with exceptional rarity include *paragangliomata, mature teratomata, yolk sac tumours, Wilms' tumour* and *Brenner tumour.*

Infiltration of the endometrium by lymphomatous or leukaemic cells is not uncommon in women suffering from the advanced stages of these diseases but, on rare occasions, lymphomata present initially as an endometrial lesion, some of these having been confined to, and apparently arisen primarily at, this site.

Metastatic tumours

Metastases do occur in the endometrium, principally from carcinomata of the breast, colon, stomach and pancreas.

Myometrium

Leiomyosarcoma

Malignant smooth muscle tumours of the myometrium are uncommon, accounting for about 50 per cent of uterine sarcomata but for only just 1 per cent of malignant uterine tumours. The neoplasm is of unknown aetiology and it is still not fully clear if it usually arises as a result of malignant change in a pre-existing leiomyoma or *de novo* from the myometrium; current opinion tends to favour the latter origin. The neoplasm develops most commonly in women in their fifth or sixth decade, about half the patients being premenopausal, and there is a high associated incidence of nulliparity. The presenting complaints are usually of abnormal vaginal bleeding, pain or the awareness of a mass.

The uterus is nearly always enlarged but the macroscopic appearances of a leiomyosarcoma are very variable, ranging from, at one extreme, a soft greyish tumour with focal areas of haemorrhage or necrosis which may form either an ill-defined intramyometrial lesion or bulge into the uterine cavity as a polypoid mass to, at the other end of the spectrum, a firm, white, well-delineated mass closely resembling a leiomyoma. The histological appearances (Fig. 10.29) are equally variable, ranging from a tumour which closely resembles a leiomyoma through an obviously malignant tumour which is, nevertheless, clearly of smooth muscle type, to a virtually anaplastic neoplasm showing considerable pleomorphism and mitotic activity. No difficulty as to the diagnosis of malignancy is encountered in the poorly differentiated tumours in which, however, the only clue to their true identity may be the finding of a few focal areas of abortive smooth muscle differentiation. In tumours that are well differentiated, the distinction between a leiomyoma and a leiomyosarcoma is based upon the degree of mitotic activity, cellularity and pleomorphism. Thus, a smooth muscle tumour with less than fifteen mitotic figures per ten high power microscopic fields and a bland cellular appearance is classed as a leiomyoma, whilst one with a count of twenty or more mitotic figures per ten high power fields is categorized as a *smooth muscle tumour of uncertain malignant potential*, this term being applied to benign-appearing neoplasms containing over fifteen

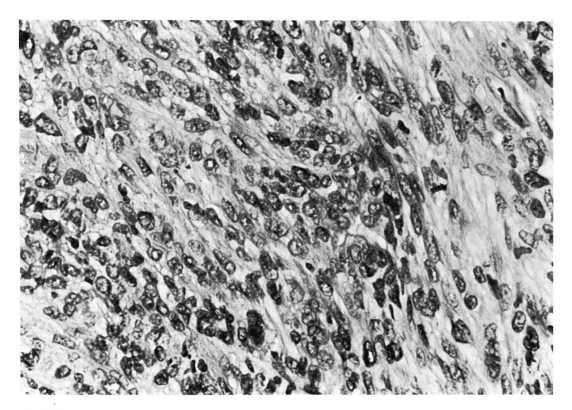

Fig. 10.29 Leiomyosarcoma of the uterus showing great variation in cellular differentiation, considerable pleomorphism and frequent mitoses (H. & E. × 270).

mitotic figures per ten high power fields and also to those in which there is a significant degree of pleomorphism, but with only two to four mitotic figures. Neoplasms containing more than four mitotic per ten micro power fields in association with cellular pleomorphism are best considered as leiomyosarcomata.

Myometrial leiomyosarcomata spread locally to invade the pelvic organs but it is uncommon for there to be lymph node metastases. Blood vessel invasion is a prominent feature of many leiomyosarcomata and it is therefore not surprising that pulmonary metastases are common, less frequent sites of blood borne secondary deposits being the kidneys and liver. The overall five-year survival rate for patients with this neoplasm is only 20–30 per cent, features indicating a gloomy outlook including the premenopausal state, poor differentiation of the tumour, vascular invasion and extrauterine extension. The tumours of uncertain malignant potential are thought to have little potentiality for local recurrence or metastasis.

Haemangiopericytomata

These are neoplasms thought to consist of a proliferation of capillaries together with surrounding pericytes. In the myometrium, such tumours grossly resemble a leiomyoma but tend to be less well defined and to lack a whorled appearance on section. Histologically, the classic appearance is of a vascular neoplasm, the blood vessels being surrounded by mantles of pericytic cells. However, variants on this theme are seen in which the tumour is composed largely of mesenchymal cells having an undifferentiated appearance, the collapsed capillaries and the circumferential arrangement of the cells only becoming apparent in sections stained for reticulin. Reticulin stains also demonstrate that the reticulin surrounds individual cells rather than cellular groups.

The haemangiopericytoma is a neoplasm of low grade malignancy and a proportion of cases will recur locally, although recurrence of uterine haemangiopericytoma occurs less commonly than is the case with similar tumours elsewhere. However, this tumour is a subject of dispute; some deny that such a neoplasm exists and others, whilst acknowledging its existence in extrauterine sites, deny that it occurs in the uterus, regarding those uterine neoplasms categorized as haemangiopericytomata as being either unusually vascular leiomyomata or low grade endometrial stromal sarcomata. This argument is far from settled, but most pathologists still recognize the uterine haemangiopericytoma as a specific entity.

Rare neoplasms

Occasional examples of myometrial *angiosarcomata*, *liposarcomata*, *alveolar soft part sarcomata*, *lymphangiosarcomata* and *soft tissue giant cell tumour* have been reported. Very exceptionally, a pure *rhabdomyosarcoma* of the myometrium is encountered.

Fallopian tube

Malignant neoplasms of the fallopian tube are uncommon, accounting for only 0.3 per cent of cases of female genital tract cancer. The vast majority of malignant tubal neoplasms are adenocarcinomata and, although a variety of other tumours have been recorded in this site, each is sufficiently rare as to be regarded as an oncological curiosity.

Adenocarcinoma

This tumour occurs most commonly during the fifth and sixth decades, the modal age of occurrence being about 52 years. An unduly high proportion of patients are nulliparous and in some studies there has been a high incidence of preceding infertility or 'one child sterility'.

Aetiology
This is completely unknown. A tube containing an adenocarcinoma is often chronically inflamed and, although it has been postulated that tubal infection predisposes to the development of an adenocarcinoma, it appears more likely that the inflammation is a secondary response to the neoplastic change. An association with tubal tuberculosis is sometimes canvassed but this is probably based upon a misinterpretation of the reactive epithelial hyperplasia which is a feature of that disease.

Clinical features
A tubal adenocarcinoma is classically associated with the triad of cramp-like iliac fossa pain, abnormal vaginal bleeding and vaginal discharge which may be watery, yellowish or serosanguinous and is occasionally extremely profuse. Most patients have one or two of the component features of this triad but few have all three. An abdominal mass may be present and the distinctive, but extremely rare, clinical picture of hydrops tubae profluens, in which a sudden gush of fluid from the vagina is accompanied by relief of pain and disappearance of a mass, is occasionally encountered.

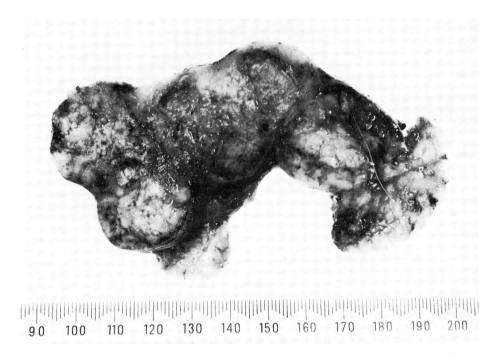

Fig. 10.30 A cut section of a fallopian tube distended by a solid mass of primary carcinoma.

Gross features

An adenocarcinoma starts as a small mucosal nodule and at this stage the tube may appear externally normal or only slightly swollen, any swelling present being most characteristically at the junction of the middle and outer thirds of the tube. More commonly, at the time of diagnosis the tube is distended by tumour to an extent that it resembles a pyo- or hydrosalpinx, although it differs from these two conditions by the frequent retention of normal fimbria and a patent abdominal ostium. Bilateral tumours are found in between 10 and 20 per cent of cases and it is not yet established whether this is due to the simultaneous development of two separate primary lesions or to metastasis in one tube from a primary tumour in the contralateral tube.

On opening the tube it is usually seen to be filled with friable, crumbling, grey tumour tissue which often shows areas of necrosis (Fig. 10.30). Overt invasion of the wall is often not apparent and perforation of the wall by tumour is unusual.

Histological features

The tumour is usually a well differentiated papillary adenocarcinoma (Fig. 10.31) and resembles closely a serous adenocarcinoma of the ovary. Less well differentiated tumours have a mixed papillary–alveolar pattern, whilst the uncommon poorly differentiated neoplasms tend to grow in a solid (or 'medullary') fashion, these variations forming the basis of the commonly employed, but not prognostically very useful, grading system:

G1 papillary pattern
G2 mixed papillary–alveolar pattern
G3 mixed alveolar–medullary pattern.

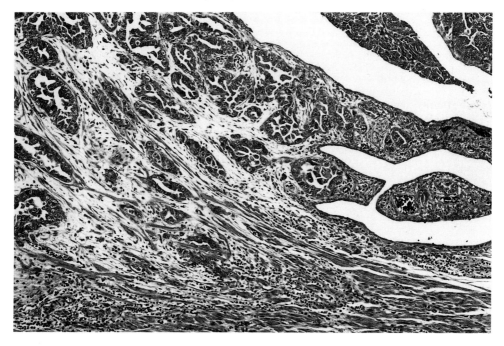

Fig. 10.31 A moderately-differentiated adenocarcinoma of the fallopian tube with an alveolar pattern. The lumen (above and to the right) contains fronds of tumour and the mucosal folds and wall of the tube (below and to the left) are infiltrated by tumour (H. & E. × 93).

Variations from this basic pattern are unusual, but rare examples of *endometrioid, adenosquamous* and *transitional cell carcinomata* have been described. The endometrioid type of carcinoma may be due to differentiation of tubal cells along an alternative müllerian pathway, but can also be due to malignant change in a focus of tubal endometriosis.

Spread and prognosis
An important mode of spread of tubal carcinoma is by direct implantation, tumour implanting via the abdominal ostium on to the peritoneum and ovary and via the uterine ostium into the uterus. In this respect, a previous salpingitis with occlusion of the fimbrial opening will tend to limit tumour dissemination. Direct spread through the tubal wall may involve adjacent structures, whilst lymphatic spread will eventually occur to the uterus and ovary and to the iliac, lumbar and para-aortic lymph nodes.

Staging of the tumour is dependent upon the extent of spread.

Stage I. Tumour confined to the tube and not penetrating the serosal surface.
Stage II. Extension of tumour to the serosal surface of the tube.
Stage III. Extension of tumour to the ovary or uterus.
Stage IV. Extension of tumour beyond the reproductive organs.

Extra-abdominal spread of a tubal carcinoma is very uncommon and this staging system is of considerable value. Thus, whilst the overall five-year survival rate for tubal adenocarcinoma is only about 25 per cent, that for Stage I cases is over 50 per cent, this figure declining rapidly to 16 per cent for Stage II cases and to below 10 per cent for Stage III and IV tumours.

The high mortality rate associated with tubal adenocarcinoma may suggest that this is a highly malignant neoplasm, but the poor prognosis is more a reflection of difficult and late diagnosis than of inherent extreme malignancy.

Squamous cell carcinoma

Very occasional squamous cell carcinomata of the tube have been described and these probably arise in foci of squamous metaplasia.

Sarcoma

Tubal sarcomata are very rare but occasional instances of *leiomyosarcoma, fibrosarcoma, angiosarcoma* and *undifferentiated spindle-cell sarcoma* have been described.

Mixed tumours

Carcinosarcomata, with or without heterologous elements, are rare in this site. They tend to occur in elderly women and form bulky masses which distend the tube. The histological features of these neoplasms are identical to those of similar type occurring in the uterus and the tumours metastasize rapidly to liver and lungs.

Choriocarcinoma

A choriocarcinoma may arise in the tube either from an ectopic pregnancy or from neoplastic transformation with trophoblastic differentiation of a germ cell which has become entrapped within the tube. The tumour tends to present clinically either as an ectopic pregnancy or with symptoms due to intraabdominal haemorrhage. At operation, a large, haemorrhagic fleshy mass is found which may have largely destroyed the tube. The histological features are identical to those described for uterine choriocarcinoma (see Chapter 17) and blood borne metastasis occurs at an early stage to lungs, liver, bone and vagina. However, there is a good response to chemotherapy.

Broad ligament

Malignant tumours in this site are rare, the least uncommon being the *leiomyosarcoma*. Instances of *liposarcoma, fibrosarcoma, neurofibrosarcoma* and *malignant mixed tumour* have also been recorded and all these various sarcomata, with the possible exception of the liposarcomata, have an extremely poor prognosis. *Adenocarcinomata* of the broad ligament may arise either from mesonephric remnants or from foci of endometriosis.

Key references

Barrowclough H and Jaarsma K W. (1980) Adenoacanthoma of the endometrium: a separate entity or a histological curiosity? *Journal of Clinical Pathology* **33**, 1064–7.

Bradgate M G, Rollason T P, McConkey C C and Powell J. (1990) Malignant melanoma of the vulva: a clinico-pathological study of 50 cases. *British Journal of Obstetrics and Gynaecology* **97**, 124–33.

Buckley C H and Fox H. (1988) Epithelial tumours of the vulva. In: *The Vulva*, pp. 263–333. Edited by C M Ridley, Churchill Livingstone, Edinburgh.

Buckley C H and Fox H. (1989) Carcinoma of the cervix. In: *Recent Advances in Histopathology 14*, pp. 63–78. Edited by P P Anthony and R N M McSween, Churchill Livingstone, Edinburgh.

Christopherson W M. (1986) The significance of the pathologic findings in endometrial cancer. *Clinics in Obstetrics and Gynaecology* **13**, 673–93.

Coleman D V and Evans D M D. (1988) *Biopsy Pathology and Cytology of the Cervix*. Chapman and Hall, London.

Ferenczy A and Winkler B. (1987) Carcinoma and metastatic tumors of the cervix. In: *Blaustein's Pathology of the Female Genital Tract, 3rd edn*, pp. 257–91. Edited by R J Kurman, Springer-Verlag, New York.

Fortune D W and Ostor A G. (1987) Mixed Müllerian tumours of the uterus. In: *Haines and Taylor, Obstetrical and Gynaecological Pathology, 3rd edn*, pp. 457–78. Edited by H Fox, Churchill Livingstone, Edinburgh.

Fox H and Buckley C H. (1988) Non-epithelial and mixed tumours of the vulva. In: *The Vulva*, pp. 235–62. Edited by C M Ridley, Churchill Livingstone, Edinburgh.

Fu Y S and Reagan J W. (1989) *Pathology of the Uterine Cervix, Vagina and Vulva*. W B Saunders, Philadelphia.

Hendrickson M R and Kempson R L. (1987) Pure mesenchymal neoplasms of the uterine corpus. In: *Haines and Taylor, Obstetrical and Gynaecological Pathology, 3rd edn*, pp. 411–56. Edited by H Fox, Churchill Livingstone, Edinburgh.

Hillborne L H and Fu Y S. (1987) Intraepithelial, invasive and metastatic neoplasia of the vagina. In: *Pathology of the Vulva and Vagina*, pp. 181–217. Edited by E J Wilkinson, Churchill Livingstone, New York.

Kurman R J and Norris H J. (1987) Endometrial carcinoma. In: *Blaustein's Pathology of the Female Genital Tract, 3rd edn*, pp. 338–72. Edited by R J Kurman, Springer-Verlag, New York.

Sedlis A. (1961) Primary carcinoma of the Fallopian tube. *Obstetrical and Gynecological Survey* **16**, 209–26.

Silverberg S G. (1988) Hyperplasia and carcinoma of the endometrium. *Seminars in Diagnostic Pathology* **5**, 135–53.

Zaino R J. (1987) Carcinoma of the vulva, urethra and Bartholin's gland. In: *Pathology of the Vulva and Vagina*, pp. 378–408. Edited by E J Wilkinson, Churchill Livingstone, New York.

Zaloudek C and Norris H J. (1987) Mesenchymal tumors of the uterus. In: *Blaustein's Pathology of the Female Genital Tract, 3rd edn*, pp. 373–408. Edited by R J Kurman, Springer-Verlag, New York.

11

Neoplasms of the ovary

The ovary gives rise to a greater range and variety of neoplasms than any other organ and this oncological profusion may prove confusing unless ovarian tumours are considered in the setting of a logical and systematic classification. Such a framework is provided by the WHO Classification of Ovarian Tumours which, since its introduction in 1973, has supplanted all preceding attempts to impose order on this host of neoplastic entities. The WHO classification defines each individual tumour type solely in histological terms, no account being taken of gross characteristics or of functional activity, and the various separate neoplasms are then grouped together on the basis of their known, or presumed, common histogenesis. The classification is, of necessity, complex, but can be simplified into six main headings:

1. Epithelial tumours
2. Sex cord stromal tumours
3. Germ cell tumours
4. Tumours of the non-specialized tissues of the ovary
5. Miscellaneous unclassified tumours
6. Metastatic tumours.

Epithelial tumours

These neoplasms constitute 60 per cent of all primary tumours of the ovary and 90 per cent of those that are malignant. The vast majority are thought to originate from undifferentiated cells in the surface, or serosal, covering epithelium of the ovary, either arising directly from that epithelium or from epithelial fragments which have become sequestrated into the ovarian cortex to form the so-called germinal inclusion cysts. The ovarian serosa is the direct descendant, and the adult equivalent, of the coelomic epithelium which, during embryonic life, overlies the nephrogenital ridge and from which are derived the müllerian (paramesonephric) ducts and the structures which arise from these namely endocervical epithelium, endometrium, and the epithelium of the fallopian tube. It is believed that undifferentiated cells in the ovarian serosa retain a latent capacity, or competence, to differentiate along the same tissue pathways as do embryonic cells and hence a neoplasm derived from these cells can differentiate along various müllerian pathways, those differentiating to form tubal epithelium constituting the *serous group of tumours*, those differentiating into endocervical epithelium being the *mucinous tumours* and yet others differentiating along endometrial lines to be classed as *endometrioid tumours*. However, two further tumours arising from the serosa fall outside this grouping of neoplasms with epithelium of müllerian type. One is the *Brenner tumour* and although in the past the nature of the epithelial cells in this neoplasm gave rise to much speculative discussion, the application of the electron microscope has shown the epithelium to be virtually identical with that of the urinary tract, the presence of uroepithelium indicating that cells in the serosa also have a potentiality for wolffian (mesonephric) as well as müllerian differentiation. The last member of the group of epithelial neoplasms is the clear cell tumour. These neoplasms used to be known

167

as mesonephroid tumours because of a historical misinterpretation of their true nature, but there is now overwhelming evidence for their müllerian nature.

The epithelial tumours of the ovary form a unitary group linked by their common derivation from the serosal epithelium. However, two codicils must be entered. First, it should not be assumed that every neoplasm in this group differentiates along only one pathway; it is not unusual to encounter tumours containing epithelia of different type, the mixed serous–mucinous type of tumour being particularly common. Second, the concept of all epithelial tumours arising from the surface epithelium is too all-embracing for a proportion of these neoplasms have a quite different histogenesis. Thus, some mucinous tumours are formed not of endocervical-type epithelium, but of gastrointestinal-type epithelium, complete with argyrophil and Paneth cells. It is possible that these *enteric-type mucinous neoplasms* occur as a consequence of gastrointestinal metaplasia of surface epithelial cells but it is equally probable that some are monophyletic teratomata, especially as all mucinous tumours found in association, and combined with, mature cystic teratomata are of the enteric type. Further, not all endometrioid or clear cell tumours are derived from the surface epithelium, a minority originating in pre-existent foci of ovarian endometriosis, whilst some Brenner tumours arise in the hilum of the ovary, possibly originating from hilar mesothelium or from structures of mesonephric origin such as the epoöphoron or epigenital tubules.

Despite these exceptions, the vast majority of epithelial neoplasms are derived from the surface epithelium and each can exist in a benign or malignant form. The malignant forms are usually collectively known as *ovarian adenocarcinoma* and, although the individual neoplasms will be separately discussed, their malignant forms share certain common characteristics which merit their being considered collectively under the general heading of ovarian adenocarcinoma. In addition to the benign and malignant types of each of these neoplasms, is a third form, namely tumours of borderline malignancy (also known as *tumours of low malignant potential* and as *proliferating tumours*); these also share many common characteristics and will be considered as a group.

Serous tumours

The benign form of these common neoplasms shows three basic patterns which may occur separately or in combination, these being the cystic, papillary and adenofibromatous forms. The cystic variety, the *serous cystadenoma*, occurs as a thin-walled, usually translucent, cyst which is commonly unilocular. These cystic neoplasms can measure anything from 1 cm to 30 cm in diameter (although they never attain the huge size which mucinous cystadenomata sometimes achieve), have a smooth glistening inner and outer surface and contain thin straw-coloured fluid. The papillary type of benign serous tumour can occur in combination with a cyst, this being the *papillary serous cystadenoma*, in which the papillae are found on either inner or outer surface, sometimes on both. The papillae may be few, small and sessile or numerous, large and pedunculated. The papillary form also occurs without any cyst formation as finger-like projections from the surface of the ovary, this being the *serous surface papilloma*, which is often bilateral (Fig. 11.1). Fragments can break off from papillary tumours and implant on the pelvic peritoneum, sometimes giving rise to ascites. Such an appearance may give a false impression of malignant spread which is dispelled only by the benign histological appearances of both the tumour and the implants. The third form, the *serous adenofibroma*, is seen as a lobulated, hard, knobbly solid mass which may develop in isolation or as a nodule in the wall of a cyst. On section, tiny cystic spaces may be seen in the largely solid mass.

Histologically, the serous cystadenoma is usually lined by a single layer of flattened or cuboidal cells but in a few instances the tubal nature of the lining epithelium may be more apparent. Certainly, the true nature of the epithelium is usually more overt in the papillary neoplasms where the central core of the papillae, formed of loose fibrous tissue, is covered by an epithelium remarkably similar to that of the tube, with recognizable secretory cells, ciliated cells and intercalary peg cells (Fig. 11.2). Psammoma

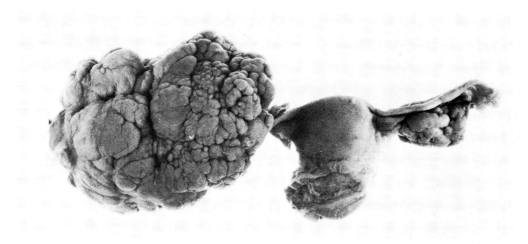

Fig. 11.1 Bilateral serous surface papillomata of the ovaries.

bodies, which are small, concentrically laminated calcospherites, are commonly found in the stroma of the papillary serous tumours. However, these structures are not specific to the serous group of neoplasms and are not, contrary to what is sometimes thought, indicative of malignancy. The serous adenofibroma is essentially a fibrous neoplasm containing small cysts, gland-like spaces or slits lined by epithelium of tubal type.

The *serous adenocarcinoma* is usually fairly large and is essentially a malignant variant of the papillary serous cystadenoma, the vast majority being partially cystic and partially solid, the solid areas being formed of closely packed, or merged, papillae which often penetrate through the outer capsule of the neoplasm. Only a very small minority of serous adenocarcinomata appear solid throughout. On section, areas of haemorrhage and necrosis are frequently seen and the fluid in the cystic portion of the tumour is often blood stained. Histologically the tumour may show a papillary, adenopapillary or diffuse pattern. The papillary, or well differentiated, type of tumour retains a clearly papillary pattern but the epithelium shows multilayering, irregular tufting, nuclear hyperchromatism, cellular pleomorphism and mitotic activity, whilst stromal invasion is readily apparent (Fig. 11.3). From this papillary form there is a spectrum of differentiation extending through to the diffuse type in which the tumour grows in solid sheets of malignant cells. However, most tumours show a mixed pattern of differentiation and indeed, unless a papillary pattern with epithelium resembling, although admittedly in a bizarre and anarchic form, that of the tube is found in some area of the neoplasm, it may be impossible to diagnose the type of tumour which has therefore to be categorized, rather unsatisfactorily, as an adenocarcinoma of indeterminate type.

Mucinous tumours

These are common, accounting for about 20 per cent of benign ovarian tumours and for about 25 per cent of ovarian adenocarcinomata. Benign mucinous tumours are usually cystic and take the form of a *mucinous cystadenoma* which, although originating as an intraovarian cyst, eventually replaces the ovary. The mucinous cystadenoma has a smooth, glistening, usually lobulated, outer surface and tends to measure between 15 and 30 cm in diameter, although these tumours occasionally attain a huge size and can completely fill the abdominal cavity. On section, the cysts have a moderately thick, parchment-like wall and are characteristically multilocular (Fig. 11.4). Not uncommonly there is one major locule accounting

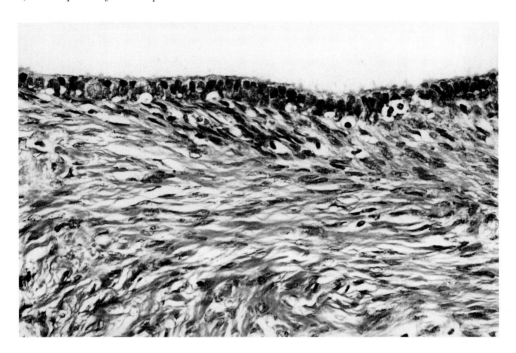

Fig. 11.2   The epithelial lining of a serous cystadenoma showing its close resemblance to tubal epithelium. The cyst wall, below, is fibrous (H. & E. × 370).

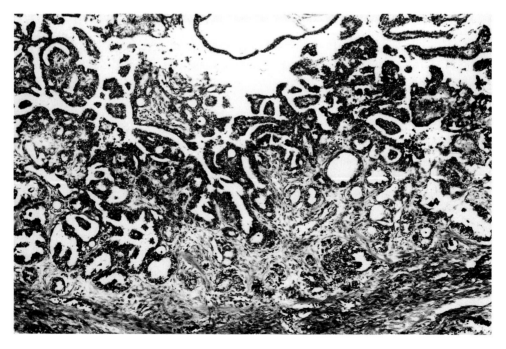

Fig. 11.3   A moderately well-differentiated serous adenocarcinoma with an adenopapillary pattern. Infiltration of the stroma is seen in the lower part of the field (H. & E. × 93).

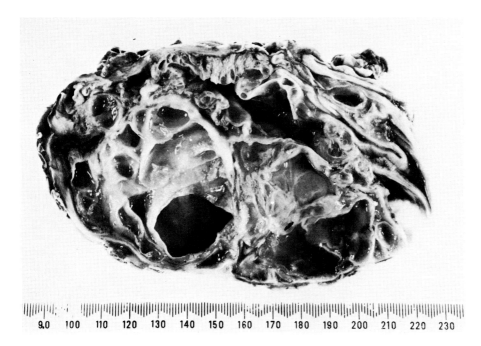

Fig. 11.4 A mucinous cystadenoma showing a typical multilocular appearance.

for most of the cyst but with a number of smaller satellite locules, whilst closely packed small locules may impart a semisolid appearance to parts of the tumour. The locules usually contain clear, tenacious mucoid material but the physical characteristics of the cyst contents vary widely and they can appear thin and watery. Histologically, the walls of the locules are formed of fibrous tissue and the cyst is lined by a single layer of tall columnar cells with slightly basophilic, glassy cytoplasm and regularly arranged, darkly staining basal nuclei, the resemblance to endocervical epithelium being acute (Fig. 11.5). However, a proportion of mucinous cystadenomata are lined by an enteric type of epithelium with goblet cells of intestinal nature, argyrophil cells and Paneth cells (Fig. 11.6). These enteric-type mucinous tumours do not differ in any other way from those lined by endocervical-type epithelium. Occasionally, the mucus within a locule ruptures into the stroma to give free pools of mucoid material, a condition as *pseudomyxoma ovarii*.

A rare type of benign mucinous tumour is the *mucinous adenofibroma*. This grossly resembles its serous counterpart but the glands within the fibrous tumour are lined by a mucinous-type epithelium.

Mucinous adenocarcinomata may be cystic and closely resemble a cystadenoma, although they usually differ from the non-malignant neoplasms by having papillary or nodular excrescences on one or both surfaces. Two-thirds of mucinous adenocarcinomata are, however, either partially or wholly solid and on section these neoplasms, although tending to exude mucoid material, often show areas of haemorrhage or necrosis. These tumours show a wide spectrum of histological appearances (Fig. 11.7), ranging from those well differentiated neoplasms with a glandular pattern, the acini being lined by cells which are still recognizably mucoid in type but with multilayering, nuclear hyperchromatism, pleomorphism, cellular atypia, mitotic activity and stromal invasion, to the poorly differentiated variety formed of sheets of pleomorphic cells in which intracellular mucus is usually present.

Spillage of cyst contents into the abdominal cavity as a result of spontaneous or surgical perforation, can complicate both benign and malignant mucinous tumours and may result in the condition of

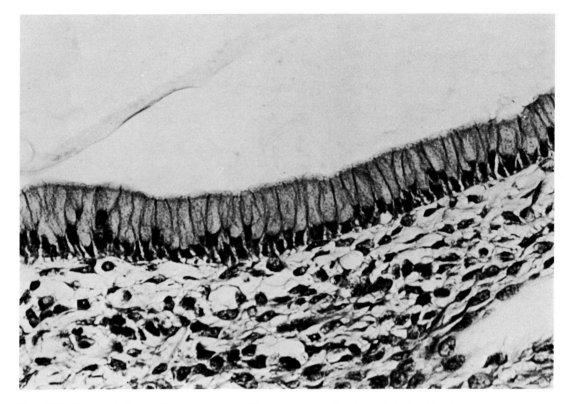

Fig. 11.5   The single layer of tall, mucus-secreting columnar cells characteristic of benign mucinous cystadenomata (H. & E. × 270).

pseudomyxoma peritoneii, in which enormous amounts of jelly-like mucoid material, often loculated, accumulate in the peritoneal cavity. It is not entirely clear if this is because of implantation and growth of tumour deposits or because of induction of mucinous metaplasia of the peritoneal serosa, but microscopic examination of the mucoid material will reveal scattered small groups of mucinous cells. Pseudomyxoma peritoneii can also complicate a mucocele of the appendix and it is well recognized that some patients with this condition have both an appendicular mucocele and a mucinous ovarian tumour, circumstances under which it is impossible to identify the primary lesion.

Endometrioid tumours

Benign endometrioid tumours are very rare, although occasional examples of an *endometrioid adenoma*, which tends to resemble an endometrial polyp, and of *endometrioid adenofibroma*, a neoplasm resembling the serous adenofibroma but in which the glands are lined by an endometrial-type epithelium, do occur. However, the rarity of benign endometrioid tumours may be more apparent than real because it is possible that many ovarian lesions classed as endometriotic cysts may, in reality, be benign endometrioid cystadenomata.

Endometrioid adenocarcinomata are common. The gross characteristics of these neoplasms are non-specific (Fig. 11.8). They generally measure between 12 and 25 cm in diameter and have a smooth outer surface. On section the tumour may be solid, partially cystic or wholly cystic, the latter variety usually showing abundant papillary ingrowth. The defining histological feature of an endometrioid adenocarcinoma is

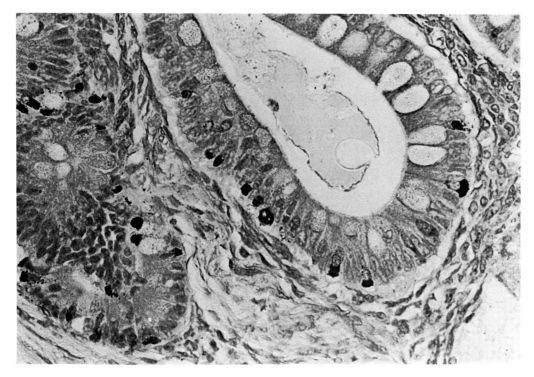

Fig. 11.6 A mucinous cystadenoma of enteric type stained by Grimelius' method to demonstrate the darkly staining argyrophil cells (Grimelius stain × 255).

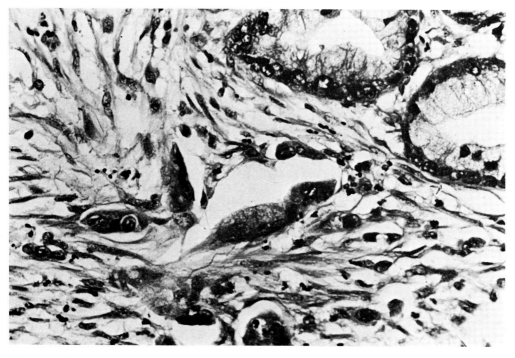

Fig. 11.7 Glandular acini of well-differentiated mucinous carcinoma lie to the right of this section, whilst infiltration of the stroma by individual malignant cells can be seen in the lower corner to the left (H. & E. × 255).

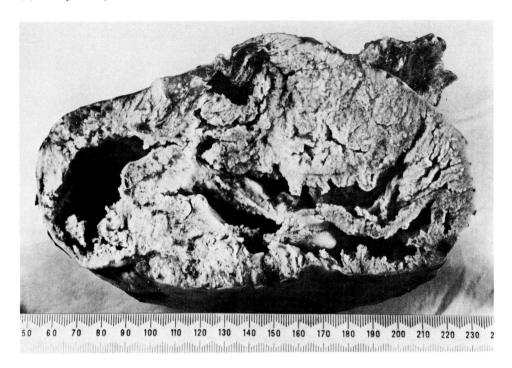

Fig. 11.8   Endometrioid carcinoma of partly solid and partly cystic appearance.

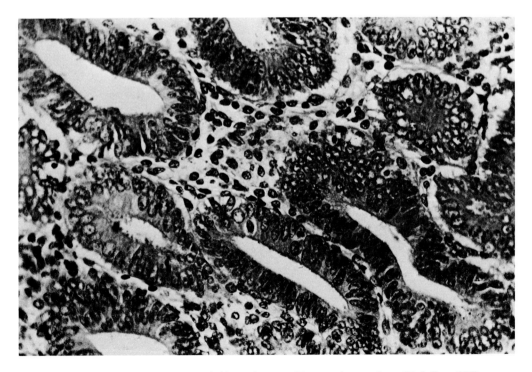

Fig. 11.9   Well-differentiated endometrioid carcinoma with an acinar pattern (H. & E. × 270).

that it mimics exactly an endometrial adenocarcinoma (Fig. 11.9). Most are well differentiated and have an acinar pattern but in a minority the cells are arranged in sheets, the endometrioid nature of the tumour being only recognizable by the presence of small foci of better differentiated glandular formations. Some tumours show a papillary pattern in a few areas and in occasional instances this pattern predominates, the papillae tending to be blunt in shape and thus differing from the more delicate branching papillae seen in serous tumours. The cells forming the acini, covering the papillae and existing in sheets are generally cuboidal or columnar with basophilic cytoplasm. In many, indeed probably most, endometrioid adeno-carcinomata, areas will be found in which the cells have a clear or vacuolated cytoplasm. Such clear cell areas may be few or form a prominent feature of the neoplasm. Many endometrioid adenocarcinomata also contain foci of squamous metaplasia and if this is extensive the neoplasm is often, unnecessarily, classed as an endometrioid adenoacanthoma. The squamous component of endometrioid tumours is usually clearly benign but is occasionally malignant, tumours showing this feature being *endometrioid adenosquamous carcinomata* and appearing histologically identical to the mixed tumours of this type found in the endometrium. This type of tumour perhaps emphasizes the fact that any neoplasm occurring in the endometrium can also arise in the ovary as a variant of an endometrioid tumour and thus rare instances of *carcinosarcoma* (with or without heterologous elements), *endometrial stromal sarcoma* and *adenosarcoma*, all identical to their more common endometrial counterparts, occur in the ovary. Even pure sarcomata such as a *rhabdomyosarcoma*, *chrondrosarcoma* or *osteogenic sarcoma* can be regarded as variants of the endometrioid tumour, these oncological exotica either representing an overgrowth of one component of a mixed tumour with obliteration of the other tissue elements or being a pure heterologous sarcoma *ab initio*.

The coexistence of endometrioid carcinoma of the ovary and adenocarcinoma of the endometrium is well recognized. Under such circumstances it may be difficult to decide whether the ovarian tumour is a metastasis or not, but the weight of evidence suggests that the two tumours are usually independent primary lesions.

Brenner tumours

Most Brenner tumours are benign and many are of microscopic size only, with the vast majority measuring less than 2 cm in diameter and only occasional examples attaining a diameter of greater than 10 cm. The neoplasm is usually well circumscribed with a smooth or bosselated surface and has a hard, slightly whorled, whitish-grey cut surface. Not infrequently, Brenner tumours occur in the wall of a mucinous cystadenoma or mature cystic teratoma and are then seen as localized, firm, white intramural nodules. A small proportion are found in association with a serous cystadenoma. Histologically, the Brenner tumour is characterized by well-demarcated nests and branching columns of epithelial cells set in a fibrous stroma (Fig. 11.10), the relative proportions of epithelial and stromal elements being very variable. The sharply demarcated epithelial nests are formed of round or polygonal cells with well delineated margins, abundant clear or weakly eosinophilic cytoplasm and ovoid or round nuclei which often show a well marked longitudinal groove. Frequently, the central areas of the cell nests become cystic, these microcystic spaces being lined by flattened endothelial-like cells, cuboidal cells or mucus-secreting columnar cells (Fig. 11.11). The fibrous stroma varies in cellularity and often shows focal but widespread hyalinization or calcification.

Malignant Brenner tumours are thought, perhaps incorrectly, to be uncommon and tend to be large and partially cystic. The solid areas may be hard and white or soft and fleshy, often with areas of necrosis, whilst the cystic portion may be unilocular or multilocular and characteristically has a shaggy or velvety lining. Histologically, the malignant Brenner tumour is characterized by a marked overgrowth of the epithelial component, with the epithelial cells showing nuclear hyperchromatism, prominent nucleoli, pleomorphism, mitotic activity and stromal invasion. The malignant cells may still appear as epithelial

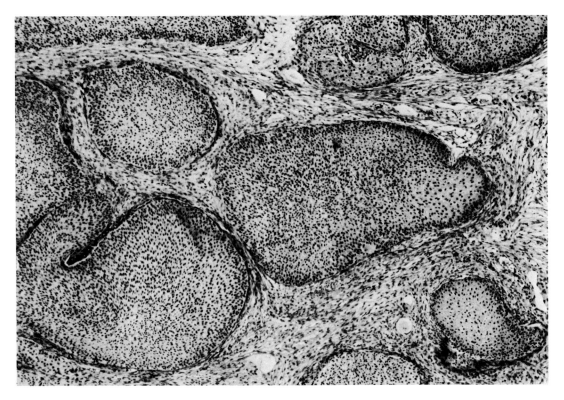

Fig. 11.10 The well-demarcated nests of epithelial cells set in a fibrous stroma characteristic of a Brenner tumour (H. & E. × 45).

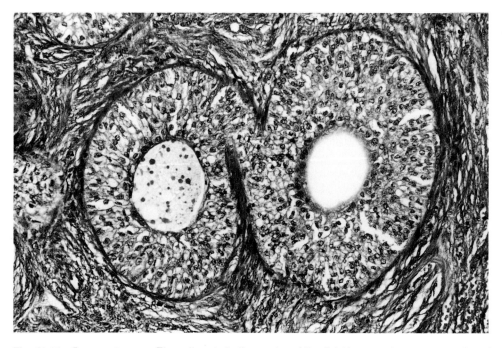

Fig. 11.11 Brenner tumour. The cell nests in the centre of the field have undergone central cystic change (H. & E. × 270).

islands set in a collagenous stroma, may grow in sheets to give an appearance strikingly similar to that of a transitional cell carcinoma of the bladder, or may form acini to resemble an adenocarcinoma. It is generally suggested that a malignant Brenner tumour should not be diagnosed unless:

Areas of benign Brenner tumour are also present in close proximity.
The presence of a mucinous cystadenocarcinoma or malignant teratoma has been excluded.
The possibility of a metastasis from a transitional cell carcinoma of the bladder is eliminated.

Clear cell tumours

Benign clear cell tumours are exceptionally uncommon and represented only by the occasionally seen *clear cell adenofibroma* which on macroscopic examination resembles the other forms of these solid neoplasms but in which the gland-like spaces are lined by cells with clear cytoplasm and hobnail-type nuclei.

Clear cell adenocarcinomata rarely measure more than 25 cm in diameter and only a minority are solid, most being cystic with solid areas. The solid portions tend to be soft and fleshy, whilst the cystic areas are commonly multilocular and often contain fluid of a mucoid nature. Histological examination reveals a complex pattern (Figs. 11.12 and 11.13) with tubular and cystic structures lined by flattened cells with large, deeply staining nuclei protruding into the lumen (hobnail nuclei), simple or complex papillae covered by a cuboidal epithelium and sheets of cells with clear cytoplasm, all usually set in a fibrous stroma.

Ovarian adenocarcinoma

The various malignant forms of the epithelial tumours of the ovary are, in clinical practice, usually grouped together as *ovarian adenocarcinoma*. These neoplasms tend to occur in women aged 45–60 and are commonly asymptomatic until they have achieved a considerable bulk. The most common complaints are of increasing abdominal girth, lower abdominal pain or discomfort and the presence of a pelvic mass. Urinary symptoms, due to pressure on the bladder, are quite frequent, whilst disturbances of the menstrual cycle or postmenopausal bleeding are relatively unusual.

The prognosis in any individual case depends upon the clinical stage at the time of diagnosis and the histological grade of the neoplasm. Until recently it was thought that histological type was of prognostic significance, with serous tumours having a much less favourable prognosis than endometrioid or mucinous neoplasms. However, multivariate analysis of prognostic features has shown that histological type is of little or no prognostic significance.

Staging of ovarian adenocarcinomata is dependent upon an understanding of the mode of spread of these neoplasms, which may be by direct contiguity, peritoneal seeding or by lymphatic or blood borne dissemination. A problem in assessing the extent of spread of ovarian adenocarcinoma is that it is quite commonly the case that bilateral ovarian tumours are present at the time of diagnosis and it is by no means clear whether this is due to the development of two independent primary lesions or to an ovarian metastasis from a unilateral lesion; it is probable that the former is more commonly the case. Peritoneal seeding is by far the most important mechanism of local spread, with implantation of secondary deposits in the pouch of Douglas, on the surface of the uterus, in the omentum and paracolic gutters and on the under surface of the diaphragm. The tube, uterus, bowel and bladder may be directly involved by contiguous invasion but vaginal deposits are usually due to an extension of tumour from a peritoneal seeding in the pouch of Douglas. Lymphatic spread is principally to the pelvic, para-aortic and mesenteric nodes, but sometimes involves the mediastinal or supraclavicular nodes. Blood borne dissemination leads

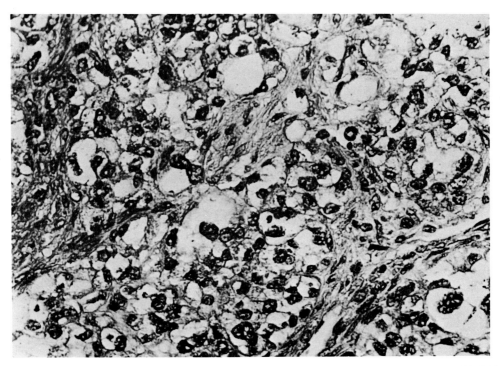

Fig. 11.12 Sheets of clear cells characteristic of the solid areas of a clear cell carcinoma (H. & E. × 255).

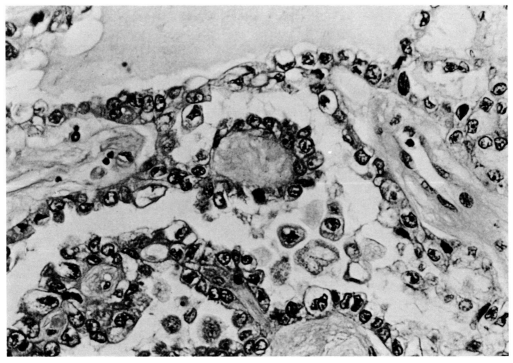

Fig. 11.13 Clear cell carcinoma showing a tubulopapillary pattern of large cells with clear cytoplasm and prominent nuclei (hobnail nuclei) (H. & E. × 255).

to deposits in the liver, lungs and, occasionally, bone. The most commonly used system of staging is that introduced by FIGO: this is rather complex but, for practical purposes, can be simplified into:

Stage 1. Tumour confined to the ovaries.
Stage 2. Tumour confined to the pelvis.
Stage 3. Tumour confined to the abdomen but not involving the liver parenchyma.
Stage 4. Tumour present outside the abdominal cavity or within the liver parenchyma.

Staging along these lines is an important guide to prognosis but it should be stressed that accurate staging requires extensive histological sampling of the omentum, lymph nodes and peritoneum of the paracolic gutters and under surface of the diaphragm. If 'aggressive' staging of this type is carried out, it will be found that many cases considered on macroscopic evidence to be Stage 1 or Stage 2 are in fact Stage 3.

The value of histological grading of ovarian adenocarcinomata is still not fully determined. It is not clear if grade is of value only in Stage 1 and Stage 2 tumours or if tumour grade is of any prognostic significance at any stage in patients treated by modern chemotherapeutic regimes. Furthermore, there is currently no agreed form of grading, some pathologists relying on the Broders' system, which indicates the percentage of undifferentiated cells, and others using an architectural grading system, i.e. classifying tumours as being of good, poor or intermediate differentiation. Irrespective of the system used, all grading has a considerable element of subjectivity and inconsistency and there is significant interpathologist variation.

Currently, ovarian adenocarcinoma has a gloomy prognosis, the overall five-year survival rate being in the region of 25 per cent. Unfortunately, little is known of the aetiology of this lethal form of neoplasia, which is the third most common cause of death from neoplastic disease in women. It has been suggested that the ground is prepared for eventual neoplasia in the surface epithelium by repeated minor trauma and certainly such trauma is inflicted regularly by ovulation. That incessant ovulation may be of importance in this respect is hinted at by evidence that both oral contraception and repeated pregnancies appear to offer some degree of protection against the risk of developing ovarian adenocarcinoma. Nevertheless, it should not be supposed that repetitive trauma is in itself responsible for ovarian neoplasia and there are grounds for believing that an exogenous carcinogen, ascending from the lower genital tract, is also implicated; it is known that both hysterectomy and tubal occlusion reduce the risk of ovarian adenocarcinoma. The exogenous carcinogen has not been identified but suspicion has fallen on talc. This substance is present in many vaginal toilet preparations and is also used to coat contraceptive diaphragms and condoms, talc crystals have been found in a number of ovarian adenocarcinomata and women using talc-containing perineal dusting powders are at increased risk of developing ovarian cancer. It is, however, by no means certain that talc is a carcinogen and it has to be borne in mind that many commercial talc preparations were, and probably still are, contaminated by asbestos, a consideration of some importance in view of the essentially mesotheliomatous nature of ovarian adenocarcinomata.

Tumours of borderline malignancy

These, also somewhat unsatisfactorily known as *proliferative tumours* or as *carcinomata of low malignant potential*, are epithelial ovarian tumours which occupy that grey area between the clearly benign and the overtly malignant. It is largely the serous and mucinous tumours that form this group; endometrioid, clear cell and Brenner tumours of borderline malignancy are rare and less clearly delineated.

A tumour of borderline malignancy may be defined as 'one in which the epithelium shows some, or all, of the characteristics of malignancy but in which there is no stromal invasion'. Thus the tumour epithelium is characterized by a variable degree of multilayering, budding, nuclear pleomorphism, cytological atypia and mitotic activity but evidence of stromal invasion is lacking (Figs. 11.14 and 11.15). It may, of course, be exceptionally difficult to exclude stromal invasion, this being particularly the case

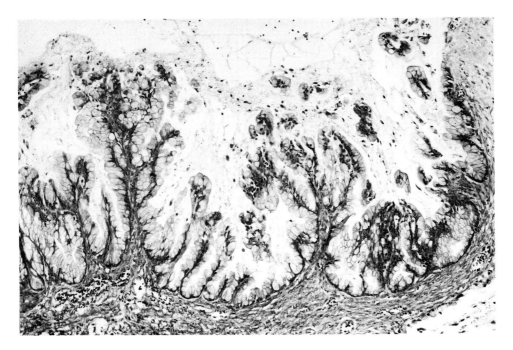

Fig. 11.14   A mucinous tumour of borderline malignancy in which the cyst lining is thrown into complex folds. The epithelial cells are multilayered and there is some loss of nuclear polarity. There is no stromal invasion (H. & E. × 93).

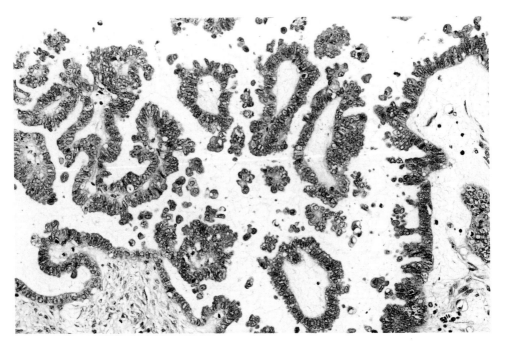

Fig. 11.15   A serous tumour of borderline malignancy showing the characteristic epithelial multilayering and budding but no stromal invasion (H. & E. × 186).

with mucinous neoplasms, and hence some pathologists will diagnose an adenocarcinoma if the epithelial abnormalities are sufficiently severe, even in the absence of demonstrable stromal invasion. However, it is felt that the lack of invasiveness of these neoplasms is a defining feature of their unique biological status and that this criterion should be retained. It will be noted that the definition of borderline tumours takes into account only the histological appearances of the ovarian neoplasm, the presence or absence of extra-ovarian spread playing no role in the definition of these neoplasms. It also has to be stressed that a diagnosis of borderline malignancy is a positive one, which is based on specific histological findings and that the use of this term is not indicative of the pathologist being unable to decide if a neoplasm is benign or malignant.

Between 10 and 15 per cent of all serous tumours fall into the borderline category and grossly these closely resemble their fully benign counterparts. In between 25 and 50 per cent of cases the tumours are bilateral, almost certainly because of a synchronous development of two primary lesions. Further, in about 35 per cent of cases, there appears to be extra-ovarian spread in the form of apparent implants in the pelvic peritoneum and omentum. However, there is considerable evidence to indicate that these apparent implants are not true metastases but develop *in situ* from foci of endosalpingiosis. This is not to deny, however, that serous borderline tumours are totally incapable of metastasizing, because examples of authentic extra-abdominal metastases from such tumours have been recorded. The overall prognosis for patients with a borderline tumour is good, with a five-year survival rate of over 97 per cent for those with Stage 1 disease and a 10-year survival rate which can be as high as 90 per cent. Patients with apparent Stage 3 disease have a survival rate of up to 85 per cent.

About 10–15 per cent of mucinous neoplasms are of borderline malignancy, these taking the form of multilocular cysts. Only 5 per cent are bilateral, whilst apparent extra-ovarian spread is noted in less than 10 per cent of cases. The nature of the extra-ovarian lesions varies with the type of mucinous tumour. Those associated with the rather small minority of mucinous neoplasms which have an endocervical-type lining are similar to those found in association with serous borderline tumours and represent *in situ* development of endosalpingiosis or endocervicosis, whilst those occurring in association with the more commonly encountered enteric-type borderline tumours take the form of pseudomyxoma peritoneii, the exact histogenesis of which is uncertain. The prognosis for women with Stage 1 mucinous tumours of borderline malignancy is extremely good, with a 98 per cent survival rate at five years and a 96 per cent survival rate at ten years. However, the outlook for the unfortunate minority with complicating pseudomyxoma peritoneal is poor; most pursue a slow but relentless downhill course, with a ten-year survival rate of less than 20 per cent.

Borderline endometrioid tumours take the form either of foci of atypical proliferation in areas of ovarian endometriosis or of adenofibromata, in which endometrial-type glandular structures showing various degrees of atypia are set in, but not invading, an abundant fibrous stroma. Clear cell tumours of borderline malignancy are also usually adenofibromata, in which the glands are lined by clear cell or hob-nail cells showing some proliferation and atypia.

A particular form of Brenner tumour, often known as a *proliferating Brenner tumour*, is regarded as this neoplasm's counterpart of the serous and mucinous tumours of borderline malignancy. These are usually large tumours which are wholly or partly cystic and tend to be multilocular, the lining of the loculi in some areas being smooth and in others having a papillary, velvety appearance. Histologically, areas of typical benign Brenner tumour are often, but not invariably present, whilst in the papillary parts of the neoplasm the Brenner epithelium is thrown into folds and the epithelial cells are arranged in layers (Fig. 11.16). The papillary folds are supported by thin connective tissue cores and the epithelial cells show varying degrees of atypia and mitotic activity. Neoplasms showing this pattern behave in a benign fashion.

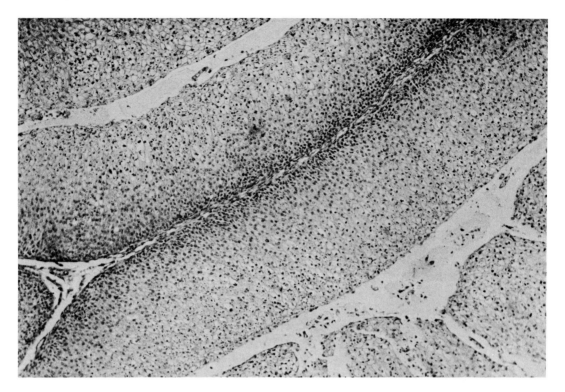

Fig. 11.16 A proliferating Brenner tumour showing the extreme thickness of the epithelium over the papillary folds and its general resemblance to low-grade transitional cell carcinoma of the bladder (H. & E. × 45).

Sex cord-stromal tumours

This group of neoplasms includes all those that contain granulosa cells, theca cells, Sertoli cells or Leydig cells either singly or in any combination. Some workers believe that all these cells are derived from the mesenchyme of the genital ridge and hence class these various neoplasms as *mesenchymomas* or *gonadal stromal tumours*. However, it appears more likely that both granulosa and Sertoli cells are derived from the primitive sex cords of the developing gonad. There is some dispute as to whether these cords are derived from the coelomic epithelium or from mesenchyme, but opinion currently favours an epithelial origin. During the early stages of embryogenesis the gonad has the potentiality for developing into either a testis or an ovary and, if it is directed to develop along 'male' lines, the sex cords will differentiate into Sertoli cells, whilst if development occurs along ovarian lines, these cells will differentiate into granulosa cells. In the adult, undifferentiated cells of sex cord origin retain this bisexual potentiality and can give rise to either granulosa or Sertoli cell neoplasms, these tumours being homologous to each other. Neoplasia of these cells is often accompanied by a stromal reaction which, in the case of granulosa cell tumours, adds a thecomatous component to the neoplasm and which in the case of Sertoli cell tumours often shows Leydig cell differentiation. Furthermore, stromal cells themselves can become neoplastic and differentiate into either thecomata or Leydig cell tumours. Overall, therefore, the term *sex cord-stromal tumours* appears the most logical for this group of neoplasms.

Granulosa and theca cell tumours

Granulosa cell tumours
Two forms of granulosa cell tumour, the adult and the juvenile are now recognized.

Adult-type granulosa cell tumours. These tumours account for about 1.5 per cent of all ovarian neoplasms. One third of adult-type granulosa cell tumours develop in women of reproductive age, the bulk of the remainder occurring in patients who have passed their menopause. Approximately 5 per cent of adult-type granulosa cell neoplasms develop in premenarchal girls. The tumours are unilateral in 95 per cent of cases and vary in size from microscopic lesions to masses measuring up to 40 cm in diameter; the average size is about 12 cm in diameter. Most adult granulosa cell tumours are predominantly solid with a smooth or bosselated outer surface. On section, they may be hard, rubbery or soft and their cut surface may be white, brown, yellow, pink or grey. Focal haemorrhage or necrosis is common and any cystic areas may contain watery serosanguineous or gelatinous fluid. A small proportion of granulosa cell tumours are predominantly cystic and may closely resemble a cystadenoma.

Histologically, the tumour cells are round, ovoid or angular with scanty eosinophilic cytoplasm and indistinct boundaries. The nuclei are vesicular, round or oval and characteristically, although not invariably, show well marked longitudinal grooving (coffee bean appearance).

The neoplastic granulosa cells may be arranged in a variety of patterns (Figs. 11.17 and 11.18) and although in any individual tumour a particular histological pattern may predominate, there is usually a combination of cellular arrangements in any single neoplasm. The tumour may show an insular, trabecular, diffuse or follicular pattern. The follicles are of three types. First, microfollicles or rosette-like structures (Call–Exner bodies) which usually contain eosinophilic material and nuclear debris. Second, macro-follicles, which are really areas of liquefaction in islands of granulosa cells. The third type of follicle is large and lined by circumferentially arranged cells, these resembling the graafian follicles of the newborn infant. The insular parts of a granulosa cell tumour are composed of large groups, or islands, of polygonal cells arranged (except at the margin) without polarity and with few microfollicles. In the trabecular regions the cells are arranged in ribbons, one, two or several layers thick, set in a stromal matrix. The cells adjacent to the stroma tend to be regimented at right angles to the axis of the ribbon, with their nuclei arranged antipodally. When the ribbons are narrow and the stroma scanty the pattern is sometimes described as 'watered silk'. The diffuse form of these neoplasms, often incorrectly called 'sarcomatoid', may be formed by polygonal or spindle-shaped cells. Cystic granulosa cell tumours have a lining which resembles that of a graafian follicle but which contains microfollicles.

There is usually little pleomorphism but about 2 per cent of these tumours contain cells with large, bizarre, hyperchromatic nuclei. Mitotic figures are usually scanty.

The stromal component of a granulosa cell tumour is variable in amount and may have a fibromatous or thecomatous appearance..

A granulosa cell tumour may produce non-specific pelvic tumour symptoms, such as pain, discomfort, dyspareunia or dysuria, but approximately three-quarters of patients have symptoms suggestive of an endocrinological disturbance. Thus, in young girls these neoplasms commonly produce isosexual pre-cocious pseudopuberty, whilst in women of reproductive age complaints of irregular vaginal bleeding are characteristic. These symptoms are due to the oestrogenic capacity of these neoplasms, a further result of which is the frequent development of simple or atypical endometrial hyperplasia and the concomitant development, in about 6–10 per cent of cases, of an endometrial adenocarcinoma. Very occasionally, granulosa cell tumours are virilizing rather than oestrogenic; these tumours usually being of the cystic variety.

A proportion of adult-type granulosa cell tumours will recur or metastasize but the magnitude of this proportion has, in the past, been minimized by an over-reliance on five-year survival rates. Granulosa cell tumours which pursue a malignant course do so in a leisurely and indolent manner, with one-third

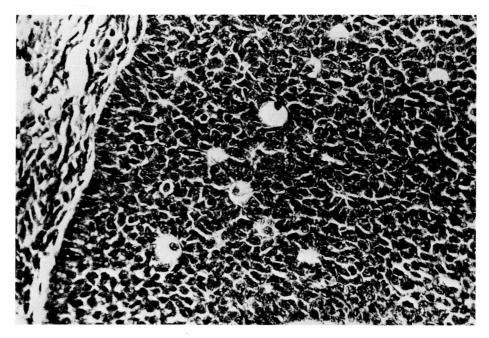

Fig. 11.17   Granulosa cell tumour of the insular and microfollicular pattern showing the uniformity of the constituent cells (H. & E. × 255).

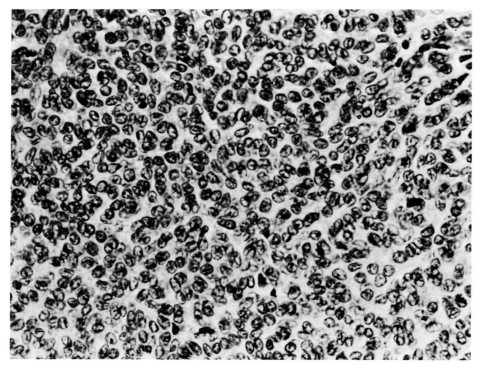

Fig. 11.18   A diffuse granulosa cell tumour in which the cells are growing in solid sheets. The typical nuclear grooving is seen in many of the cells (H. & E. × 255).

of recurrences presenting more than five years after initial treatment and one-fifth after ten years; indeed, recurrences can develop after as long a period as 25 years. A true estimate of the malignancy of these neoplasms can only be achieved by prolonged surveillance, probably life-long, but for at least 20 years. In a number of such studies, the corrected 20-year survival rate for women with adult-type granulosa cell neoplasms has been in the region of 50–60 per cent. It is clear, therefore, that all granulosa cell tumours should be regarded as being at least potentially malignant and it has to be stressed that, on pathological grounds, no tumour of this type can be unequivocally classed as fully benign. Conversely, the only absolute indication of a poor prognosis is the presence of extra-ovarian spread at the time of initial diagnosis. Other prognostic indicators are more debatable and although there has been a measure of agreement that the larger the neoplasm the greater the tendency towards a poor outcome, it has not been clearly established that this factor is prognostically significant for those tumours confined to the ovary. The type of histological pattern seen in the tumour is not prognostically relevant and it has not been proved that a high mitotic count is of strict relevance for those tumours without extra-ovarian spread. Atypia is not, in itself, indicative of a poor prognosis.

Juvenile granulosa cell tumours. About 85 per cent of granulosa cell neoplasms which occur before puberty have a distinctive histological appearance which has therefore been considered to be typical of the juvenile granulosa cell tumour. However, neoplasms showing this pattern are not confined to the prepubertal years, for whilst 45 per cent occur in the first decade of life and 32 per cent in the second decade, 20 per cent develop in the third decade and 3 per cent after the age of 30 years. The tumour usually arises in otherwise normal children, although there is a suggestion of a specific, though weak, association with Ollier's disease and Maffucci's syndrome.

The tumours are usually unilateral and are largely solid, although cystic forms are occasionally encountered.

Histologically, there is a nodular or, less commonly, a diffuse pattern of tumour cells set in an oedematous, loose stroma. The nodules may be solid but usually contain a number of sharply etched, rounded or irregular follicles which bear some resemblance to normal developing follicles; these are lined by one or more layers of granulosa cells and their lumens commonly contain mucinous material (Fig. 11.19). Cystic spaces, often relatively large, may be present and have a multilayered lining of granulosa cells. Thecal cells may lie in the stroma adjacent to the granulosa cell nodules but the two cell types can be intermingled in a haphazard fashion. Luteinization is often a striking feature of these neoplasms, whilst the granulosa cell nuclei tend to be hyperchromatic and lack the characteristic longitudinal grooving of an adult-type granulosa cell tumour. A degree of cytological atypia is not uncommon and mitotic figures, sometimes of abnormal form, are frequently plentiful.

Approximately 5 per cent of juvenile granulosa cell tumours behave in a malignant fashion, these usually, but not invariably, being those showing the greatest degree of atypia and mitotic activity. However, the indolent course pursued by malignant adult-type granulosa cell tumours is not mirrored by the malignant juvenile forms; these tend to recur rapidly and disseminate widely throughout the abdominal cavity within two years of initial diagnosis.

Thecoma

Thecomata are only a third as common as granulosa cell tumours and, although of very variable size, commonly measure 8–10 cm in diameter. They are well demarcated, non-encapsulated and have a smooth or lobulated outer surface (Fig. 11.20). On section they are predominantly solid (although small cystic areas are often seen), of hard or rubbery consistency and have a characteristic yellowish colour, although the tumour is rarely yellow throughout. Most characteristically, there are islands of yellowish tissue separated by septa of grey fibrous tissue. Histologically the tumour is formed of plump, pale, ovoid or spindle-shaped cells with indistinct borders, small ovoid nuclei and abundant cytoplasm. These cells are arranged in interlacing bundles or anastomosing trabeculae irregularly traversed by bands of less cellular

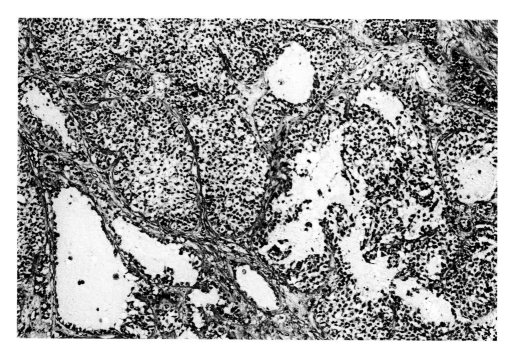

Fig. 11.19   A juvenile granulosa sinus tumour showing solid areas and irregular cystic follicles lined by granulosa cells (H. & E. × 93).

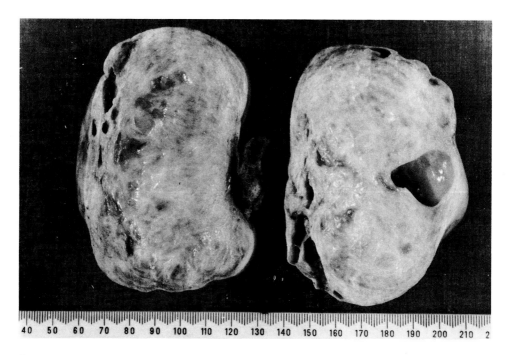

Fig. 11.20   A solid thecoma with areas of cystic degeneration.

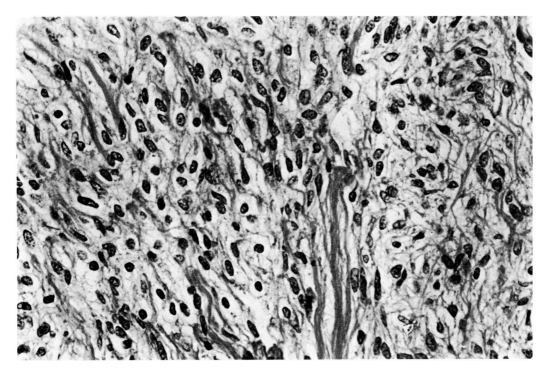

Fig. 11.21 The typical plump cells with clear cytoplasm and ovoid nuclei which are characteristic of a thecoma (H. & E. × 270).

fibrous tissue (Fig. 11.21). Plaques of hyalinized collagen are frequently present, fat is usually demonstrable within the cytoplasm of the tumour cells and focal luteinization is occasionally encountered.

These neoplasms arise from the ovarian mesenchyme and occur most commonly in postmenopausal women. They are oestrogenic and produce symptoms similar to those found in women with a granulosa cell tumour; a few androgenic thecomata producing clinical virilization have been described.

Thecomata are, with few exceptions, benign, although rare examples of malignant thecoma have been reported. The diagnosis of malignancy in a thecoma rests upon the presence of cellular pleomorphism and of abnormal mitotic figures.

Androblastoma

An androblastoma is a neoplasm composed of Sertoli cells, Leydig cells, or the precursors of either, alone or in any combination. These tumours were previously classed as *arrhenoblastomas*, but this name implies that they are invariably virilizing. This is not the case and the term *androblastoma* is preferred not only because it lacks any connotation of endocrinological activity but also because it emphasizes that these tumours recapitulate phases in the development of the male gonad.

Sertoli cell tumour

The rare Sertoli cell tumours are usually intra-ovarian, small (average diameter 9 cm), solid and have an orange or yellow cut surface.

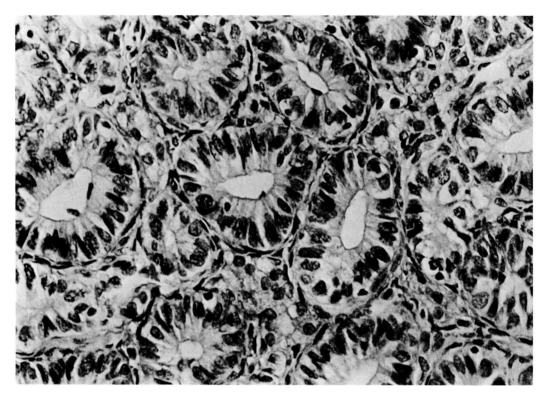

Fig.11.22   Sertoli cell tumour. The section shows closely packed tubules lined by tall columnar cells, with basal nuclei and pale cytoplasm (H. & E. × 270).

Histologically, Sertoli cell neoplasms have a predominantly tubular or trabecular pattern (Fig. 11.22). The hollow tubules are generally uniform, rounded or ovoid and lined by a single layer of cuboidal or low columnar cells with clear cytoplasm and basal nuclei. The lining cells often have well defined apical margins but in some instances their apical cytoplasm trails off towards the lumen to form intertwining fibrils. The trabeculae are usually elongated and are sometimes admixed with Sertoli cells arranged in a diffuse pattern. The Sertoli cells commonly contain cytoplasmic lipid droplets and, in a proportion, the tumour cells are markedly distended by fat, a pattern sometimes given the term 'folliculome lipidique'.

Patients with a Sertoli cell neoplasm usually present with symptoms suggestive of an endocrinological disturbance and over 70 per cent of these neoplasms appear to be oestrogenic, the patients complaining of excessive, prolonged or irregular bleeding or of postmenopausal haemorrhage and the endometrium often showing evidence of oestrogenic stimulation. A further 20 per cent of these tumours appear to be androgenic and produce clinical virilization, whilst only about 10 per cent are lacking in obvious functional activity.

Virtually all Sertoli cell tumours are benign but one such neoplasm, occurring in a young girl, rapidly recurred and led to death within five months. In this particular tumour there was a typical tubular pattern in some areas but elsewhere there were aggregates of pleomorphic cells showing mitotic activity.

Leydig cell neoplasm
Tumours of this type can be regarded as a form of androblastoma but are more conveniently considered as a type of steroid cell neoplasm (see page 207).

Sertoli–Leydig cell tumours

These neoplasms contain a mixture of Sertoli and Leydig cells, although there are increasingly strong grounds for believing that the Leydig cell component is not truly neoplastic but is due to a Leydig cell differentiation in stromal cells that are reacting to the presence of a Sertoli cell neoplasm. They are rare, accounting for only 0.2 per cent of all ovarian neoplasms and occur most commonly between the ages of 11 and 45 years, the mean age of patients being 25 years. A few familial cases of Sertoli–Leydig cell tumours have been described; these women also had a high incidence of associated thyroid abnormalities, such as goitres and adenomata.

Sertoli–Leydig cell tumours are unilateral in 98 per cent of cases and are of variable size, averaging about 10 cm in diameter. The neoplasms have a smooth external surface and are usually solid and firm, the cut surface often having a yellowish tinge. Cystic change is sometimes apparent but areas of necrosis or haemorrhage are uncommon except in poorly differentiated neoplasms.

Sertoli–Leydig cell tumours are traditionally, and probably usefully, categorized according to their degree of differentiation. The well differentiated neoplasms (Fig. 11.23) are formed by clearly defined tubular structures (which may be hollow or solid) lined by Sertoli cells. These tubules are set in a fibrous stroma which contains a variable number of cells resembling Leydig cells; it is unusual for Reinke's crystals to be identifiable in these cells. Tumours of intermediate differentiation tend to have a lobular pattern and contain Sertoli cells arranged in islands, trabeculae, sheets or cords; solid or hollow tubules are occasionally encountered. This Sertoli cell element is set in a fibrous or oedematous stroma in which Leydig cells are found singly, in clumps or in sheets. The Leydig cells are seen most conspicuously at the periphery of the cellular lobules and at the margin of the tumour as a whole. Poorly differentiated Sertoli–Leydig cell tumours are formed largely of sheets of closely packed spindle-shaped cells, this tissue bearing

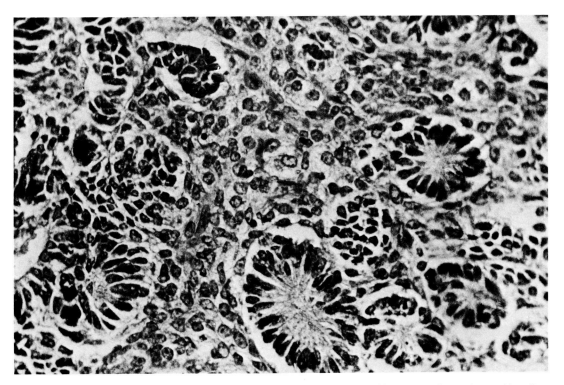

Fig. 11.23 A well-differentiated Sertoli–Leydig cell tumour with groups of large round or polygonal Leydig cells between tubules lined by Sertoli-like cells (H. & E. × 270).

a close resemblance to the stroma of the undifferentiated gonad. However, set in this undifferentiated sex cord–stromal tissue are occasional poorly formed tubules or irregular epithelial cords and in most cases there are also a few clusters of Leydig cells.

Sertoli–Leydig cell tumours can occur at any age but the majority develop in women aged between 10 and 35 years. Abdominal symptoms are not uncommon but endocrinological disturbances tend to dominate the clinical picture. Well differentiated Sertoli–Leydig cell tumours are commonly androgenic and produce clinical virilization, but occasional instances appear to have been solely, or predominantly, oestrogenic. Over 90 per cent of women with less well differentiated tumours are virilized to some extent and oestrogenic activity is not seen with the poorly differentiated forms.

The biological behaviour, and hence the prognosis, of Sertoli–Leydig cell tumours is still not fully defined although it is now reasonably clear that well-differentiated neoplasms always behave in a benign fashion. However, the outlook for patients with tumours of intermediate or poor differentiation is less clear. In one series of 64 tumours showing intermediate or poor differentiation, the corrected ten-year survival rate was 92 per cent, but in another large study the survival rate for patients with neoplasms of intermediate differentiation was 89 per cent whilst that for poorly differentiated tumours was only 41 per cent. Nevertheless, it is clear that most Sertoli–Leydig cell tumours which behave in a malignant fashion fall into the poorly differentiated category. In those tumours which do pursue a malignant course, metastases or recurrence are usually apparent within 12 months of initial treatment and most women with malignant tumours are dead within two years. Metastases usually occur in the omentum, abdominal lymph nodes or liver but deposits have been noted in sites such as lung, bone and brain.

Retiform Sertoli–Leydig cell tumours

Approximately 10 per cent of Sertoli–Leydig cell tumours contain, at least in part, areas which show a pattern of growth resembling that of the rete testis. The retiform areas may be only a minor component of such neoplasms, can represent a moderate proportion of the tumour or can be a predominant, even exclusive, feature of a Sertoli–Leydig cell neoplasm. Tumours with prominent retiform components tend to occur in children and in women who are, on average, younger than are those whose tumours lack a retiform element (average age 17 years).

Retiform neoplasms tend to be larger and are more often cystic than more conventional Sertoli–Leydig cell tumours. Histologically, the retiform areas of these tumours are characterized by a network of elongated, irregularly shaped, not uncommonly slit-like, tubules and spaces. The tubules are sometimes dilated and contain eosinophilic material, thus having a slight resemblance to thyroid follicles. Papillary structures are also present in most cases, projecting into the tubules and cysts. These papillae may be short, with a hyalinized core, large or polypoid, with fibrous or oedematous cores or have a complex branching pattern. The stroma may be fibrous or of a loose mesenchymal nature and often shows foci of hyalinization. The Sertoli–Leydig cell component of these tumours is invariably of intermediate or poor differentiation.

Retiform Sertoli–Leydig cell tumours appear to have a relatively poor prognosis. In one series of 21 such neoplasms, five patients succumbed to their tumours at intervals ranging from six months to 17 years after initial therapy.

Sertoli-Leydig cell tumours with heterologous elements

Heterologous elements are present in about 20 per cent of Sertoli–Leydig cell tumours; most commonly gastrointestinal-type epithelium, and less frequently, muscle or cartilage. Very rarely, cells resembling hepatocytes or neuroectodermal elements may be seen. There has been debate as to whether neoplasms of this type are teratomatous in nature or whether the heterologous elements develop by a process of neometaplasia. On balance, the latter view appears the more convincing.

In tumours containing gastrointestinal-type epithelium the enteric component may be inconspicuous, although in some cases it predominates, the Sertoli–Leydig cells occurring in the wall of what appears to be an unexceptional mucinous neoplasm. The mucinous epithelium is usually benign but occasionally shows a pattern of borderline malignancy whilst, rarely, it may be frankly malignant. The enteric epithelium often contains argyrophil cells and small foci of carcinoid tumour may develop. Heterologous skeletal muscle or cartilage in Sertoli–Leydig cell tumours is always immature and the muscle component sometimes develops into a rhabdomyosarcoma.

Sertoli–Leydig cell tumours containing heterologous gastrointestinal epithelium have a good prognosis and in a study of 31 such neoplasms only two behaved in a malignant fashion and proved fatal. By contrast, neoplasms containing heterologous muscle or cartilage are associated with a poor outlook; in a series of 10 patients with such tumours only two survived.

Gynandroblastoma

This diagnosis has commonly been applied in an indiscriminate manner but should be restricted to neoplasms in which both Sertoli–Leydig and granulosa-thecal components are present, both in substantial quantities and in typical and unequivocal form. There must also be a true intermingling of the two cell patterns; for there have been instances of a granulosa cell tumour and a Leydig cell neoplasm occurring as separate and discrete entities within the same ovary.

With the application of these precise criteria only a very small number of acceptable cases of gynandroblastoma have been reported. All these appeared to behave in a benign fashion but not enough examples have accumulated for the true biological behaviour of these neoplasms to be defined.

Sex cord tumour with annular tubules

These are neoplasms with a very distinctive histological appearance (Fig. 11.24), being formed of sharply circumscribed, rounded or ovoid nests of epithelial cells set in a fibrous stroma. The epithelial cells have clear or eosinophilic cytoplasm, indistinct margins and regular, round, occasionally grooved, nuclei. The cell nests contain acidophilic, PAS-positive, hyaline bodies which may coalesce to form complex networks within the epithelial nests. The hyaline material, which is occasionally so abundant as to obliterate most of the cellular elements in some or even most nests, appears to be basement membrane protein. The epithelial cells are characteristically palisaded around the periphery of the cell nests and around the hyaline bodies so as to give two basic patterns — there may be a simple, closed, ring-shaped tubule or a complex pattern in which cells envelope numerous single or confluent hyaline bodies. Between the epithelial islands is ovarian-type stroma which may show extensive hyalinization.

There has been considerable debate as to whether the epithelial cells in a sex cord tumour with annular tubules are of granulosa or Sertoli cell type but they are best regarded as immature cells or sex cord origin which have a potentiality for differentiating into either granulosa or Sertoli cells.

The original descriptions of the sex cord tumour with annular tubules stressed the association between these neoplasms and Peutz–Jeghers syndrome but as more cases have accumulated it has become clear that they can also occur in women with no stigmata of this syndrome. Furthermore, it has become apparent that those tumours associated with Peutz–Jeghers syndrome differ both clinically and pathologically from those arising in otherwise normal women. Thus, sex cord tumours with annual tubules occurring in women with Peutz–Jeghers syndrome are usually bilateral, commonly only of microscopic size, frequently calcified, not associated with granulosa or Sertoli cell tumoural overgrowth and never behave in a malignant fashion. By contrast, histologically identical tumours developing in women lacking the stigmata of Peutz–Jeghers syndrome are unilateral, usually large, rarely calcified and are associated not infrequently

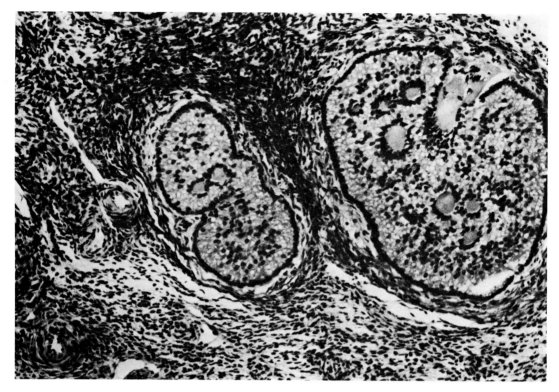

Fig. 11.24 Sex cord-stromal tumour with annular tubules. Nests of epithelial-like cells showing palisading at the periphery of the nests and around hyaline bodies (H. & E. × 108).

with an overgrowth of either granulosa cells or Sertoli cells; about 15 per cent of these neoplasms behave in a malignant fashion.

Unclassified sex cord-stromal tumours

Between 5 and 10 per cent of tumours which are clearly of sex cord-stromal type defy any more specific diagnosis. Difficulties in precise categorization are particularly likely to arise in sex cord-stromal tumours occurring in pregnant women, the combination of oedema and luteinization contributing markedly to the diagnostic difficulties.

Germ cell tumours

Tumours derived from germ cells may be *dysgerminomata*, which show no evidence of differentiation into either embryonic or extra-embryonic tissues, can differentiate along embryonic lines to give the various forms of *teratoma* or may differentiate along an extra-embryonic pathway, either into trophoblast to give a *choriocarcinoma* or into yolk sac structures to produce the varying forms of *yolk sac tumour*. However, it is becoming increasingly clear that many germ cell tumours are of mixed type with various patterns or permutations of dysgerminoma, teratoma, choriocarcinoma and yolk sac tumour being found admixed within a single neoplasm.

Undifferentiated germ cell tumours

The *dysgerminoma* accounts for 1 per cent of malignant ovarian tumours. It is a neoplasm formed of cells which, at both the light and electron microscopic levels, resemble primordial germ cells and which show no evidence of differentiation into either embryonic or extraembryonic structures; as such, the tumour is identical to the seminoma of the testis. The neoplasm generally averages about 15 cm in diameter, is often lobulated but is sometimes smoothly spheroidal and has a pinkish-grey or slightly yellowish cut surface. Areas of haemorrhage or necrosis are common and small foci of cystic degeneration are occasionally seen. Dysgerminomata are macroscopically bilateral in 10 per cent of cases, while in a further 10 per cent an apparently unilateral neoplasm is associated with microscopic foci of tumour in a grossly normal contralateral ovary. The tumour cells are large, uniform, round, ovoid or polyhedral, with well-defined limiting membranes, abundant, slightly eosinophilic cytoplasm and large, round, vesicular, central nuclei. The cells are commonly arranged in alveoli separated by delicate fibrous septa but may form cords or strands embedded in a fibrous stroma or sheets with little evidence of any stroma (Fig. 11.25). A lymphocytic infiltration of the stroma, sometimes with germinal follicle formation, is a characteristic feature, as are the presence of granulomata and of scattered multinucleated giant cells which stain positively for hCG. Occasional dysgerminomata are of the 'anaplastic' type and show considerable pleomorphism and mitotic activity; the prognostic significance, if any, of these features has not yet been determined.

Dysgerminomata commonly arise in patients aged between 10 and 30 years, their development usually being announced by non-specific symptoms such as abdominal pain or enlargement; isosexual precocious

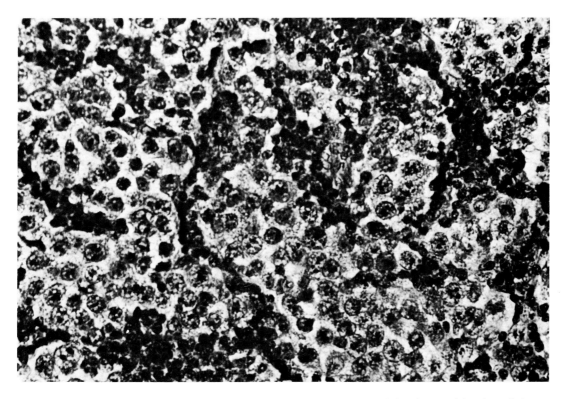

Fig. 11.25 Dysgerminoma. The tumour cells are large, round or oval and closely resemble primordial germ cells. Note the lymphocytic infiltrate (H. & E. × 270).

pseudopuberty is sometimes seen in young girls. Although it is often thought that these neoplasms arise particularly in patients with developmental abnormalities of the genital tract, the vast majority of dysgerminomata are found in otherwise fully normal adolescent girls and young women.

Dysgerminomata are malignant neoplasms. Rupture of their enveloping 'capsule' often leads to direct implantation of tumour deposits on the pelvic peritoneum and omentum, whilst lymphatic spread occurs relatively early to the para-aortic, retroperitoneal, mediastinal and supraclavicular nodes. Haematogenous spread occurs at a late stage to the liver, lungs, kidneys and bone. The tumours are markedly radiosensitive and the five-year survival rate for patients with a freely movable encapsulated tumour is in the region of 100 per cent. This figure falls to about 80 per cent for patients with higher stage disease. Histological features suggestive of a relatively good prognosis are a marked lymphocytic infiltration, a low mitotic figure count and minimal atypia of the tumour cells.

Germ cell tumours showing extraembryonic differentiation

Choriocarcinoma

Most ovarian choriocarcinomata are combined with other malignant germ cell elements and thus form one component of a mixed tumour. Very occasionally, a pure choriocarcinoma of the ovary is encountered but, in women of reproductive age, such a neoplasm is not necessarily of germ cell origin. It is usually impossible to determine if the malignant trophoblast has arisen from the placental tissue of a primary ovarian pregnancy, from malignant transformation of originally benign trophoblast transported from an intrauterine site to the ovary, as a metastasis from an intrauterine choriocarcinoma which has subsequently regressed or from neoplasia of germ cells. In prepubertal girls and in postmenopausal women this problem does not, of course, arise and here an origin from ovarian germ cells, which are showing extra-embryonic differentiation into trophoblast, can be accepted.

The tumour is of variable size, sometimes nodular, and has a variegated appearance on section with extensive areas of necrosis and haemorrhage. The histological features of an ovarian choriocarcinoma are identical to those of a uterine gestational choriocarcinoma, with both malignant cytotrophoblast and syncytiotrophoblast being present. The tumour produces human chorionic gonadotrophin (hCG) and hence precocious isosexual pseudopuberty is a common feature in premenarchal girls. The prognosis is very poor, with rapid pelvic invasion, intra-abdominal spread and extensive lymphatic and haematogenous dissemination. The ovarian choriocarcinoma responds relatively poorly to the chemotherapeutic regime which is so successful with gestational uterine choriocarcinoma. To some extent, this poor response may be due to the fact that many of the tumours classed as ovarian choriocarcinomata are probably mixed germ cell neoplasms.

Yolk sac tumours

The *yolk sac tumour* is one which is thought to represent germ cell differentiation along extraembryonic lines into extra-embryonic mesoblast and yolk sac endoderm. This concept was originally based upon a comparison of the morphological characteristics of the tumour to those of the rodent yolk sac and has been subsequently confirmed by the shared ability of these neoplasms and yolk sac structures to secrete α-fetoprotein.

These tumours form large, encapsulated, smooth or nodular masses of rubbery consistency. The cut surface is yellowish-grey with conspicuous areas of haemorrhage and necrosis together with small gelatinous cysts (Fig. 11.26). Their histological appearances (Fig. 11.27) are complex; for although a number of patterns are usually present, in some tumours one or two of these may predominate. A loose, vacuolated, labyrinthine network containing microcysts lined by flattened cells is a characteristic feature, as is the presence of Schiller–Duval bodies, which have a mesenchymatous core containing a central capillary and an epithelial investment of cuboidal or columnar cells. Gland-like structures are often

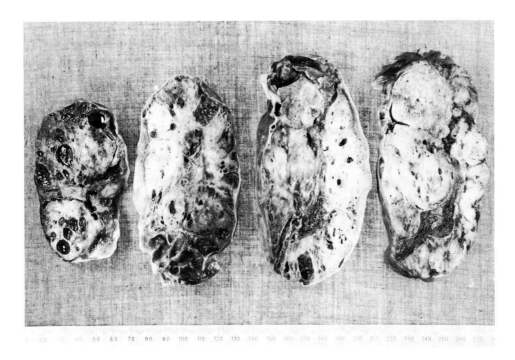

Fig. 11.26 Serial slices through a yolk sac tumour showing the variegated solid and cystic appearance.

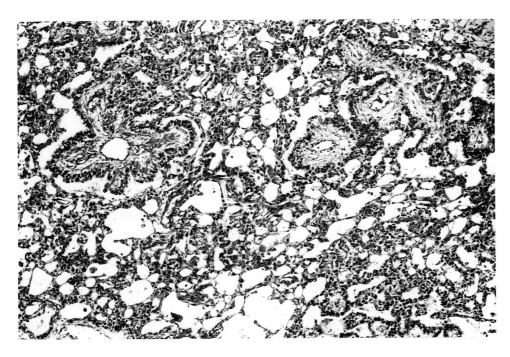

Fig. 11.27 A yolk sac tumour with a microcystic and glandular alveolar pattern. Schiller–Duval bodies are seen in the upper half of the field (H. & E. × 120).

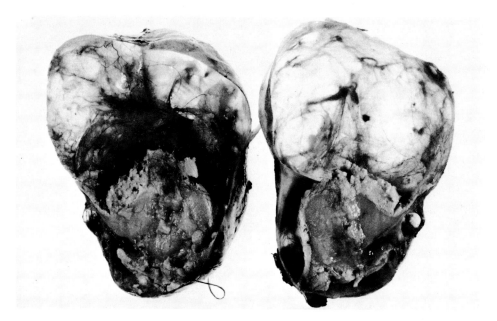

Fig. 11.28   A mature cystic teratoma. The mamillary body at the lower pole contains adipose tissue and is covered by hair-bearing epithelium, whilst the upper pole is occupied by a thin-walled cyst.

present, as are elongated anastomosing channels lined by flattened, cuboidal or hobnail cells, whilst groups or sheets of stellate cells of indifferent nature may be a conspicuous feature. Small cysts, lined partially by columnar cells and partially by flattened mesothelial cells, are seen in many yolk sac tumours. These are known as polyvesicular vitelline structures and the biphasic lining epithelium is thought to correspond to the transformation of primary yolk sac endoderm into secondary endoderm. Sometimes, this particular histological feature predominates or is the sole pattern present, neoplasms having this microscopic appearance being known as *polyvesicular vitelline tumours*. Eosinophilic, PAS-positive hyaline droplets are present in nearly all yolk sac tumours and are formed of α-fetoprotein and other proteins. Occasionally, yolk sac tumours show evidence of differentiation into cells that resemble those of a hepatocellular carcinoma while, exceptionally, a pattern resembling that of an endometrioid adenocarcinoma is encountered.

Yolk sac tumours occur predominantly in girls aged between 14 and 20 years and commonly present with non-specific symptoms, an endocrine disturbance not being a feature of the pure yolk sac tumour. These tumours are highly malignant and, in the past, their rapid spread in the abdomen and to distant sites led invariably to early death. However, in recent years promising results have been obtained with chemotherapy and the prognosis is now relatively hopeful, with a survival rate of 80 per cent for Stage 1 cases and a 50 per cent survival rate for those with more advanced disease. The progress of the tumour and the development of recurrences can be monitored by serial estimations of serum α-fetoprotein levels.

Germ cell tumours with embyronic differentiation

These neoplasms, all grouped as *teratomata*, are conventionally classified into:

(i)   benign cystic teratoma
(ii)   benign cystic teratoma with malignant change
(iii) solid teratoma
(iv)   monodermal teratoma.

The physical appearance of a neoplasm is a poor basis for tumour classification, especially as most 'solid' teratomata are partially cystic, whilst 'cystic' teratoma may contain solid areas. In practice, however, the cystic and solid teratomata are distinctive clinical and pathological entities and the conventional nomenclature is only misleading if it is wrongly taken to imply that cystic teratomata are always benign and solid teratomata invariably malignant. It is also now recognized that the terms 'benign' and 'malignant' are not truly applicable to teratomata, the prognosis of any individual neoplasm being determined not by the usual criteria of malignancy but by the degree of maturity of the constituent tissues. Those in which all the components are fully mature run a benign course and increasing degrees of tissue immaturity are associated with a progressive tendency towards malignant behaviour. Hence teratomata are classed as either 'mature' or 'immature', the term 'malignant' being reserved for those cases in which malignant change has occurred in mature tissues, as happens in some cases of mature cystic teratoma.

Mature cystic teratoma
These neoplasms, usually known in the gynaecological vernacular as 'dermoids', form between 10 and 20 per cent of all ovarian tumours and account for 97 per cent of ovarian teratomata. Just over 10 per cent are bilateral, most measure between 5 and 15 cm in diameter and some are pedunculated. They are round or ovoid with a smooth or slightly wrinkled outer surface and, when freshly removed, are soft and fluctuant. As they cool their contents solidify and they become heavy and 'doughy', characteristically showing pitting indentation when pressed with the thumb. On opening, teratomata are usually unilocular and have a smooth or granular inner surface. There is commonly a focal hillock-like protuberance into the cyst lumen, this being variously known as Rokitansky's tubercle, the nipple or the mamillary body. The cysts nearly always contain brownish-yellow, greasy, pultaceous material of sebaceous nature and hair (Fig. 11.28). Teeth are present in about a third and may be found lying free in the cyst, embedded in the walls or attached to a rudimentary jaw bone. Osseous tissue may be apparent and is occasionally recognizable as a specific bone such as a temporal, occipital or jaw bone. Sometimes the sebaceous material within the cyst becomes inspissated to form solid, rounded, yellowish lumps, sometimes known as 'butter-balls', whilst very rarely the tissues within a cystic teratoma become organized into a fetiform structure.

Histologically, squamous epithelium is present in nearly every case as a lining to the cyst, and skin appendages are also extremely common (Fig. 11.29). Fat, respiratory-type epithelium, bone, cartilage, neural tissue, gastrointestinal-type epithelium, thyroid and salivary gland tissue are frequent components. Breast tissue is not usually obvious except in some tumours removed from pregnant women. The appearances may be altered by partial or total ulceration of the squamous epithelium with a resulting granulomatous reaction, of foreign body type, in the cyst wall. If the squamous epithelium is completely lost the diagnosis may be dependent upon the finding of 'sieve-like' areas in the cyst wall. These are present in about a third of cases and are a highly characteristic and specific finding, although their true nature is unknown.

Mature cystic teratomata can occur at any age but 90 per cent are found in women of reproductive age. A high proportion are asymptomatic incidental findings and when symptoms do occur they are usually those of a non-specific pelvic mass. There is a relatively high incidence of accompanying menstrual disturbances; the basis for this is currently unknown.

Some patients present with complications, of which torsion is the most common, occurring in about 10 per cent of cases and presenting as acute abdominal pain. This catastrophe is predisposed to by the pedunculation and 'heaviness' of the tumour and can lead to gangrene and rupture of the cyst wall.

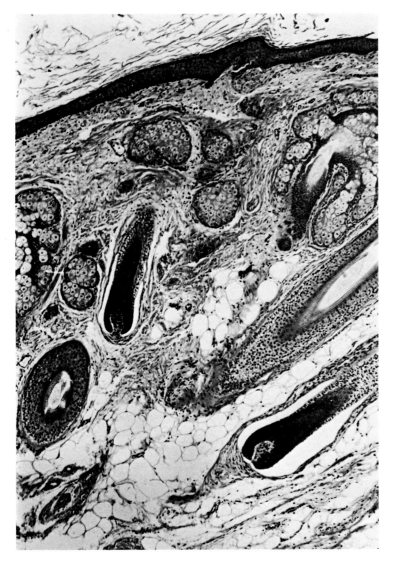

Fig. 11.29 The lining of a mature cystic teratoma showing squamous epithelium, sebaceous glands, hair follicles and adipose tissue (H. & E. × 45).

Occasionally, a torted cyst becomes detached from its pedicle and adheres to another organ to assume a parasitic existence.

Rupture of a cystic teratoma occurs in under 1 per cent of cases and is predisposed to by torsion, infection or trauma. Nevertheless, despite the thick wall of the cyst, a significant proportion of cystic teratomata that rupture appear to do so for no obvious reason. There may be sudden perforation into the peritoneal cavity with the patient presenting as an acute abdominal emergency, or a slow leakage of cyst contents into the peritoneal cavity with the production of a chronic chemical peritonitis characterized by dense peritoneal adhesions, 'oily' ascites and the presence of multiple peritoneal, omental and serosal nodules which contain greasy sebaceous material and hairs. Less commonly, a mature cystic teratoma ruptures into a viscus such as the bladder, intestine or uterus.

Infection of a cystic teratoma, either by lymphatic or haematogenous spread, direct extension from a focus of pelvic sepsis or from injudicious tapping, is uncommon, whilst a very rare complication is the development of a haemolytic anaemia which can be cured only by the removal of the ovarian neoplasm. The cause of this anaemia is unknown but may be due to the presence of tumour antigens that stimulate antibodies which cross-react with red blood cells or to tumour production of anti-red cell antibodies.

Malignant change in mature cystic teratoma. Malignant change supervenes in between 1 and 2 per cent of mature cystic teratomata. About 85 per cent of malignant neoplasms arising in mature cystic teratomata are squamous cell carcinomata and the only others occurring with any frequency are adenocarcinomata or carcinoid tumours. On occasion a wide range of other tumours can develop in mature cystic teratomata and examples of malignant melanoma, basal cell carcinoma, osteogenic sarcoma, chondrosarcoma, neuroblastoma, glioblastoma and sebaceous carcinoma have been recorded.

A mature cystic teratoma that has undergone malignant change may show little or no evidence of this macroscopically, although, more commonly, on opening the cyst the malignant tissue forms a papillary or polypoid mass of whitish tissue growing into the lumen. Less commonly, there may be only a localized thickening or plaque in the wall.

Malignant change occurs most commonly in women aged 40–60 years and spread of a squamous cell carcinoma from a cystic teratoma is principally by direct extension to pelvic structures; direct implantation onto the omentum and lymphatic spread are comparatively unusual. The overall five-year survival rate is only 15–20 per cent and the most important factor governing prognosis is whether or not the cyst wall is perforated by tumour at the time of operation, the five-year survival rate if the cyst wall is intact being over 70 per cent but falling to 6 per cent if the wall is perforated by tumour. The prognosis for patients who develop an adenocarcinoma in a mature cystic teratoma is extremely poor.

Mature solid teratomata

These are rare tumours which tend to form bulky masses and to occur principally in children and adolescents. Despite their name, the tumours are characteristically partially cystic and the cystic areas may contain pultaceous material and hairs. Histologically, the tumour is formed solely of mature tissues, such as squamous epithelium, cartilage, bone and glial tissue, arranged in an orderly fashion, the appearances resembling those seen in the much more common cystic mature teratoma (Fig. 11.30). Tissues derived from all three germ layers are usually present and neural tissue may be a conspicuous feature. However, the presence of any immature neuroepithelial tissue refutes the diagnosis of mature teratoma and all solid teratomata require very extensive sampling before the presence of immature tissue components can be confidently excluded.

Mature solid teratomata are benign. However, the prognostic picture may be clouded by the finding of multiple peritoneal and omental implants in association with a mature solid teratoma. Histological examination reveals that these implants are formed of mature glial tissue and this condition of *peritoneal gliomatosis* is non-progressive and apparently due to extrusion of mature glial tissue through a defect in the capsule of the teratoma.

Immature solid teratoma

These are rare tumours occurring most commonly during the first two decades. They form large masses which are well circumscribed with a bosselated, lobular or nodular surface. On section they are predominantly solid but usually contain a number of small microcystic areas. Areas of haemorrhage and necrosis are common. Microscopic examination reveals a melange of mature and immature tissue components, although the appearances are often dominated by immature mesenchymal or neuroepithelial tissue (Fig. 11.31). It should be stressed that in this context the term 'immature' refers to embryonic-type tissue and not to tissues showing the more conventional features of malignancy. The immature teratoma is a malignant tumour which implants upon the pelvic peritoneum, metastasizes to retroperitoneal and

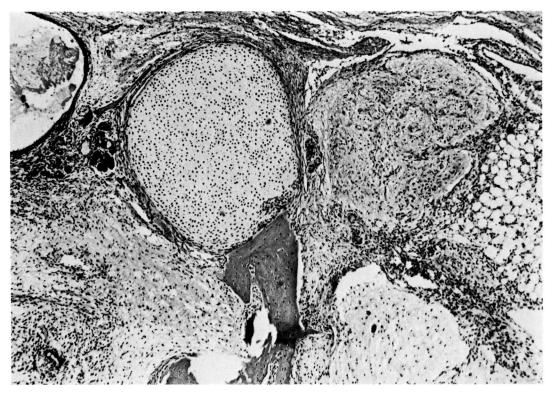

Fig. 11.30 Mature solid teratoma. This particular section shows mucinous and serous glandular acini to the upper left, cartilage and bone centrally and mature nervous and adipose tissue to the right (H. & E. × 45).

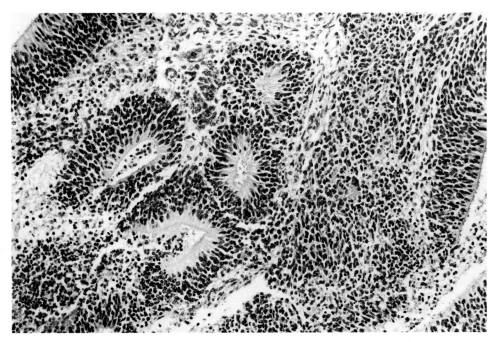

Fig. 11.31 An immature teratoma in which the immature neuroepithelial tissue forms rosette-like structures (H. & E. × 186).

para-aortic lymph nodes and is disseminated via the bloodstream to the liver and lungs. The prognosis in any particular case is determined by the degree and extent of tissue immaturity and a widely used classification of immature teratomata is as follows.

Grade 1. Minor foci of immature tissue: rare mitotic activity.
Grade 2. Moderate quantities of immature tissue: moderate mitotic activity.
Grade 3. Large quantities of immature tissue.

This grading system is of considerable prognostic value but in recent years attention has been focused upon the amount of immature neuroepithelium present in the tumour as a prognostic guide, quantitation of the amount of tissue of this type adding a further degree of prognostic precision.

Until recently, the prognosis of immature solid teratomata of the ovary was extremely poor, the overall five-year survival rate being less than 20 per cent. However, current chemotherapeutic regimes are holding out the promise of a much improved long-term survival rate with sustained complete remissions being obtained in 90 per cent of cases.

Monodermal teratomata
Although teratomata are usually thought of as containing a mixture of tissues, some consist entirely, or predominantly, of only one tissue. These teratomata are germ cell tumours, which have differentiated along only one extra-embryonic pathway, or have originally been more conventional teratomata in which one tissue component has overgrown and obliterated the other elements of the neoplasm. The most common monodermal teratoma is the enteric type of mucinous cyst which, as discussed previously, is formed solely of gastrointestinal-type epithelium.

Thyroid tissue is present in many teratomata but the diagnosis of *struma ovarii* should be confined to those neoplasms in which thyroid tissue is the sole, or overwhelmingly predominant, tissue (Fig. 11.32). These tumours are uncommon and form unilateral, encapsulated, smooth, lobulated masses with prominent surface vessels. On section, the tumour tissue has a 'meaty' appearance and there may be a well marked colloid sheen. Many struma ovarii are combined with a mature cystic teratoma or, less commonly, a mucinous cystadenoma of enteric type, and appear as circumscribed masses or nodules in the wall or septa of a cyst. Histologically, the struma ovarii is formed of tissue identical to that of the normal thyroid gland, with well formed acini lined by a cuboidal epithelium and containing eosinophilic colloid. Struma ovarii is a benign neoplasm but in about 10 per cent of cases there is a complicating ascites which may be very marked; a proportion of women also develop a hydrothorax. Malignant change can, and does, occur in a struma ovarii but this is extremely rare. The histological diagnosis of malignant struma ovarii is occasionally straightforward, with the development of a typical, usually papillary, adenocarcinoma, but it is usually fraught with difficulty, with often the only unequivocal evidence of malignancy being the development of metastases, spread being via the lymphatics to regional lymph nodes and by the bloodstream to the lungs and bones. Peritoneal and omental deposits of malignant struma ovarii are not uncommon and these may have a deceptively benign appearance. This condition of *peritoneal strumatosis* is characteristic of indolently malignant tumours and is compatible with long survival.

The thyroid tissue in a struma ovarii is physiologically identical with normal thyroid tissue and a number of examples of hyperthyroidism due to a struma ovarii have been reported. In most of these cases the patient has a coincidental occurrence of a struma ovarii and genuine primary hyperthyroidism, with the thyroid tissue in the ovary being as susceptible as that in the cervical thyroid to long-acting thyroid stimulator. The resulting hyperthyroidism will not be cured surgically until both cervical and ovarian thyroid tissue have been removed. Only very rarely does a struma ovarii appear to have functioned autonomously to produce a true pelvic hyperthyroidism. Several rather unconvincing examples of Hashimoto's disease in a struma ovarii have also been reported.

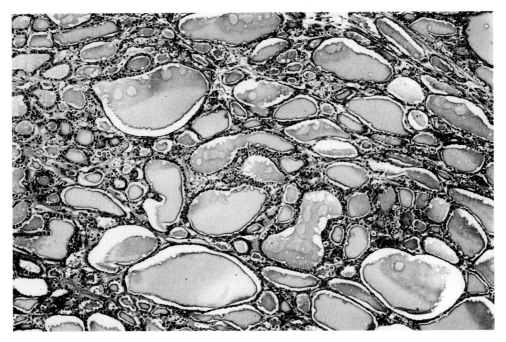

Fig. 11.32 Struma ovarii. The section shows mature thyroid tissue (H. & E. × 93).

Ovarian *carcinoid tumours* are uncommon and most occur in association with a mature cystic teratoma or enteric type of mucinous cystadenoma. However, a few are pure and unmixed with any other tissue element and these can be confused with a metastasis from an intestinal carcinoid tumour. The pure carcinoid tumours are usually about 10 cm in diameter, have a smooth or bossed outer surface and are solid, their cut surface appearing yellow, orange, grey or white. Histologically, the tumour cells are small and polyhedral, with slightly granular eosinophilic cytoplasm, and are closely packed, either being arranged in solid islands or as trabecular cords or strands (Fig. 11.33). Argyrophil cells are commonly present but argentaffin cells are uncommon. Most ovarian carcinoids occur in women aged over 50 years and, whilst many patients have only non-specific pelvic tumour symptoms, about 40–50 per cent, those whose tumours show an insular pattern, will have some or all of the symptoms of the classic carcinoid syndrome, with facial flushing, diarrhoea and pulmonary or tricuspid stenosis. This syndrome is due to the ability of these tumours to elaborate substances such as 5-hydroxytryptamine, bradykinin and prostaglandins and it should be noted that, because these substances pass directly into the systemic, rather than into the portal, circulation, the incidence of carcinoid syndrome is much higher with ovarian tumours of this type than it is with intestinal carcinoid neoplasms. These tumours are of low grade malignancy and tend to pursue an indolent course, patients with known metastases in abdominal lymph nodes or liver living in apparently good health for many years. Most patients do not have metastases at the time of operation and for them the prognosis is extremely good. A rare form of ovarian carcinoid is the *mucinous carcinoid tumour*. This is formed of nests and glands which contain an admixture of mucus-secreting goblet cells and small cuboidal argyrophil cells. These neoplasms behave in a more aggressive fashion than do conventional carcinoid tumours and tend to spread mainly via the lymphatics.

The *strumal carcinoid* is an extremely rare neoplasm and is a form of combined struma ovarii and carcinoid tumour. The thyroid component differs in no way from that found in a conventional struma ovarii, but this merges into a carcinoid pattern in which the cells are arranged in trabeculae or ribbons. It has been suggested that the carcinoid component of this neoplasm is derived from the parafollicular

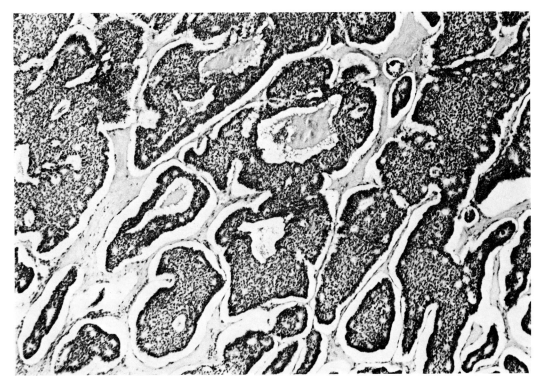

Fig. 11.33 Ovarian carcinoid tumour. The islands of small, regular cells with round or oval nuclei and granular cytoplasm are typical of this lesion (H. & E. × 45).

cells of the thyroid tissue and that it is thus homologous with the medullary carcinoma of the thyroid gland.

Other rare monodermal teratomata include the pure *primary malignant melanoma* of the ovary, the *melanotic neuroectodermal* (or *retinal anlage*) *tumour, epidermoid cysts*, which are lined by squamous epithelium but lack any skin appendages, and the ovarian *sebaceous gland tumour*.

Mixed germ cell tumours

A significant proportion of germ cell tumours show a mixed pattern, with combinations such as dysgerminoma–yolk sac tumour, dysgerminoma–choriocarcinoma, dysgerminoma–immature teratoma, immature teratoma–yolk sac tumour being encountered. Increasing use of the immunoperoxidase technique for demonstrating hCG, as a marker for trophoblastic differentiation, and α-fetoprotein as a marker for yolk sac differentiation, have shown that a proportion of germ cell tumours which appear histologically pure are in fact of mixed type, this applying particularly to dysgerminomata and immature teratomata. It is probable that most of the tumours previously classed as 'teratocarcinomata' were examples of mixed malignant germ cell neoplasms, and this misleading term should be avoided.

A particular, but very rare, type of mixed germ cell neoplasm is that known, perhaps inappropriately, as *embryonal carcinoma*, which occurs in young girls, is associated with a high incidence of precocious isosexual pseudopuberty and is formed of sheets of pleomorphic epithelial-like cells which appear to be a mixture of primitive embryonic cells, primitive trophoblast and primitive yolk sac cells. This is a highly malignant neoplasm which invades and metastasizes at an early stage.

Tumours of non-specialized tissues

Tumours can develop from any of the non-specialized ovarian mesenchymal tissues and *haemangiomata, haemangio-endotheliomata, lymphphangiomata, neurilemmomata* and *ganglioneuromata* of the ovary have all been described. Ovarian *leiomyomata* are fairly uncommon, have the same pathological characteristics as their more common uterine counterparts and may arise either from the musculature of the ovarian vessels, from smooth muscle fibres of the uterine ligaments which pass into the ovary or from smooth muscle fibres which are normally present in the ovarian stroma. Ovarian *fibromata* constitute about 4 per cent of all ovarian neoplasms and occur as well defined, but not encapsulated, nodular masses which show a very considerable range in size. They have a smooth, lobulated or nodular external surface and on section are formed of uniformly white or whitish-grey tissue; microcystic change and calcification are not uncommon. Histologically, a fibroma is formed of bundles of spindle-shaped cells with narrow ovoid nuclei running parallel to their long axes (Figs. 11.34 and 11.35). These cells are arranged in interlocking bundles but the appearances may be markedly altered by oedema, hyalinization or myxoid change. Fibromata probably arise from stromal mesenchymal cells and are most commonly found in women aged 40 to 60 years. Although most fibromata present with non-specific symptoms, a few undergo torsion and cause an acute onset of abdominal pain, whilst ascites complicates about 15 per cent of cases, although it is only found in association with tumours having a diameter greater than 6 cm. Fluid may also accumulate in the pleural cavity, to give a typical Meigs' syndrome (found in 1–2 per cent of cases) and occasionally in the legs, anterior abdominal wall or vulva. The cause of this fluid accumulation is obscure and the usual explanation proffered, that it is due to exudation of fluid from the neoplasm, is unconvincing. Rarely, an ovarian fibroma forms part of the basal cell naevus syndrome or Gardner's syndrome.

The vast majority of ovarian fibromata are fully benign but occasional examples show an increased cellularity with a variable degree of mitotic activity. Such neoplasms are subdivided into *cellular fibromata* and *fibrosarcomata*. Cellular fibromata are characterized by increasing cellularity, a minor degree of pleomorphism and a mitotic count of less than 4 per 10 high power microscopic fields, whilst fibrosarcomata show more marked pleomorphism and a higher mitotic count. The prognosis for patients with a cellular fibroma is generally good but a minority, about 20 per cent, of these tumours recur, particularly if removal has been incomplete. By contrast, fibrosarcomata are highly malignant and are associated with a very poor prognosis.

A distinct entity, differing from a fibroma, is the *sclerosing stromal tumour*, which usually develops during the second or third decades and forms a well circumscribed mass which, on section, is predominantly solid, greyish-white and firm but with areas of necrosis and microcystic change. Microscopy reveals a pseudolobular pattern in which cellular nodules are separated from each other by bands of hyaline or oedematous connective tissue. In the cellular areas there is a mixture of fibroblasts, lipid-containing rounded cells and oval polyhedral cells. This neoplasm is thought to arise from the ovarian stroma, is occasionally associated with clinical features suggestive of an oestrogenic effect and is invariably benign.

Miscellaneous unclassified tumours

Certain ovarian neoplasms either cut across, or cannot be fitted into, a logical histogenetic classification of ovarian tumours. These include the mixed germ cell–sex cord-stromal tumours, the steroid cell neoplasms, small cell carcinomata, hepatoid carcinoma and ovarian lymphomata.

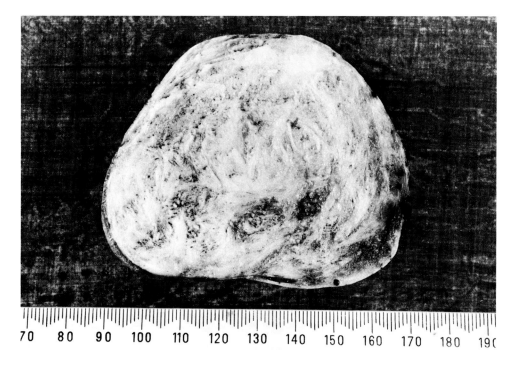

Fig. 11.34 A solid ovarian fibroma in which a nodular and whorled pattern can be seen.

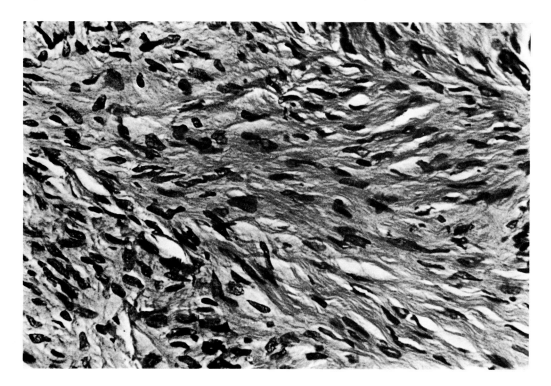

Fig. 11.35 Fibroma. The section shows cells with elongated and fusiform nuclei (H. & E. × 255).

Mixed germ cell–sex cord stromal tumours

The *gonadoblastoma* is an uncommon neoplasm usually found in a dysgenetic gonad in individuals who, although phenotypically female, have either an XY or an XY/mosaic chromosomal constitution. Most gonadoblastomata measure less than 5 cm in diameter and many are of only microscopic size. The tumour forms a smooth, rounded mass and on section is solid and grey with patchy yellowish areas; calcification is often obvious on cutting the tumour. In about one-third of cases the gonadoblastomata are bilateral.

The essential histological feature of a gonadoblastoma is the presence of large germ cells admixed with smaller cells which resemble immature Sertoli or granulosa cells (Fig. 11.36). The cells tend to be arranged in nests which are surrounded by a collagenous stroma. The small ovoid cells of sex cord type may be arranged in a microfollicular pattern around blobs of hyaline material, may form an investment around groups of germ cells or surround individual germ cells in a coronal fashion. The stroma between the cell nests often, but not invariably, contains Leydig-type cells and foci of calcification are extremely common.

Gonadoblastomata occur predominantly in patients with either a pure or a mixed gonadal dysgenesis and the gonad in which they arise is almost invariably a streak or a testis (albeit usually an immature or atrophic testis), only very rare instances having occurred in normal ovaries. The patients are either non-virilized phenotypic females (40 per cent), virilized phenotypic females (45 per cent) or phenotypic males with anomalous external genitalia (15 per cent) and nearly all will have a Y chromosome.

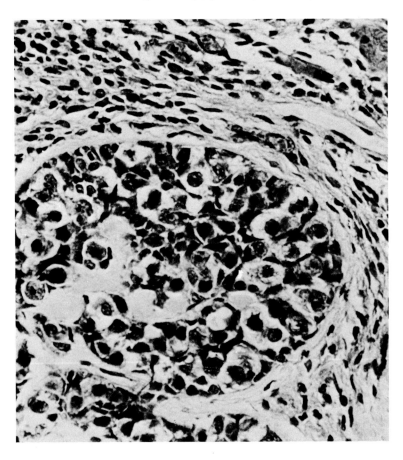

Fig. 11.36 Gonadoblastoma showing a typical nest of germ cells and smaller ovoid cells of sex cord type (H. & E. × 300).

The gonadoblastoma is a benign tumour and indeed there is some doubt as to whether it is truly neoplastic, there being good grounds for believing that it is a hamartomatous malformation of testicular tissue. Nevertheless, malignant germ cell neoplasms will eventually develop in about 50 per cent of cases, an incidence that has provoked a description of the gonadoblastoma as a 'germ cell tumour *in situ*'. In preceding gonadoblastoma. However, the germ cell tumour may also, on occasion, be an immature teratoma, a choriocarcinoma, a yolk sac tumour or any combination of these. It is because of this propensity towards germ cell neoplasia that prophylactic gonadectomy is often recommended in patients with a dysgenetic gonad and a Y chromosome.

A very rare form of mixed germ cell–sex cord tumour has been described in recent years. This tends to develop in children, occurs in otherwise normal females with a normal karyotype and normal ovaries and is formed of a mixture of germ cells and immature Sertoli or granulosa cells arranged in solid tubules or in trabecular cords. These tumours do not resemble a gonadoblastoma and appear to be benign.

Steroid cell tumours

The term 'steroid cell tumour' is used to describe a group of neoplasms having an endocrine type architecture and being formed of cells resembling luteal, Leydig or adrenocortical cells.

It is believed that all steroid cell tumours are derived from the ovarian stroma which is presumed to have the capacity to differentiate along a variety of pathways. The Leydig cell tumours present a particular difficulty in classification, because although some such neoplasms appear to develop from ovarian stromal cells, a majority arise from pre-existing hilar cells. The inclusion of Leydig cell tumours in this category of steroid cell tumours is therefore a matter of expediency rather than of fact. Adrenal-type tumours do not, as is often thought, arise from ovarian adrenal rests, for intraovarian rests of this nature have never been demonstrated. The adrenocortical nature of the cells in these neoplasms has been confirmed by ultrastructural studies and by the fact that some patients with tumours of this type develop many of the features of Cushing's syndrome.

Leydig cell tumours

A pure Leydig cell tumour can arise either from pre-existing hilar cells or, much less commonly, from ovarian stromal cells. The neoplasms appear as unilateral, small (usually less than 5 cm in diameter), well circumscribed, solid, brown, orange or yellow masses, those arising from hilar cells presenting as nodules within the mesovarium and those of stromal origin occurring within the medullary portion of the ovary. If the tumours are small a distinction can usually be drawn between hilar and stromal types but large neoplasms often cannot be specifically categorized in these terms. A somewhat arbitrary distinction is drawn between Leydig cell tumours of hilar cell origin and nodular hyperplasia of the hilar cells, which occurs in pregnancy and after the menopause, the latter being frequently multiple and rarely exceeding 2 mm in diameter.

Histologically, Leydig cell neoplasms (Fig. 11.37) are formed of uniform rounded or polygonal cells with abundant granular or vacuolated eosinophilic cytoplasm and large central nuclei. These cells are arranged in nests, sheets and cords and a characteristic feature is the presence, in some areas, of nuclear 'pooling' or aggregation. There is some controversy as to whether it is permissible to make a diagnosis of a Leydig cell tumour in the absence of Reinke's crystals. The crystals, when present, are very unevenly distributed and are absent from hilar Leydig cells in many adult ovaries. Thus, making an insistence on their presence as a diagnostic criterion appears too stringent. It would be a reasonable compromise not to insist on the finding of the crystals for those mesovarian tumours which are clearly of hilar cell origin but to retain this diagnostic requirement for those tumours of stromal origin and for those whose large size will not permit their recognition as either hilar or non-hilar.

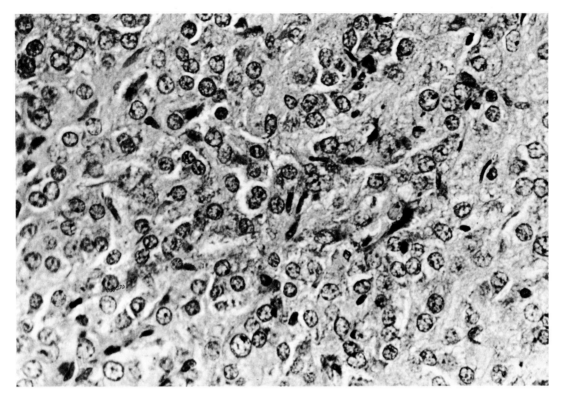

Fig. 11.37 A Leydig cell tumour composed of sheets of cells with regular, large round nuclei and granular, vacuolated cytoplasm; note the nuclear grouping or pooling (H. & E. × 270).

Leydig cell tumours usually occur in women aged 50–70 years and 80 per cent of patients present with varying degrees of defeminization or virilization. A small proportion of these neoplasms are oestrogenic, whilst a few appear to be endocrinologically inert.

The vast majority of ovarian Leydig cell tumours are benign but a small percentage, probably less than 5 per cent, pursue a malignant course and give rise to widespread metastases. Those which behave in this fashion may or may not show histological features suggestive of malignancy.

Adrenal-like steroid cell tumours
Adrenal-like steroid cell tumours are commonly small, usually unilateral and are formed of large polygonal or rounded cells with well defined borders and abundant, usually lipid-containing, clear, vacuolated or foamy cytoplasm. The cells are arranged in nests or columns around a rich capillary network (Fig. 11.38). The histological mimicry of an adrenocortical adenoma by these neoplasms is usually quite striking. Most behave in a benign fashion but about 5 per cent recur locally in the pelvis or metastasize to lymph nodes, liver or omentum. In some of these latter cases their malign nature has been recognizable histologically but others have not shown any features to suggest their aggressive nature.

Steroid cell tumours of indeterminate type
These are neoplasms which, whilst clearly falling into the steroid cell category, cannot be further categorized in more specific terms. The tumours range in size up to 45 cm in diameter but have an average diameter of 8–9 cm: most are solid with a yellow or orange cut surface but some are reddish or brown. Histologically, polygonal or rounded cells are arranged in nests or columns separated by a rich

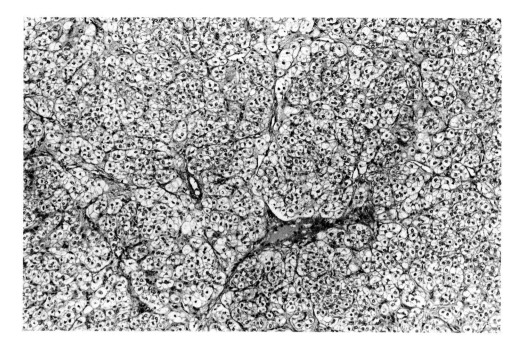

Fig. 11.38 An adrenal-like steroid cell tumour. The tumour lobules are composed of cells with copious clear or foamy cytoplasm and small, regular nuclei (H. & E. × 93).

vascular network. The tumour cells have granular or foamy cytoplasm, sharp-cut cell borders and central nuclei.

About 40 per cent of steroid cell tumours of indeterminate type are clinically malignant and, although the only absolute evidence of malignancy in these neoplasms is the presence of metastases, certain pathological features correlate well with malignant behaviour. Thus, nearly 80 per cent of tumours measuring more than 7 cm in diameter are malignant, whilst neoplasms smaller than this appear to be invariably benign, two-thirds of the neoplasms showing marked nuclear typia and 80 per cent of those with two or more mitotic figures per 10 high power fields pursue a malignant course.

Small cell carcinoma

These neoplasms occur in young women and are highly aggressive. They present as unilateral, large, predominantly solid masses, commonly showing foci of haemorrhage and necrosis. Histologically, the small cell carcinoma is formed of small, closely packed cells with scanty cytoplasm and small nuclei containing a large nucleolus. The cells may be arranged in sheets, islands or cords and large follicle-like structures are commonly present.

The true nature of these neoplasms is currently unknown, although many patients have an associated hypercalcaemia. The tumours spread rapidly, respond poorly to chemotherapy and usually lead to death within months rather than years.

Hepatoid carcinoma

This very rare neoplasm occurs in relatively elderly women. Histologically, it resembles a hepatocellular carcinoma; it is highly malignant.

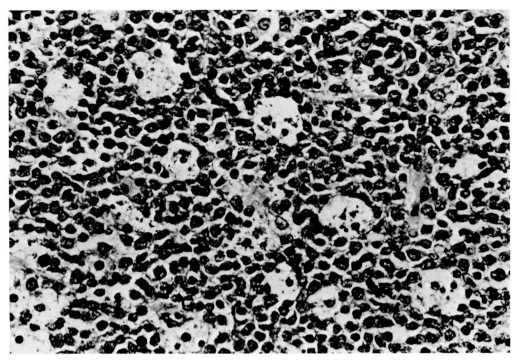

Fig. 11.39   Burkitt's lymphoma. Pale macrophages contrast sharply with the darkly staining undifferentiated stem cells (H. & E. × 255).

Wolffian tumours

These very uncommon ovarian neoplasms are histologically identical to the tumours, thought to be of wolffian origin, which occur in the broad ligament (page 104).

Malignant lymphoma

The ovary may, of course, become involved in a disseminated malignant lymphoma and autopsy studies have demonstrated that nearly a quarter of women with malignant lymphoma have lymphomatous infiltration of their ovaries. Such infiltration is commonly asymptomatic but occasionally these patients do develop a palpable ovarian mass which can cause local symptoms.

Primary extranodal malignant lymphoma originating in the ovary is extremely rare and presents as a bossed or lobulated solid tumour which usually completely replaces the ovary. The lymphoma is usually of non-Hodgkins type and the origin of these neoplasms is obscure in so far as the ovary does not normally contain lymphoid tissue.

A particular type of lymphoma with a predilection for the ovary is *Burkitt's lymphoma*. This is basically a lymphoma in which the predominant cell is an undifferentiated or primitive stem cell. Macrophages are frequently interspersed amongst the tumour cells to give a 'starry sky appearance' (Fig. 11.39), although this pattern is not specific to Burkitt's lymphoma. The disease occurs principally, but not solely, in sub-Saharan Africa and the ovaries are involved in 70–80 per cent of female cases; the ovarian tumours, which form large masses, being only one facet of a clinical picture which includes tumours of the jaw, kidneys and thyroid. In African patients the ovarian tumours are the principal cause of symptoms in nearly 40 per cent of cases and in non-African patients the disease may be confined to the ovary.

Metastatic tumours

The ovary is a common site of metastasis, particularly from primary sites in the breast, gastrointestinal tract and uterus. Thus ovarian metastases are found in nearly a third of women dying from malignant disease and metastatic deposits have been noted in the ovary in 50 per cent of women with gastric carcinoma, in 40 per cent of fatal cases of breast carcinoma and in 30 per cent of cases of colonic carcinoma. Of more importance to the clinician is the proportion of apparently primary malignant ovarian tumours that eventually turns out to be metastases. This figure is difficult to estimate but is probably between 10 per cent and 20 per cent.

Women with ovarian metastatic carcinoma may present with symptoms referable solely to the ovarian neoplasm, but rather more commonly such symptoms are combined with others that are due to the primary tumour.

The pathology of metastatic ovarian disease is usually straightforward but has been bedevilled by the loose and inconsistent usage of the term '*Krukenberg tumour*'. This term has been variously applied to any ovarian metastasis from the stomach or gastrointestinal tract, to any metastatic ovarian tumour, to a pathological entity characterized by solid ovarian tumours formed of mucus-secreting signet-ring cells set in a hyperplastic cellular stroma and to any neoplasm showing these histological characteristics irrespective of its gross appearance. In fact, the diagnosis of a Krukenberg tumour is a purely histological one and any metastatic mucus-secreting adenocarcinoma, whether it be from a primary origin in the stomach, colon, breast or gall bladder, may fall into this group. The true Krukenberg tumour is commonly bilateral and forms a solid mass with smooth or nodular contour, cystic change being very uncommon (Fig. 11.40). On section the tumours are formed of firm, solid, white or yellow tissue which is often coarsely lobulated. Histologically, the true Krukenberg tumour is formed of plump, rounded epithelial cells set in a dense cellular stroma. The epithelial cells occur singly, in clumps or sheets or may form tubules, a proportion are mucus containing and have their nuclei displaced laterally to give a signet-ring appearance (Fig. 11.41) The stromal cells are plump, spindle-shaped, show a moderate degree of pleomorphism and mitotic activity and are often, incorrectly, described as having a 'pseudosarcomatous' pattern. Those metastatic tumours of non-Krukenberg type are less frequently bilateral than true Krukenberg tumours and tend to show extensive haemorrhage, necrosis and cystic change. Histologically, they demonstrate a variety of patterns and tend to resemble the primary tumour. The stroma does not show any unusual features apart from occasional instances of luteinization.

The age of patients with a true Krukenberg tumour tends to be unusually low, most being aged between 30 and 50 years, approximately half being aged less than 40 years and a significant proportion being in their twenties. Women with a non-Krukenberg type of ovarian metastasis tend, on average, to be about ten years older than this.

The outlook for patients with a metastatic tumour of their ovaries is gloomy, less than 10 per cent surviving for two years.

A vexing question is whether a typical Krukenberg tumour can arise as a primary neoplasm of the ovary. A number of such cases have been reported and there seems no good reason why a primary mucus-secreting adenocarcinoma of the ovary should not occasionally assume the histological appearances of a Krukenberg tumour. Nevertheless, such a diagnosis should be made with extreme caution for the absence of a primary extraovarian tumour may be very difficult to prove and instances have been described of patients with a presumed primary Krukenberg tumour whose carcinoma of the stomach did not become clinically apparent until four-and-a-half years after removal of the ovarian neoplasm. Indeed, the diagnosis of primary Krukenberg tumour of the ovary should not be entertained until the patient has lived in good health for at least five years after removal of the ovarian tumour or has been shown at autopsy to have no primary extraovarian tumour.

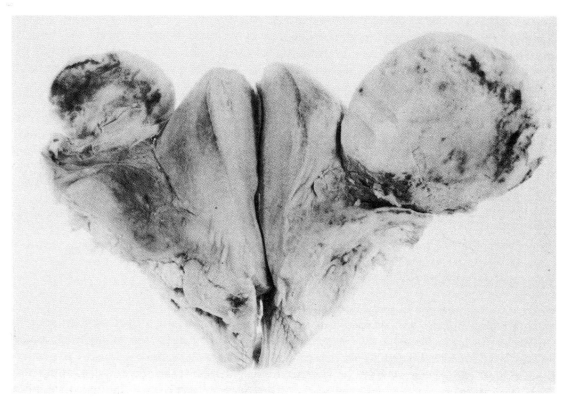

Fig. 11.40 Bilateral ovarian Krukenberg tumours from a woman with adenocarcinoma of the stomach.

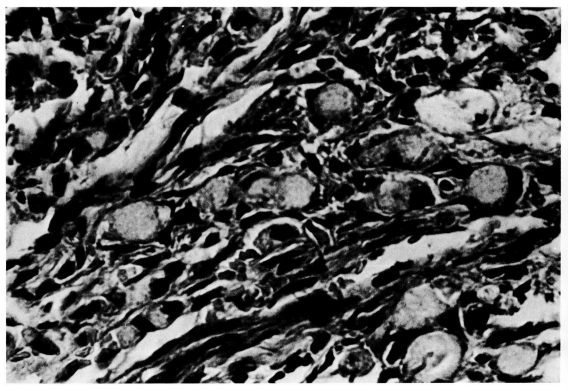

Fig. 11.41 A Krukenberg tumour showing mucus-secreting signet-ring cells lying between cellular fibrous bands (H. & E. × 450).

Key references

Fox H. (1989) The concept of borderline malignancy in ovarian tumours: a reappraisal. *Current Topics in Pathology* **78**, 111–34.

Langley F A and Fox H. (1987) Ovarian tumours: classification, histogenesis and aetiology. In: *Haines and Taylor, Obstetrical and Gynaecological Pathology, 3rd edn*, pp. 542–55. Edited by H Fox, Churchill Livingstone, Edinburgh.

Nogales F. (1987) Germ cell tumours of the ovary. In: *Haines and Taylor, Obstetrical and Gynaecological Pathology, 3rd edn*, pp. 637–75. Edited by H Fox, Churchill Livingstone, Edinburgh.

Roth L M and Czernobilsky B. (eds) (1985) *Tumors and Tumor-like Conditions of the Ovary*. Churchill Livingstone, New York.

Russell P. (1984) Borderline epithelial tumours of the ovary: a conceptual dilemma. *Clinics in Obstetrics and Gynaecology* **11**, 259–77.

Russell P. (1987) Common epithelial tumours of the ovary. In: *Haines and Taylor, Obstetrical and Gynaecological Pathology, 3rd edn*, pp. 556–622. Edited by H Fox, Churchill Livingstone, Edinburgh.

Scully R E. (1979) *Tumors of the Ovary and Maldeveloped Gonads*. Atlas of Tumor Pathology, 2nd Series, Fascicle 16. Armed Forces Institute of Pathology, Washington D C.

Serov S F, Scully R E and Sobin L H. (1973) *International Histological Classification of Tumours, No. 9. Histological Typing of Ovarian Tumours*. World Health Organization, Geneva.

Silverberg S G. (1989) Prognostic significance of pathologic features of ovarian carcinoma. *Current Topics in Pathology* **78**, 85–109.

Talerman A. (1987) Germ cell tumors of the ovary. In: *Blaustein's Pathology of the Female Genital Tract, 2nd edn*, pp. 659–721. Edited by R J Kurman, Springer-Verlag, New York.

Teilum G. (1971) *Special Tumors of the Ovary and Testis*. Munksgaard, Copenhagen.

Young R H and Scully R E. (1984) Ovarian sex cord-stromal tumours: recent advances and current status. *Clinics in Obstetrics and Gynaecology* **11**, 93–134.

12

Tumour-like conditions of the ovary

A number of non-neoplastic lesions of the ovary can mimic an ovarian neoplasm clinically. Thus, large luteal or follicular cysts, particularly the large solitary follicular cysts sometimes occurring in pregnancy or the puerperium, may be mistaken for a tumour, as can theca-lutein cysts, ovarian abscess, endometriosis or ovarian pregnancy. Doubt as to the true nature of such lesions rarely survives histological examination, but there are a number of non-neoplastic abnormalities in which the differentiation from a true tumour is less easy.

Stromal hyperplasia and hyperthecosis

Some degree of proliferation of the ovarian stroma occurs in many menopausal and post-menopausal women and hence the term *stromal hyperplasia* is restricted to those cases in which this process is unduly marked. Stromal hyperplasia results in bilateral enlargement of the ovaries, which may each measure up to 7 cm in diameter. The ovaries have a rounded contour and on section most of the parenchyma appears to be replaced by firm pinkish-grey or yellow-grey tissue. Histologically, there is replacement of normal ovarian tissue by diffuse or multinodular masses of hyperplastic stromal cells which are present principally in the medulla but extend out, in multiple tongue-like fashion, into the cortex. The hyperplastic cells are generally similar to those of the normal stroma but are rather plumper and contain, in a patchy fashion, lipid. There is an association between ovarian stromal hyperplasia and endometrial adenocarcinoma.

If clusters or nests of luteinized cells are seen scattered throughout the hyperplastic stroma (Fig. 12.1), a further diagnosis of stromal hyperthecosis can be made and this condition, of combined stromal hyperplasia and hyperthecosis, is sometimes associated clinically with some degree of virilization.

Stromal luteoma

This lesion is often regarded as a neoplasm but is more likely to be a tumour-like mass occurring as a result of overgrowth of a group of luteinized cells in ovarian stromal tissue showing hyperplasia and hyperthecosis. The stromal luteoma can measure up to 3 cm in diameter, may be yellow, brown or white and is usually single, although occasionally there may be multiple nodules either in one or both ovaries. The luteoma is non-encapsulated and is formed of large round or polyhedral cells arranged in sheets, nests or cords. Both the ovary containing the luteoma and the contralateral gonad will show stromal hyperplasia and the foci of stromal lutein cells that characterize stromal hyperthecosis. This lesion usually occurs in postmenopausal women and may be associated clinically with either a variable degree of

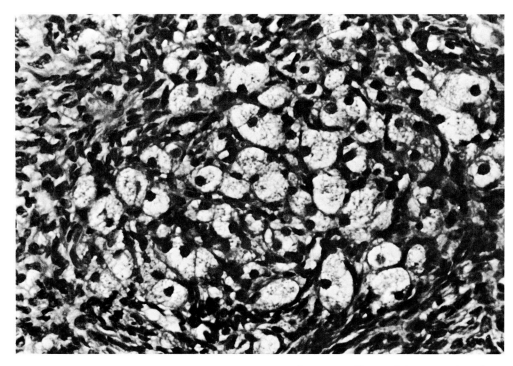

Fig. 12.1 A cluster of luteinized cells in hyperplastic ovarian cortex. The nuclei are round, uniform and excentric and the cytoplasm is pale and vacuolated or granular (H. & E. × 255).

masculinization or with vaginal bleeding. Endometrial hyperplasia is a common accompaniment of this lesion and appears to be due to extraglandular conversion of excess androgens to oestrogens.

Luteoma of pregnancy

This, as its name implies, is found only in pregnancy or the puerperium. The luteomata are bilateral in 50 per cent of cases and, whilst having an average diameter of about 8 cm, can reach a size of 20 cm across. They form rounded, non-encapsulated, but well demarcated masses and may appear as a single mass or as multiple nodules (Fig. 12.2). On section they are fleshy or soft and range in colour from greyish-yellow to yellow-orange. Histologically, the pregnancy luteoma is formed of large polyhedral cells arranged in sheets, cords or nodules (Fig. 12.3). The cells have large central round nuclei, which are occasionally hyperchromatic and pleomorphic, and abundant eosinophilic, finely granular cytoplasm.

The pregnancy luteoma is thought to arise either from foci of stromal luteinization or from the thecal cells of atretic follicles, and is not derived from the corpus luteum of pregnancy, which is discrete and separate from the luteoma. The stimulus for this unusual degree of growth is uncertain but it is clear that the condition is of a hyperplastic rather than a neoplastic nature for it regresses rapidly after pregnancy has terminated.

Most pregnancy luteomata are incidental findings at caesarean section or postpartum tubal ligation but they occasionally attain a sufficient size to present as an adnexal mass. A few luteomata appear to be androgenic and produce mild maternal virilization during late pregnancy and, very rarely, partial masculinization of the external genitalia of a female child.

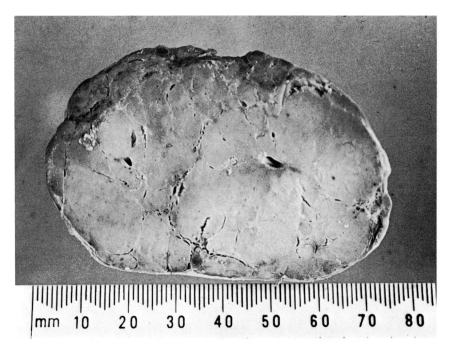

Fig. 12.2   A luteoma of pregnancy which was removed from a patient in whom a puerperal abdominal mass had been found. The cut surface of this was a yellow–tan colour.

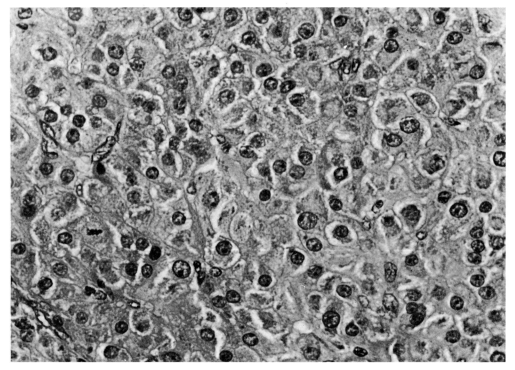

Fig. 12.3   A section of a luteoma of pregnancy showing sheets of regular polyhedral cells with large central, somewhat pleomorphic nuclei (H. & E. × 255).

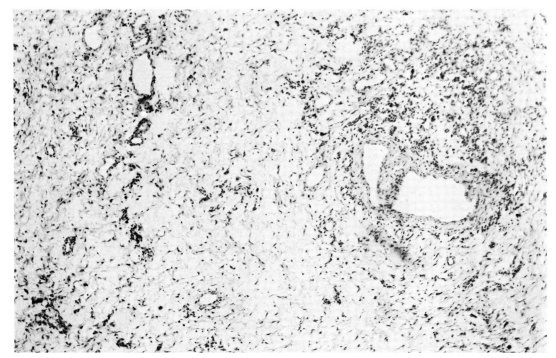

Fig. 12.4   Massive oedema of the ovary, demonstrating the interstitial oedema and venous dilatation so typical of this condition (H. & E. × 45).

Massive oedema of the ovary

This is a rare condition which usually involves only one ovary, although it is occasionally bilateral, there is a marked tendency for the right rather than the left ovary to be involved. Massive ovarian oedema occurs during early life, the age range of reported cases being from 5 to 33 years, with a median age of 20 years. The condition usually presents with acute or chronic abdominal pain but patients occasionally present with menstrual disturbances or virilization without accompanying pain. The ovary is considerably enlarged, up to 35 cm in diameter, and on section tends to have a moist, oedematous shiny cut surface which exudes fluid. Histological examination shows marked diffuse interstitial oedema (Fig. 12.4) with dilatation of lymphatic and venous channels, the oedema being most marked in the medulla and tending to spare the outer cortex. Luteinized stromal cells are often present in the oedematous areas.

   This condition is probably due to intermittent incomplete torsion of the mesovarium with obstruction of venous and lymphatic drainage; the torsion not being of a sufficient degree as to produce ischaemic necrosis. In a proportion of cases the torsion and oedema of the ovary appear to be secondary to an ovarian fibromatosis. It is thought that the oedema acts as a mechanical stimulus to stromal luteinization and that these luteinized cells are responsible for the endocrine effects.

Massive haemorrhagic infarction

Occasionally, an otherwise normal ovary undergoes complete torsion and infarction, this being most likely to occur in infants and young girls in whom the ovaries are particularly mobile. The infarcted ovary, discovered at operation for severe abdominal pain, is enlarged, measuring up to 15 cm in diameter, and on section shows massive haemorrhagic infarction. It will be appreciated that this condition is aetiologically very similar to massive oedema and, indeed, a few cases of massive oedema in one ovary with massive haemorrhagic infarction of the other ovary have been described.

Key references

Clement P B. (1985) Tumorlike conditions of the ovary. In: *Tumors and Tumor-like Conditions of the Ovary*, pp. 109–27. Edited by L M Roth and B Czernobilisky, Churchill Livingstone, New York.

Hayes M C and Scully R E. (1987) Stromal luteoma of the ovary: a clinicopathological analysis of 25 cases. *International Journal of Gynecological Pathology* **6**, 313–24.

Rice B F, Barclay D L and Sternberg W H. (1969) Luteoma of pregnancy: steroidgenic and morphologic considerations. *American Journal of Obstetrics and Gynecology* **104**, 685–94.

Roth L M, Deaton R I and Sternberg W H. (1979) Massive ovarian edema: a clinicopathologic study of five cases including ultrastructural observations and review of the literature. *American Journal of Surgical Pathology* **1**, 11–21.

Scully R E. (1979) Lesions resembling ovarian tumours. In: *Tumors of the Ovary and Maldeveloped Gonads*, pp. 364–99. Atlas of Tumor Pathology, 2nd Series, Fascicle 16. Armed Forces Institute of Pathology, Washington, D C.

Snowden J A, Harkin P S R, Thornton S G and Wells M. (1989) Morphometric assessment of ovarian stromal proliferation — a clinicopathological study. *Histopathology* **14**, 369–79.

Sternberg W H and Barclay D L. (1966) Luteoma of pregnancy. *American Journal of Obstetrics and Gynecology* **95**, 165–81.

Vasquez S B, Sotos J F and Kim M H. (1982) Massive edema of the ovary and virilization. *Obstetrics and Gynecology* **59**, 95s–9s.

Young R H and Scully R E. (1984) Fibromatosis and massive edema of the ovary, possibly related entities: a report of 14 cases of fibromatosis and 11 cases of massive edema. *International Journal of Gynecological Pathology* **3**, 153–78.

13

Pathology of contraception and of hormone therapy

Pathology of contraception

The intrauterine contraceptive device (IUCD) induces changes which are largely limited to the genital tract, but the administration of steroid contraceptives is associated with a combination of both local and systemic effects.

Intrauterine contraceptive device

Three basic types of IUCD are currently encountered, the inert plastic device, which is rarely used nowadays but may still be found in women who have been wearing a device for many years, copper-coated plastic devices, which are in current vogue, and, less commonly, progestagen impregnated devices. About 50 per cent of women wearing an IUCD have no symptoms attributable to the presence of the device but others may have intermenstrual spotting, menorrhagia, uterine colic or dysmenorrhoea. These symptoms tend to diminish when the device has been in place some time. A small proportion of women using a device complain of symptoms, such as irregular bleeding, associated with pelvic pain and vaginal discharge, which suggest a complicating uterine infection. Penetration of the uterine wall at the time of insertion, occurs in between 0.3 and 0.4 per cent of patients (Fig. 13.1), the incidence of this complication varying somewhat with the type of device used and the experience of the operator. In some instances uterine perforation produces few symptoms and the presence of the device within the abdominal cavity remains undetected. This may lead eventually to peritoneal adhesions and intestinal obstruction, the copper-containing devices tending to produce the most severe peritoneal reaction. Occasionally, the device may be recovered from within the intestine or bladder.

Endometrium
Insertion of an IUCD invariably introduces bacteria from the vagina into the uterus and these produce a mild, asymptomatic, transient endometritis. A mild, superficial inflammatory cell infiltrate, limited to the contact sites of the device, and characterized by intraglandular polymorphs and intrastromal lymphocytes, macrophages and occasional plasma cells is usually attributed to mechanical irritation and persists whilst the device remains in place (Fig. 13.2). It is not unusual in such endometria to find a general, slight increase in the mononuclear cell population. Compression of the endometrial stroma and epithelium occurs in most cases at the site of contact and focal pseudodecidual change can be seen in the stroma. The endometrium lying between the device coils or arms may be normal but it is sometimes thrown into oedematous folds. In some endometria these folds form polypoidal projections with focally congested and inflamed tips. A few women have a more severe endometritis, which is usually polymicrobial, with extension of the inflammatory infiltrate beyond the contact sites of the device and with widespread intraglandular polymorph exudation (Fig. 13.3) and a plasmalymphocytic infiltration of the stroma which extends more deeply into the endometrium and is indicative of infection (Fig. 13.4). Vascular thrombosis,

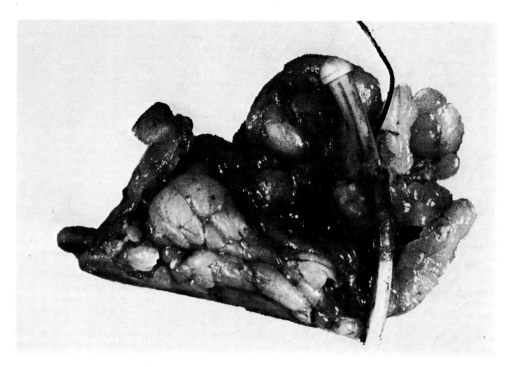

Fig. 13.1   A Gravigard Copper-7 IUCD embedded in a piece of omentum, the uterus having been perforated.

stromal fibrosis, impairment of cyclical endometrial maturation, foreign-body type granulomata and ulceration may occasionally develop. Focal squamous metaplasia is a rare occurrence.

Reactive changes can occur in the endometrial epithelium in response to the inflammation and this can produce cells which appear so atypical in a cervical smear that a suspicion of adenocarcinoma may be raised if the cytopathologist is not aware of the presence of an IUCD (Fig. 13.5).

In patients with an IUCD, the cyclical changes usually occur normally in the absence of infection but on occasions the endometrial glands immediately subjacent to the contact site show a pattern of maturation which differs slightly from that in the adjacent areas.

In women wearing a progestagen-impregnated device there are, in addition to the local irritative effects described above, changes attributable to the progestagen. The appearances are similar regardless of the phase of the menstrual cycle, the duration of IUCD use or the type of progestagen-containing device. Stromal pseudodecidualization, which is usually most marked in the first months after insertion, and glandular atrophy are typical. Stromal calcification, small polyps and thick-walled fibrotic blood vessels, similar to those seen in endometrial polyps, may develop after several years of use. Cells with slight nuclear atypia, resembling those in the Arias–Stella phenomenon, are occasionally seen in glands lined by otherwise inactive cells.

It should be noted that IUCD usage is not causally related to the development of either atypical hyperplasia or adenocarcinoma of the endometrium.

Cervix

Microglandular hyperplasia, of a degree less florid than that seen in oral contraceptive users, occurs in women with an IUCD. Furthermore, reserve cell hyperplasia, squamous metaplasia and an active non-

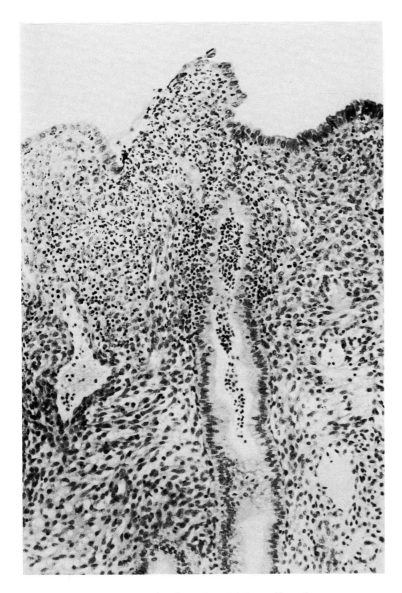

Fig. 13.2 Focal inflammation in endometrial curettings from a woman wearing an IUCD. Note the early superficial ulceration (H. & E. × 108).

specific chronic cervicitis are almost constant features. These changes are usually focal and there is a suspicion that they are due to local mechanical irritation from the tail of the device. There is no evidence of a direct relationship between the use of an IUCD and the development of cervical neoplasia.

Myometrium
No specific pathological changes occur in the myometrium of IUCD users but, in the presence of a severe endometritis, inflammation may extend into the muscle wall.

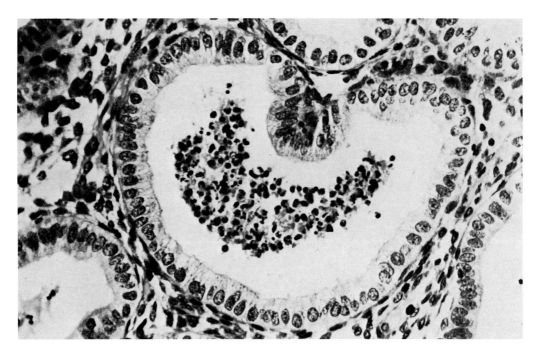

Fig. 13.3 A typical collection of intraglandular polymorphs and cellular debris in an endometrium (H. & E. × 255).

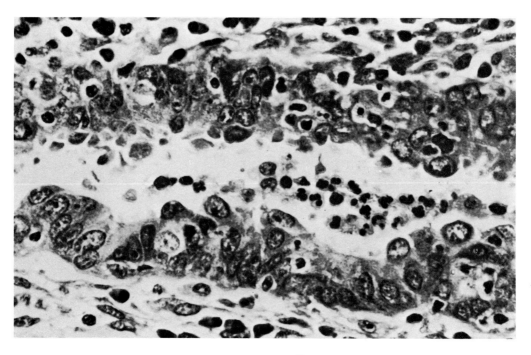

Fig. 13.4 Severe endometritis in an inert device wearer. The gland contains polymorphs and the stroma is infiltrated by plasma cells and lymphocytes (H. & E. × 255).

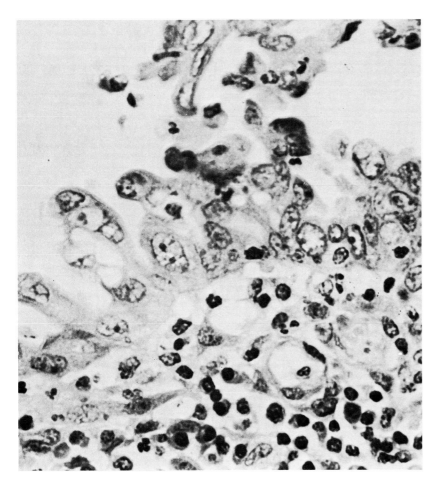

Fig. 13.5 The surface epithelium of this inflamed endometrium from a woman using a copper IUCD shows marked cellular atypia characterized by pleomorphism and cytoplasmic vacuolation (H. & E. × 450).

Pelvic inflammatory disease

Pelvic inflammatory disease (PID) occurs up to seven times more frequently in IUCD users than in non-users, the proportion of users developing PID varying from 1 per cent to 8 per cent in different patient populations but being highest in young, sexually active, nulliparous women.

Some degree of chronic endosalpingitis is present in almost half of the fallopian tubes examined from patients using an IUCD. Acute endosalpingitis is less common but is still three times more frequent than in non-users and will, in about 10 per cent of cases, progress to severe tubo-ovarian inflammation with abscess formation (Fig. 13.6). Rather strangely, unilateral tubo-ovarian abscess is particularly characteristic of PID in users of a device. The infecting organisms are commonly anaerobic and multiple and reach the pelvis via the genital tract; instances of infection by relatively exotic organisms, such as Actinomyces (Fig. 13.7) and Aspergillus, have been reported in inert device users. However, the presence of Actinomyces-like organisms in a cervical smear, in the absence of symptoms, is not indicative of infection. About a quarter of those women who develop severe PID will be rendered sterile as a result of the disease.

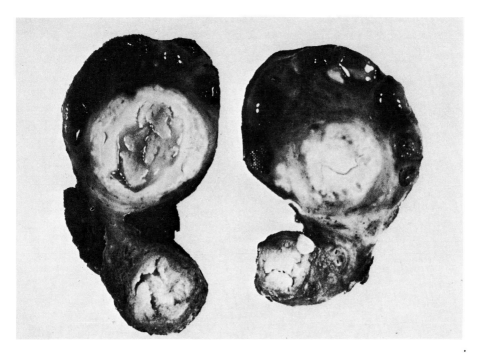

Fig. 13.6   A vertical section through an ovary (above) and a fallopian tube of a woman using an IUCD. There is an intraovarian pyogenic abscess and an acute endosalpingitis.

Pregnancy

A small proportion of women using an IUCD, particularly in the first year of use, will have an intra-uterine pregnancy (Fig. 13.8). Approximately one-quarter will give birth to a live child, but about half will be terminated and about one-fifth will abort spontaneously. In the past, a mid-trimester septic abortion was a particular feature of pregnancy occurring in women using a Dalkon shield; this device is no longer used and septic abortion is now distinctly uncommon. If pregnancy continues until term, the infant is usually normal, there being no observed increase in the incidence of congenital abnormalities.

A high proportion, between 4 and 10 per cent, of IUCD users who become pregnant have an ectopic gestation, this being a very considerably higher incidence than in non-users. There is a particular increase in the incidence of intra-ovarian pregnancy for, whilst in non-IUCD users an ectopic pregnancy occurs once in the ovary for every 150–200 times in the tube, this ratio is 1 in 9 for IUCD wearers. It should not be assumed from these figures that IUCDs actually cause ectopic gestation; the real reasons for this high incidence of extrauterine pregnancy are less simplistic than this. It should first be recognized that an IUCD does not prevent conception but inhibits successful implantation of the fertilized ovum; it is therefore highly probably that the incidence of successful conception is not only very much higher in IUCD users than in those women employing other forms of contraception but also than in those taking no precautions against pregnancy, this latter group actually reducing the number of conceptions by becoming pregnant. In the IUCD user, the vast majority of fertilized ova that reach the uterus will fail to implant. The device has only a restricted capacity for inhibiting tubal implantation and will therefore reduce only to a limited extent the number of tubal gestations. In addition, women using an IUCD have, as has been previously mentioned, an increased risk of tubal damage secondary to PID. This is a proven cause of tubal ectopic gestation. Indeed, it has been claimed that, among IUCD wearers, a tubal ectopic gestation occurs only in those women with PID. An IUCD has no effect on ovarian implantation and

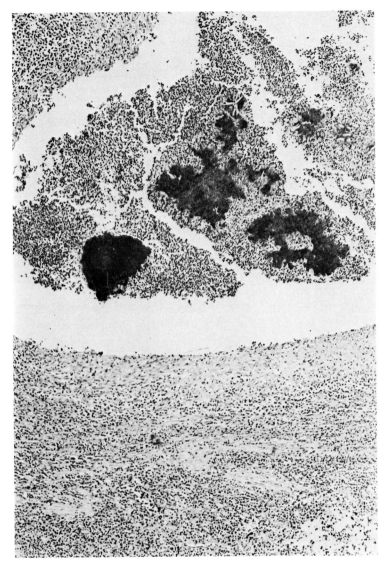

Fig. 13.7 An ovarian abscess from a woman wearing an inert IUCD. The abscess wall (below) is lined by an acute non-specific inflammatory exudate and granulation tissue and the abscess cavity (above) contains colonies of *Actinomyces* (H. & E. × 45).

will therefore not influence the number of intra-ovarian pregnancies, the incidence of which is not increased as a proportion of the total number of conceptions.

Steroid contraception

Steroid contraceptives fall into two main groups, those in which an oestrogen and progestagen are given in combination and those containing only a progestagen.

Modern steroid contraceptives contain a minimum effective dose of hormone and many of the more florid and bizarre histological changes and systemic problems encountered with earlier regimes are no

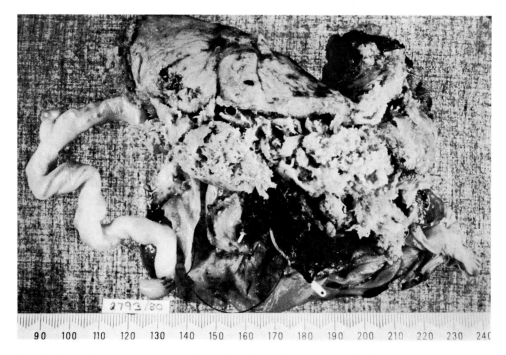

Fig. 13.8   A full-term placenta in which a Gravigard Copper-7 is embedded.

longer seen. Indeed, much of the information which has been gathered over the years on the effects of steroid contraceptives has been collected from women who have at some time taken high-dose preparations and is probably no longer applicable to the present generation of low-dose steroid contraceptive users and those using the modern, new progestagens which have a greater contraceptive specificity and can be used at low dosage.

Most women follow a regimen in which between 20 and 50 micrograms of oestrogen, usually ethinyloestradiol, combined with a progestagen is taken for 21 days out of every 28. The proportion of hormone in the preparation may be identical throughout the 21 days or there may be a phased formulation in which the hormone content of the pill is increased in the middle of the cycle. On the seven hormone-free days either a placebo is taken or there are 7 pill-free days. Combined steroid contraceptives effect contraception by abolishing ovulation.

Some women, particularly those over the age of 35 years, heavy smokers and those in whom oestrogens induce severe side-effects, may use a progestagen-only contraceptive. The progestagen, which is taken every day, may be administered in one of several ways, the effects upon the genital tract being independent of the mode of administration. It is not as reliable a contraceptive as is the combined steroid contraceptive, pregnancy rates of 2–7 per 100 woman-years or 2 per cent per annum being reported. Further experience with the newer progestagens may enable this risk to be reduced.

Endometrium

In the first few months in which a combined steroid contraceptive is used, the pattern of endometrial changes may be cyclical but after prolonged usage the regenerative capacity of the endometrium may be diminished, because of the inhibitory effect of the progestagen upon the oestrogen-stimulated growth; cyclical changes may be minimal or absent. The morphological effects of combined steroid contraceptives,

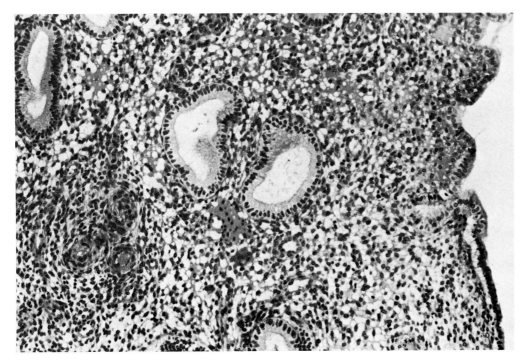

Fig. 13.9 A shallow endometrium with straight or poorly coiled tubular glands showing minimal secretory activity. The stroma is rather oedematous and there is focal decidual change. Fourteenth day of cycle in a woman on combined steroid contraceptives (H. & E. × 102).

whilst being generally similar whatever the precise hormone combination and dosage, show sufficient variation for the relative importance of the oestrogen and progestagen in the combination to be evident.

Following hormonal withdrawal bleeding at the end of each cycle of hormone usage, the endometrium regenerates and there is a brief proliferative phase lasting five or six days, during which the endometrium remains shallow, this being followed by a short, inadequate secretory phase in which the glands remain narrow and tubular and the stroma shows only a mild transient oedema (Fig. 13.9). In the latter half of the cycle there is regression of the secretory change and the endometrium becomes inactive (Fig. 13.10). The precise appearance of the endometrium depends upon the particular hormone combination being used and is more variable in phased contraceptive users. Bleeding occurs from this inactive, rather shallow endometrium, this is often scanty.

The endometrium usually remains shallow whilst combined steroid contraceptives are in use but with modern, low dose preparations the profound atrophy reported in the past is not encountered (Fig. 13.11). There is also evidence that the use of combined steroid contraceptives reduces a woman's risk of developing endometrial adenocarcinoma by 60 per cent after four years of use compared with 'never-users' and that the beneficial effect persists after the menopause providing that the woman is not given unopposed oestrogen hormone replacement therapy. Maximum protection is afforded to those who have used the pill for many years and are nulliparous.

A very variable endometrial picture is encountered in women using a progestagen-only contraceptive. The dose is small and the contraceptive effect depends not upon suppression of ovulation but upon alterations in tubal transport and in the quality of the cervical mucus. Ovulation is suppressed in only about 50 per cent of cycles and, as a consequence the underlying, endogenous hormone pattern, suppression may vary from cycle to cycle and from patient to patient. In addition it is usual to give the same dose of

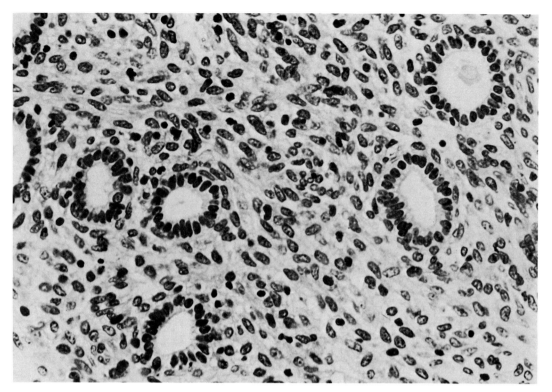

Fig. 13.10 Regressed endometrium from a patient using Logynon. The glands show neither secretory nor proliferative activity and the stroma is compact (H. & E. × 270).

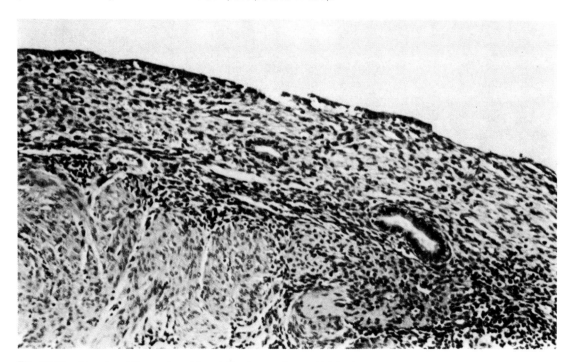

Fig. 13.11 Atrophy of the endometrium following prolonged high-dose combined steroid contraceptives. Appearances such as this are rarely encountered nowadays (H. & E. × 108).

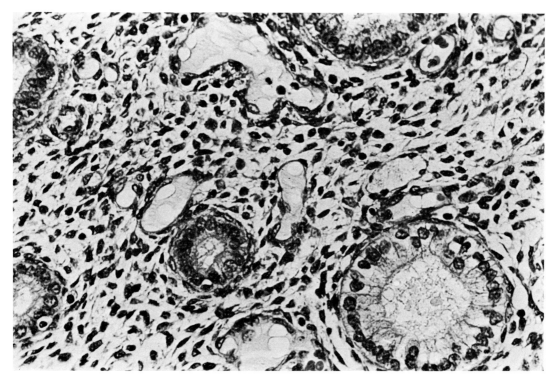

Fig. 13.12 Endometrium from a woman on progestagen-only contraception. The glands are straight and tubular and show variable secretory activity. Dilated capillaries are conspicuous in the stroma (H. & E. × 270).

progestagen every day, or to administer it systemically by depot injection rather than in a cyclical fashion, and amenorrhoea or breakthrough bleeding with intermittent healing therefore occurs.

The most commonly encountered pattern is one in which glands of rather variable size and secretory activity are set in a spindle-celled stroma containing thin-walled vascular channels and showing little or no evidence of decidualization (Fig. 13.12). After prolonged usage the endometrium often appears atrophic.

Myometrium

Myometrial hyperplasia and changes in uterine leiomyomata, characterized by enlargement, necrosis, oedema and bizarre cellular changes, have been reported in women using both combined steroid contraceptives and progestagen-only contraception. It is our experience that such changes are infrequently seen and their more frequent reporting in the older literature is probably a reflection of the higher dose preparations in use at the time. There is certainly no evidence that steroid contraceptive usage is associated with an increased incidence of malignant change in myometrial leiomyomata.

Cervix

The cervical response to steroid contraceptives may be classified as physiological or pathological. The development of an ectopy, hypersecretion of mucus, increased vascularity, stromal oedema and focal, decidua-like change are features which may be regarded as physiological responses to hormone administration.

A significant proportion of steroid contraceptive users develop cervical microglandular hyperplasia of a type similar to that found in pregnant women. This may be only apparent on histological examination but in some cases is of sufficient degree to form a polypoidal mass, visible to the naked eye, within the endocervical canal or on an ectopy. Microglandular hyperplasia may be accompanied by intermenstrual or postcoital bleeding and it is of vital importance to distinguish the benign, self-limiting lesion from an adenocarcinoma. It should be remembered that both microglandular hyperplasia and stromal decidual changes associated with contraceptive steroid use may cause an abnormal cervical vascular pattern visible to the colposcopist.

It has proved difficult to establish whether there is any relationship between steroid contraceptive use and the development of cervical intraepithelial or invasive neoplasia. Studies of various types have yielded conflicting results because of the difficulty of analysing the multitude of social factors associated with the use of such a highly effective non-barrier method of contraception, e.g. age at first coitus and sexual promiscuity. However, there is some evidence of a higher incidence of cervical intraepithelial and invasive carcinoma among women who have used steroid contraceptives for a long period than among women who have never used steroid contraceptives.

Ovary
Steroid contraceptives prevent the maturation of ova and after several successive cycles there is a substantial reduction in the size and number of developing follicles and an absence of corpora lutea. The number of follicle cysts is also reduced. After several years there is atrophy of the cortex and a reduced ovarian size.

There is evidence from case-control studies that prolonged inhibition of ovulation by steroid contraception provides a significant degree of protection against the development of malignant epithelial neoplasms of the ovary.

Fallopian tube
After two or three years of continuous steroid contraceptive use, tubal epithelial atrophy may be apparent.

Vagina
In patients using the low oestrogen combined steroid contraceptives, dyspareunia may accompany the vaginal dryness consequent upon diminution of cervical and vaginal secretion resulting from relative oestrogen deprivation.

In women with pre-existing vaginal adenosis (a very small proportion of the population), steroid contraception may induce a vaginal microglandular hyperplasia similar in type to that seen in the cervix. It is of paramount importance that this be distinguished from a clear cell carcinoma.

Breast
Cystic hyperplastic mastopathy, in which epithelial atypia is absent or minimal, occurs less frequently in steroid contraceptive users than in non-users, although there is no reduction in those forms of mastopathy showing severe cellular atypia.

Investigations into the effect of steroid contraceptives on the risk of breast carcinoma have produced conflicting results. Most studies have failed to show any significant impact of steroid contraceptives upon the risk of breast carcinoma whilst others have noted an increased risk if the hormones are taken early in life or before the first pregnancy but no risk if the contraceptives are taken later in life. A recent study suggests that, in the small group of women who develop breast cancer under the age of 36 years, there may be a relative increased risk of 1.74 of carcinoma of the breast developing when steroid contraceptive use has exceeded eight years. There is also some evidence that progesterone-only contraception may protect against the development of carcinoma of the breast.

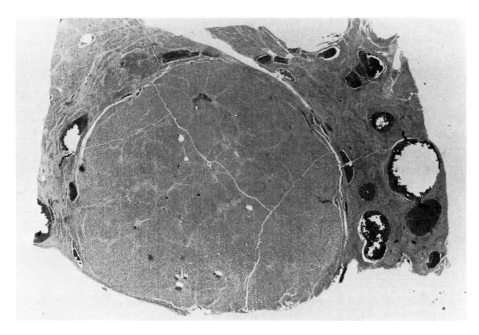

Fig. 13.13 A section through a hepatic adenoma showing the uniformity of the lesion and dilated vessels (peliosis) in the surrounding parenchyma (H. & E. × 5.6).

Liver

Steroid contraceptives appear to affect hepatic secretory function and transient rises in serum bilirubin and transaminase levels often occur in the first few cycles of usage. A small proportion of women develop intrahepatic cholestasis and jaundice which is reversible on stopping the hormones. Steroid contraceptives should be avoided in women who have a pre-existing hepatic disorder, such as Dubin–Johnson or Rotor syndrome, or who have had idiopathic jaundice of pregnancy.

An increased risk of both hepatic adenoma (Fig. 13.13) and hepatocellular carcinoma is reported in steroid contraceptive users, although it should be stressed that such tumours, even when their incidence is notably raised, are still very uncommon and that a causal relationship between steroid contraceptives and neoplasia has not been finally established. Regression of some of the lesions diagnosed as adenomas suggests that they may be reactive rather than neoplastic. The risk of developing a neoplasm appears to vary in proportion to the dose of the oestrogen in the preparation and the duration of its use.

Focal nodular hyperplasia of the liver is a hamartoma, which is usually identified incidentally at laparotomy or postmortem but which, in steroid contraceptive users, may enlarge, undergo necrosis or haemorrhage and can rupture (Figs. 13.14 and 13.15). Similar changes may rarely occur in hepatic adenomata.

Pituitary

It has been maintained that the use of steroid contraceptives is associated, in a small proportion of women, with the development of prolactin-secreting pituitary microadenomata which may, after cessation of contraceptive usage, impair fertility or cause amenorrhoea associated, in some instances, with galactorrhoea. However, considerable doubts have recently been cast upon the validity of this association.

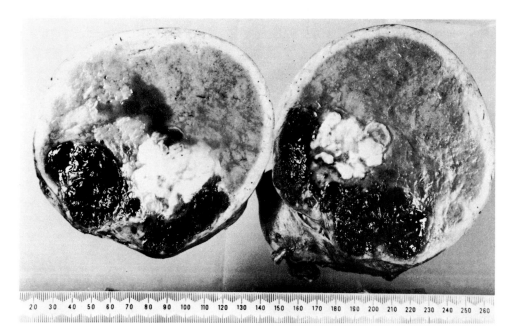

Fig. 13.14 The cut surface of a pedunculated mass of focal nodular hyperplasia. It has undergone partial necrosis and focal haemorrhage. The specimen was removed from a postpartum patient who had used combined oral steroid contraceptives until shortly before her pregnancy.

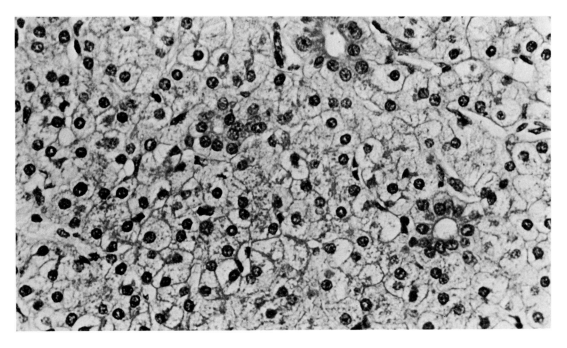

Fig. 13.15 Focal nodular hyperplasia is characteristically composed of hepatocytes and bile ducts (H. & E. × 270).

Post-pill amenorrhoea

It is doubtful whether this condition exists as a true entity. A delay in, or lack of, the return of the menses is more likely in women whose original menstrual cycle is irregular and infrequent and may, therefore, be indicative of underlying hypothalamic–pituitary dysfunction. It is a problem in less than 1 per cent of users.

Other systemic effects

A mild increase in systemic blood pressure is not uncommon but in about 1 per cent of women there is a significant increase and this is more likely in women who have a past history of hypertension in pregnancy. Glucose intolerance also develops in a small proportion of steroid contraceptive users but there is, as compared to non-users, no increase in the incidence of clinical diabetes mellitus. However, diabetes is usually regarded as a contraindication to continuation of the medication.

High dose steroid contraceptives used to be associated with an increased risk of thromboembolism but the deliberate reduction in oestrogen in the preparations has reduced the incidence of thromboembolic disease. However, current use of steroid contraception increases the risk of acute myocardial infarction among women who also smoke (relative risk 20.8 for heavy smokers and 41.0 for heavy smokers who have a history of pregnancy-induced hypertension).

Increased plasma levels of cholesterol, very low density lipoproteins, high density lipoproteins, triglycerides and protein-bound iodine (PBI) have been reported and there may be reduced levels of low density lipoproteins, vitamin B6, vitamin B12, folic acid, ascorbic acid and riboflavin. These changes, whilst statistically significant in most cases, result in values which remain within the normal range.

Pathology of non-contraceptive hormone therapy

Oestrogens alone, or in combination with a progestagen, are given for the relief of menopausal symptoms, as postmenopausal hormone replacement therapy and in the management of various hypogonadal states such as Turner's syndrome. Progestagens are administered for the treatment of menorrhagia, endometrial hyperplasia, some forms of adenocarcinoma and endometriosis. In the past, and particularly in the United States, diethylstilboestrol (DES) was extensively used in the hope of preventing abortion but this form of therapy has been abandoned since it was shown that prenatal exposure to DES causes vaginal adenosis which, in turn, predisposes to the development of clear cell carcinomata of the cervix and vagina during, or within a few years of, puberty.

Endometrium

Prolonged unopposed oestrogen therapy, whether administered continuously or cyclically, is associated with a high incidence of simple glandular hyperplasia of the endometrium and, less commonly, with complex or atypical hyperplasia. There is also no doubt that there is an increase in the incidence of endometrial adenocarcinoma in women given unopposed oestrogen therapy, this being in the order of a two-fold increase for short term therapy (up to one year) and in the region of ten- to fifteen-fold after long term administration (i.e. more than five years). The mean age at which an endometrial adenocarcinoma develops is lower in oestrogen users than in non-users and the tumours are usually well differentiated. The overall five- and ten-year survival rates for oestrogen users who develop adenocarcinoma are higher than are those in non-users but this difference disappears if the grade of the neoplasm is taken into account. It should be added that there is no evidence that cyclical rather than continuous administration of oestrogens will significantly reduce the risk of neoplasia, that the effect of the oestrogen is cumulative, that the risk of carcinoma is greatest with conjugated oestrogens and

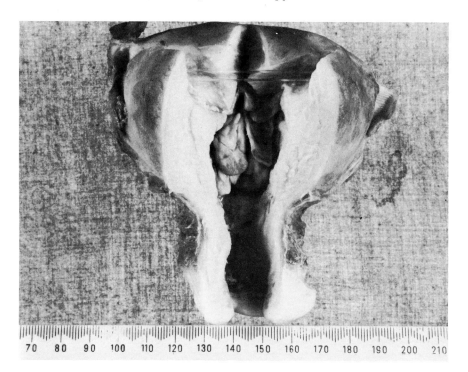

Fig. 13.16 A uterus opened to show the polypoidal endometrium of a patient who has received a high dose of progestagen for a short period of time.

diethylstilboestrol and that the administration of a progestagen for a minimum of ten days per cycle will protect the endometrium against the carcinogenic effect of oestrogens.

Tamoxifen is a triphenylethylene compound which, as a consequence of competing for and blocking oestrogen binding sites, has antioestrogenic properties. It is convenient to consider its effects here because in a small proportion of women it appears, somewhat paradoxically, to induce an oestrogen-like effect which has been described both experimentally and clinically. Endometrial proliferative activity, the induction of progesterone receptors, the development of endometrial hyperplasia and adenocarcinoma have all been described.

Administration of pure progestagen is not associated with any risk of endometrial adenocarcinoma, the picture initially being one of stromal pseudodecidual change and K-cell (granulated lymphocyte) infiltration with initial glandular secretion, or hypersecretion, but rapid glandular exhaustion (Figs. 13.16 and 13.17). After prolonged use the endometrium becomes shallow and inactive. The endometrium usually recovers rapidly after the cessation of therapy and we do not usually see the profound, permanent atrophy with stromal hyalinization which has been previously described. When the progestagen has been used in the treatment of endometrial hyperplasia secretory changes may be superimposed, the appearances sometimes being known as 'secretory hyperplasia'. With continued therapy simple hyperplasia may regress completely but atypical hyperplasia may regress only partly, leaving islands of architecturally atypical glands.

Tumour growth may be suppressed in hormonally responsive endometrial adenocarcinomas and areas of regression or degeneration may be apparent.

Danazol, which is a synthetic, weakly progestagenic, anti-gonadotrophic androgen, is used in the treatment of endometriosis and usually renders the endometrium moderately atrophic *ab initio*.

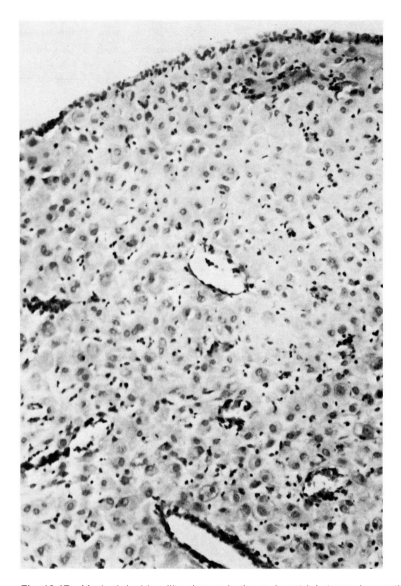

Fig. 13.17 Marked decidua-like change in the endometrial stroma in a patient given a high dose of progestagens for treatment of endometriosis. Note the atrophic glands and scattered K-cell infiltrate (H. & E. × 108).

Postmenopausal hormone replacement therapy is recommended for the prevention of osteoporosis and in the treatment of menopausal symptoms. Oestrogen alone may be given safely for this purpose in women who have had a hysterectomy but it is usually considered more prudent to administer a progestagen sequentially to protect against the development of an endometrial adenocarcinoma in women who have retained their uterus. The endometrium in women using a sequential hormone replacement regimen shows cyclical changes, the precise appearance of which depends upon the proportion of oestrogen and progestagen in the combination.

Ovary

There is no clear evidence of a relationship between ovarian neoplasia and the use of oestrogens, but a rise in the incidence of endometrioid carcinoma of the ovary in the United States has coincided with an increase in the use of hormonal replacement therapy.

Breast

Although there is little evidence of a relationship between therapeutic oestrogens and breast carcinoma in the short term, there is some evidence that the risk of mammary carcinoma appears to increase after twelve years use. Furthermore, women with benign breast lesions appear to have an increased risk of developing malignancy if oestrogens are administered.

Key references

Beral V, Hannaford P C and Kay C. (1988) Oral contraceptive use and malignancies of the genital tract. Results from the Royal College of General Practitioners'; Oral Contraception Study Group. *Lancet* ii, 1331–5.

Buckley C H. (1987) Pathology of contraception and of hormonal therapy. In: *Haines and Taylor, Obstetrical and Gynaecological Pathology*, pp. 839–73. Edited by H Fox, Churchill Livingstone, London.

Croft, P and Hannaford P C. (1989) Risk factors for acute myocardial infarction in women: evidence from the Royal College of General Practitioners' oral contraception study. *British Medical Journal* **298**, 165–8.

Drife J O. (1989) The contraceptive pill and breast cancer in young women. *British Medical Journal* **298**, 1269–1270.

Eyong E and Elstein M. (1989) Clinical update on a new progestogen-gestodene. *British Journal of Family Planning* **15**, 18–22.

Fornander T, Rutqvist L E, Cedermark B. *et al.* (1989) Adjuvant Tamoxifen in early breast cancer: occurrence of new primary cancers. *Lancet* i, 117–9.

Huggins G R and Zucker P K. (1987) Oral contraceptives and neoplasia: 1987 update. *Fertility and Sterility* **47**, 733–61.

Nuovo M A, Nuovo G J, McCaffrey R M, Levine R U, Barron B and Winkler B. (1989) Endometrial polyps in postmenopausal women receiving Tamoxifen. *International Journal of Gynecological Pathology* **8**, 125–31.

Prentice R L and Thomas D B. (1987) On the epidemiology of oral contraceptives and disease. *Advances in Cancer Research* **49**, 285–401.

Robinson G E. (1989) Older women taking modern pills. *British Journal of Family Planning* **15**, 11–3.

Schlesselmann J J. (1989) Oral contraceptives in relation to cancer of the breast and reproductive tract — an epidemiological review. *British Journal of Family Planning* **15**, 23–33.

Singh M M, Ingham H R, Wadehra V and Morris K. (1989) Endometrial culture in IUCD users with actinomycosis-like organisms (ALOs) on cervical smears. *British Journal of Family Planning* **15**, 3–6.

UK Family Planning Research Network. (1989) Pregnancy outcome associated with the use of IUCDs. *British Journal of Family Planning* **15**, 7–10.

UK National Case-Control Study Group. (1989) Oral contraceptive use and breast cancer risk in young women. *Lancet* i, 973–82.

Vessey M. (1989) Oral contraception. In: *Contraception: Science and Practice*, pp. 52–68. Edited by M Filshie and J Guillebaud, Butterworth, London.

14
Pathology of infertility

Infertility is an extremely complicated problem and it is thought that the fault lies entirely with the female in only about one-quarter of infertile couples; in a further quarter, female abnormalities are a contributory factor. In this chapter, only the pathology of female infertility will be discussed and it must be borne in mind that this limitation gives a very incomplete picture of the complex and often multifactorial topic of reproductive failure.

Classification of infertility

The simplest classification of infertile women is into those who are ovulatory and those who are anovulatory, or who ovulate infrequently and inconsistently. Anovulatory infertility is due to malfunction of the hypothalamus, pituitary or ovary, whilst ovulatory infertility is usually a result of disease of the genital tract, it being remembered that some cases of apparent ovulatory infertility are really due to repeated early abortion rather than to any failure of conception.

Anovulatory infertility and disturbances of ovulation

Control of ovulation is complex and depends upon the integrity of the hypothalamic–pituitary–ovarian axis and its ability to coordinate and regulate the pulsatility, timing and magnitude of gonadotrophin secretion in response to feedback mechanisms operated by the ovarian hormones. Suprahypothalamic centres also play a role in this complicated system and, indeed, the anovulation which not infrequently accompanies psychological illness is probably due to disturbances at this level.

Hypothalamic–pituitary factors

Gonadotrophin deficiency
Inadequate production of gonadotrophins may be simply one component of a panhypopituitarism or it can occur as an isolated phenomenon. A generalized pituitary failure may be secondary to hypothalamic disease or to damage such as that caused by a hypothalamic or optic glioma, by compression from a pinealoma or cranioparyngioma or by Hand–Schüller–Christian disease, but it is more commonly due to destruction of the pituitary by irradiation, trauma, surgery, nonfunctional large tumours, post-partum ischaemic necrosis or infarction due to sickle cell anaemia. In all such cases the hypogonadism is simply one facet of the clinical picture of multiple hormonal deficiencies. A clearer picture of gonadal dysfunction is seen in cases of isolated gonadotrophin deficiency, which can be due to a failure of the hypothalamus either to synthesize or release luteinizing hormone-releasing hormone (LRH), to a primary failure of the pituitary to synthesize luteinizing hormone (LH) or FSH or to defective pituitary subunit synthesis or coupling. The most common form of isolated gonadotrophin deficiency is Kallmann's syndrome (also

known as olfactory–genital dysplasia or hypogonadotrophic eunuchoidism), in which hypogonadism is associated with anosmia, due to partial or complete agenesis of the olfactory lobes, and, often but not invariably, anomalies of orofacial development. In this condition the hypogonadism appears to be due to deficient LRH secretion by the hypothalamus and patients can be induced to develop secondary sex characteristics and to ovulate by administration of exogenous LRH. Some individuals with a deficiency of hypothalamic LRH secretion have no other stigmata of Kallmann's syndrome but their response to exogenous LRH differentiates these women from those with a primary fault in pituitary synthesis of LH or FSH, who will show no response to LRH stimulation.

Gonadotrophin deficiency occurs occasionally, although not in isolation, in the empty sella syndrome in which there is a defective, incomplete or vestigial diaphragm sellae with extension of the subarachnoid space into the sella, this being accompanied by compression and flattening of the pituitary.

Hyperprolactinaemia

Prolactin is secreted by the lactotrophs of the anterior pituitary which appear as acidophils in histological preparations but are more specifically identified by immunofluorescence or immunoperoxidase techniques. Normal prolactin secretion is controlled by the hypothalamus, by means of the tuberoinfundibular dopamine system which exerts an inhibitory action.

The actions of prolactin are numerous but it appears to inhibit ovulation, when present in excess, by interfering with the pulsatility of LH secretion and by blocking the effects of gonadotrophins on the ovary.

The most common cause of hyperprolactinaemia is a prolactin-secreting pituitary adenoma. Such adenomata are surprisingly common and about 70 per cent of chromophobe adenomata produce prolactin. Patients with acidophil adenomata producing acromegaly are also often hyperprolactinaemic but this is more commonly due to hypothalamic or pituitary stalk compression than to tumour secretion of prolactin. A tumour in which the maximum diameter is less than 10 mm is termed a microadenoma and it has been estimated that such microadenomata account for approximately one-third of all cases of hyper-prolactinaemia and for between 5 and 7 percent of all cases of amenorrhoea. There is no evidence that such microadenomata may be induced by oestrogens, particularly when taken as a component of the contraceptive pill, but it has been postulated that in some women the blood supply of a circumscribed region of the pituitary is derived not from hypophysial portal vessels but from arteries in the lower infundibular stem or infundibular process. Such an isolated group of cells would not be subjected to the inhibitory action of unfundibular dopamine in the hypophysial portal blood and would therefore act as an explant independent of hypothalamic regulation.

Hyperprolactinaemia may also accompany hormonally inert pituitary tumours if the expanding neoplasm compresses the pituitary stalk or hypothalamus and thus interrupts the inhibitory action of dopamine; damage to the pituitary stalk by trauma, surgery or irradiation will produce similar results. Hypothyroid patients are also commonly hyperprolactinaemic, this reflecting the prolactin-releasing action of TRH.

Ovarian factors

Ovulatory failure due to ovarian factors falls into three main categories. Those in which there is a congenital or acquired absence of germ cells, as in gonadal dysgenesis or radiation damage. Those in which germ cells are present but fail to mature normally either because they are unresponsive to gonadotrophins or because an enzymatic deficiency precludes response. Those in which follicular maturation may occur, albeit incompletely, inadequately or inconsistently, but in which the process of ovulation is, in some way defective, as in autoimmune oöphoritis, luteinized unruptured follicle syndrome, polycystic ovary syndrome and luteal phase insufficiency.

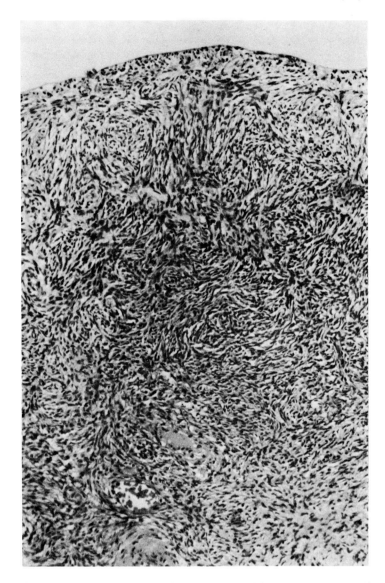

Fig. 14.1 An ovarian biopsy from a woman of 26 years who had suffered a premature menopause. In sharp contrast to the gonadotrophin-resistant ovary, there is a complete absence of primordial follicles (H. & E. × 108).

Gonadal dysgenesis

Gonadal dysgenesis (discussed in Chapter 2) is usually associated with infertility, because although dysgenetic gonads have a virtually normal complement of germ cells during embryonic life, these have usually disappeared by the time of puberty, the postpubertal streak gonad showing a total absence of ova or follicular derivatives. Complete loss of ova is certainly the rule in patients with a pure XO karyotype, but those with an XO mosaic chromosomal pattern may retain a few ova into early adult life, sometimes menstruate and, very occasionally, become pregnant.

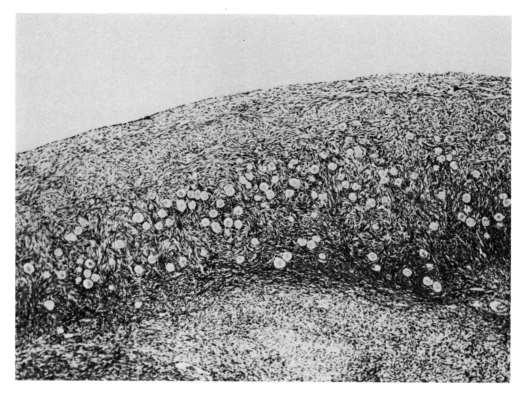

Fig. 14.2   The typical ovary of gonadotrophin-resistant syndrome. There is a total absence of follicular development but a large number of primordial follicles are present (H. & E. × 45).

Premature ovarian failure

A few otherwise apparently normal women suffer a premature menopause (i.e. before the age of 35). Gonadotrophin levels are high but ovarian biopsy shows a complete absence of primordial and developing follicles (Fig. 14.1), the lack of these structures allowing for differentiation from the gonadotrophin-resistant ovary. It is possible that these patients have a primary paucity of germ cells, accelerated follicular atresia or, in the case of women with galactosaemia, deficient germ cell migration to the gonad. In some patients there appears to be a genetic basis. Claims by some to have found organ-specific antiovarian antibodies in this syndrome have not been substantiated.

Ovulatory failure due to ovarian damage

Pelvic irradiation, e.g. for the treatment of cervical carcinoma, results in the loss of germ cells with narrowing and fibrosis of the ovarian cortex. Such complete destruction of follicles is not inevitable following chemotherapy and normal fertility is retained in a proportion of young women or children treated in this way.

Infections of the ovary may occur without loss of follicles, subsequent infertility resulting from damage to the fallopian tubes or the development of peritoneal adhesions (see later) but occasionally, following mumps, there may be significant follicular damage and cortical fibrosis leading to a premature menopause.

Gonadotrophin-resistant ovary syndrome ('savage syndrome')
This syndrome, usually congenital but occasionally acquired, is characterized by anovulation, low oestrogen values and high levels of gonadotrophins. Ovarian biopsy reveals plentiful primordial follicles, primary follicles and occasional secondary follicles but little or no evidence of follicular maturation. There is no response to exogenous gonadotrophins (Fig. 14.2). The gonadotrophins secreted by these patients are normal in all respects. It appears possible, in some cases, that ovarian unresponsiveness is due to non-immune receptor or postreceptor defect, whilst in others autoimmunity is implicated and antibodies inhibiting the binding of gonadotrophins to the follicle cells are found.

17-hydroxylase deficiency
This rare enzyme deficiency results in decreased adrenal and gonadal synthesis of steroid hormones. Defective ovarian oestrogen production leads to sexual infantilism associated with hypergonadotrophism. There is a failure of normal follicular maturation and it is not uncommon for the ovary to contain multiple small follicular cysts. There appears to be a particular tendency for the ovaries of patients with this syndrome to undergo torsion and infarction.

Autoimmune ovarian failure
Antibodies directed against steroid-producing cells in the ovary are found in a proportion of women with autoimmune Addison's disease. These cross-react with steroid-synthesizing cells in the adrenal cortex and are not found in any other form of premature ovarian failure. The presence of anti-steroid antibodies is clearly associated with a decline in ovarian function. Amenorrhoea and anovulation are the rule, the failure to ovulate being secondary to the local deficiency of oestrogen synthesis. Immunofluorescent studies have shown these antibodies to have a rather variable pattern of staining of the developing follicle, theca interna and corpus luteum, suggesting that a number of antibodies are produced which react with different antigens in the ovarian steroid-synthesizing cells. Histological examination of ovaries from women with this type of ovarian failure shows either atrophy and fibrosis or lymphocytic infiltration, the latter being most prominent around developing follicles.

Luteinized unruptured follicle syndrome
In this condition the follicle ripens normally but fails to release the ovum. Luteinization of the granulosa and theca layers proceeds normally and an ovum-containing corpus luteum is formed. Hormonal activity within the ovary appears to be undisturbed and secretory changes occur in the endometrium; there thus appears to be a primary defect in the ovum-releasing mechanism. This syndrome can be suspected if normal endometrial cyclical activity and a normal cyclical biochemical profile is not accompanied by stigmata of ovulation on laparoscopic examination of the ovarian surface.

Failure of ovum release despite follicle rupture
This phenomenon is sometimes a problem in women subjected to artificial ovarian stimulation as well as in spontaneous cycles.

Polycystic ovary syndrome
The polycystic ovary syndrome is best defined in endocrinological and pathophysiological terms because the corresponding clinical and pathological features of the disorder are very variable. The classic description

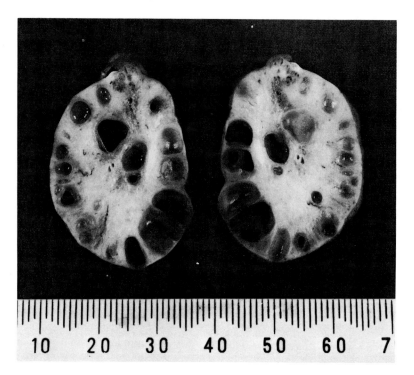

Fig. 14.3 Sections through an ovary from a woman with polycystic ovary syndrome. Although the ovary is not enlarged, the multiple, subcapsular follicular cysts are typical of this syndrome.

of the syndrome includes bilateral ovarian enlargement with fibrosis of the superficial cortex, hyperplasia and luteinization of the theca interna and an absence of ovulation. These morphological findings are accompanied by the clinical triad of amenorrhoea, hirsuties and obesity (the Stein–Leventhal syndrome).

The ovaries commonly show a moderate degree of enlargement which is due to the presence of multiple, small (less than 1 cm diameter) cortical, atretic follicular cysts lined by several layers of granulosa cells, which are the only consistent morphological feature of the syndrome, and an increase in stroma (Figs. 14.3 and 14.4). However, the ovaries are of normal size in 40 per cent of cases. The characteristic pearly-white fibrous thickening of the superficial cortex is found in only about half of polycystic ovaries, usually those in which the androgen levels are elevated. Recent or old corpora lutea, indicative of active ovulation, are present in 25 per cent of polycystic ovaries. Hyperthecosis and thecal luteinization are common, although not invariable, features.

Clinical features are equally variable. Anovulatory infertility occurs in about 75 per cent of cases, 70 per cent of whom also have some degree of hirsuties. Obesity is found in only about 40 per cent of cases whilst approximately 25 per cent appear to ovulate normally and one in eight has regular cyclical bleeding.

The pathophysiology of this syndrome is complex. There is an excess production of androgens, by both the ovaries and the adrenal cortex, and peripheral extraglandular conversion of the excess androstenedione leads to chronically elevated, acyclic oestrogen levels which act on the normal hypo-thalamic-pituitary complex to produce an increased pituitary sensitivity to LRH with subsequent low, constant FSH release and erratically, or inappropriately elevated, non-pulsatile LH secretion. The basic aetiology of this syndrome remains obscure; possibly there is, in some cases, a congenital enzyme

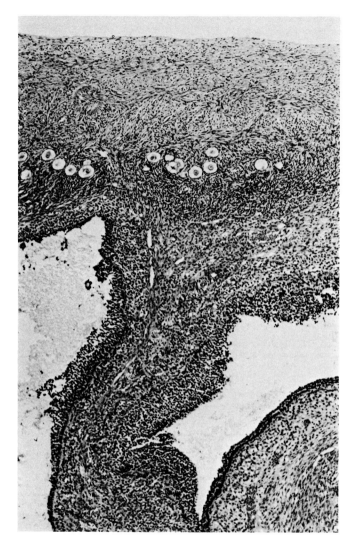

Fig. 14.4   A section from the ovary shown in Fig. 14.3. It shows moderate capsular thickening, primordial follicles and follicular cysts lined by granulosa cells (H. & E. × 45).

deficiency in both ovarian and adrenal steroid-synthesizing systems, but it is also possible that the primary abnormality is an excess production of adrenal androgens, the pituitary and ovarian abnormalities being secondary to this.

Luteal phase insufficiency
Luteal phase insufficiency is associated with infertility and recurrent early spontaneous abortion. It occurs when there is insufficient production of progesterone following ovulation and it is believed to be due to a defective corpus luteum. The insufficiency may be expressed as a failure of progesterone to reach physiological levels following ovulation or as a premature decline in progesterone levels following the early demise of the corpus luteum. It is most commonly the consequence of inadequate preovulatory

follicular stimulation by FSH leading to a paucity of follicular oestrogen. The endometrial changes associated with luteal phase insufficiency are described in Chapter 3. It is unlikely that the abnormal morphology of the endometrium is the cause of the infertility, a more likely explanation being disturbances of tubal transport and ovum support.

Ovarian neoplasms

Both oestrogen-secreting ovarian tumours, such as granulosa cell neoplasms or thecomata, and androgenic neoplasms, such as androblastomata, can cause anovulation, largely because of their effects on the ovarian hormonal feedback mechanism.

Ovulatory infertility

In ovulatory infertility the integrity of the hypothalamic–pituitary–ovarian axis is maintained and both gonadotrophin and oestrogen levels are usually within normal limits.

Tubal factors

It is only too easy to regard the fallopian tube simply as a conduit and to consider the tubal contribution to infertility solely in terms of mechanical obstruction. In reality, the tube has a complex physiological role to play and current interest in salpingeal physiology centres on topics such as the contractility of tubal muscle fibres, the dynamics and character of tubal secretion, the significance of the ampullary–isthmic junction, the isthmic noradrenergic sphincter, tubal ciliary activity and the response of the tube to ovarian hormones and to prostaglandins. It is probable that disturbances of any of these functions can contribute to infertility, but pathological studies of the tube have lagged well behind in the exploration of these pathophysiological concepts and accounts of tubal factors in infertility are still limited largely to the effects of postinflammatory damage.

Congenital abnormalities of the tube are rare but absence of the müllerian structures may occur in Rokitansky–Küster–Hauser or testicular regression syndrome. Segmental atresia of the isthmus is reported and congenital malformations associated with intrauterine exposure to diethylstilboestrol are well documented.

Salpingitis

Tubal inflammation is discussed in Chapter 5. The overall effects of inflammation on tubal function are complex and can be divided into those which are the result of ascending endosalpingitis, such as luminal scarring and obstruction, fimbrial damage, ostial occlusion, follicular salpingitis and hydrosalpinx, and those which may be seen following haematogenous granulomatous salpingitis, all of which are highly important factors in infertility.

Extratubal inflammation

Perisalpingeal adhesions may follow tubal involvement in local pelvic inflammatory disease such as an appendicular abscess or diverticulitis. The resulting kinking or distortion of the tube is commonly unilateral and is likely to be an important factor in infertility only when it is bilateral.

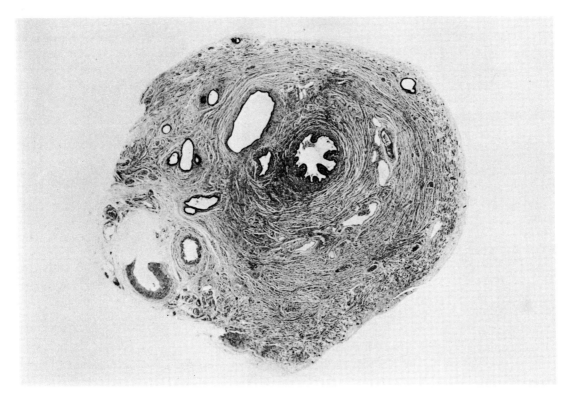

Fig. 14.5 A transverse section of a fallopian tube with salpingitis isthmica nodosa showing an excentric lumen and a series of intramural spaces lined by tubal epithelium (H. & E. × 5.4).

Salpingitis isthmica nodosa

This is characterized by the presence of tiny nodules in the isthmic area of the tubes. Histologically, there is marked hypertrophy of the muscle at this site and the thickened wall is honeycombed by branching spaces lined by tubal-type epithelium (fig. 14.5). A slit-like lumen is sometimes apparent and serial sections show a continuity between the lumen and the intramural epithelial structures. Despite its name, it is unlikely that this condition is due to local inflammation. However, it is clearly related to tubal obstruction, whether functional or mechanical, and may, therefore, follow inflammation elsewhere in the tube. It appears to be a form of localized diverticular disease and is distinct from cornual adenomyosis. It is clearly associated with tubal ectopic gestation (see Chapter 15) as well as infertility.

Endometrial factors

Endometrial biopsy plays an important role in the investigation of the infertile woman. Endometrial abnormalities encountered in such patients may be due to intrinsic endometrial disease, such as endometritis, but more commonly reflect abnormalities of gonadal function, e.g.anovulation or luteal phase defect. The timing of endometrial biopsy, in terms of the menstrual cycle, is of crucial importance for whilst anovulatory cycles or luteal phase defect are most apparent in biopsies taken during the late stages of the cycle, a chronic non-specific endometritis is most easily recognized in samples obtained during the preovulation phase when the presence of a physiological premenstrual inflammatory cell infiltrate does not cloud the issue. On the other hand, tuberculous endometritis is best diagnosed during the premenstrual phase, when any tubercles present are most fully developed, and delayed endometrial shedding can be recognized only in biopsies obtained during the late menstrual phase. Accurate diagnosis in the infertile woman is dependent upon receiving detailed information as to the patient's obstetric, menstrual, contraceptive and medication history. The biopsy should be of adequate size and not taken from the relatively hormonal-insensitive areas of the endometrium, such as that of the basal layer or the lower uterine segment.

Endometritis

An acute endometritis is not a significant factor in infertility for this condition is usually of short duration and resolves completely.

Non-specific chronic endometritis is discussed in Chapter 5. The incidence of infertility in women with a chronic endometritis has been variously estimated as being between 2 and 10 per cent and any reduction in reproductive capacity is probably due either to the disturbed cyclical activity of the endometrium or to associated tubal inflammatory disease.

Tuberculous endometritis, now uncommon in the United Kingdom but still rampant in many parts of the world, is almost invariably accompanied by infertility. In tuberculosis, as with non-specific endometritis, there appears to be an unresponsiveness of the endometrium to ovarian hormones, and infertility may be attributed either to this or to the tubal tuberculosis which invariably accompanies endometrial infection.

Mycoplasmal infection is a recognized cause of infertility, whilst schistosomal infection of the endometrium is commonly associated with infertility in countries in which this disease is endemic.

Asherman's syndrome

This condition is also known as intrauterine synechiae, fibrotic endometritis or traumatic hypomenorrhoea-amenorrhoea, and is characterized by the presence of adhesions between the two surfaces of the endometrial cavity (Fig. 14.6). These may be single or multiple and can, in extreme cases, completely obliterate the cavity. The adhesions usually occur as a complication of puerperal or postabortal curettage and are particularly prone to develop in women subjected to curettage three or four weeks after childbirth. Rarely, adhesions may follow myomectomy or caesarean section but whether trauma alone is an adequate explanation for the formation of adhesions or whether there must also be superadded infection is a moot point. Certainly, the condition can complicate intrauterine infections, particularly tuberculous endometritis, in the absence of any history of instrumentation. Infertility is common and the diagnosis, suspected because of mechanical difficulties experienced during curettage, is confirmed by hysterography. The bands joining the two endometrial surfaces are seen histologically to consist of a core of partially fibrotic or hyalinized endometrial stroma covered on all aspects by cells similar to those of the endometrial surface epithelium (Fig. 14.7). Occasionally, the bands contain smooth muscle fibres or calcific foci. The endometrium away from the adhesions may be normal, with retention of cyclic activity, or can show a mosaic pattern of well developed secretory change, inadequate secretory change and inactive glands but, despite normal ovarian function, it may be inactive and atrophic; quite frequently, there is a moderately severe non-specific chronic endometritis.

The actual cause of infertility in women with this syndrome is not fully established. The adhesions may be sufficiently extensive as to obstruct sperm passage, interfere with implantation or cause early, unrecognized abortion of an implanted blastocyst, but the accompanying abnormalities in the uninvolved endometrium may well be of equal importance. Complete endometrial inactivity is usually associated with adhesions in the lower uterine segment with stenosis of the internal os, and a neural inhibitory mechanism may be a possible cause of this refractoriness to ovarian hormones. Corporeal adhesions are

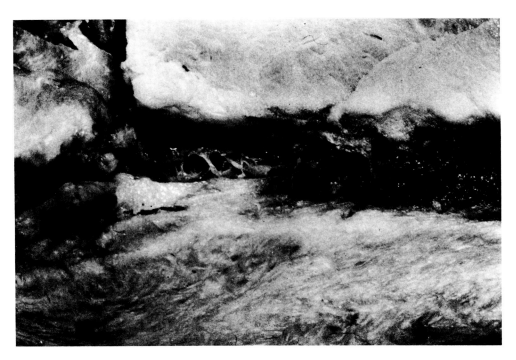

Fig. 14.6   A vertical section through the uterus of a patient with Asherman's syndrome. The lumen is almost completely obliterated by the presence of synechiae which can be seen linking the anterior wall (above) with the posterior wall.

more commonly associated with a normal endometrial response to ovarian hormones, any reduction in menstrual bleeding being directly proportional to the extent of endometrial scarring.

Absent gonadal function

In patients with non-functioning ovaries, the endometrium is thin and atrophic. The glands are few, small, narrow and lined by low cuboidal cells which show no proliferative activity, whilst the stroma is fibrotic. If this state of affairs persists for a prolonged period, the endometrium may become completely resistant to ovarian hormones.

Anovulatory cycles

If ovulation fails to occur the follicle usually persists for several weeks and the endometrium is thus subjected to continuing oestrogenic stimulation without any supervening progestational phase. The development of a secretory endometrium is presumptive evidence of ovulation, but it has to be emphasized that the absence of secretory activity and the persistence of a proliferative pattern cannot be taken as absolute proof of anovulation unless this finding is noted in endometrial biopsies taken after the third week of the cycle. This codicil is necessary because some women normally have a prolonged follicular phase lasting up to twenty-one days and hence only persistence of a proliferative endometrium beyond this stage of the cycle can be taken as evidence of anovulation.

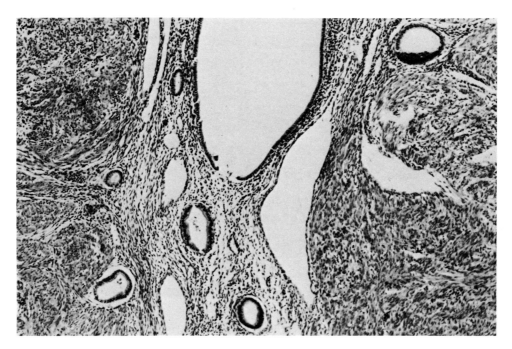

Fig. 14.7   A histological section from the uterus of a patient with Asherman's syndrome. A stromal band covered by epithelium links the adjacent uterine walls which are lined only by basal endometrium (H. & E. × 50).

Pseudocorpus luteum insufficiency
Very exceptionally, the clinical and histological features of a corpus luteum defect may be found in a woman with normal luteal activity. In such a case, exogenous progesterone has no effect on the endometrial abnormalities, which appear to be due to a local deficiency of progesterone receptors.

Myometrial factors

Leiomyomata
The role of leiomyomata in female infertility is a disputed one, because although 40 per cent of women with multiple leiomyomata are infertile, this could mean only that both infertility and myometrial leiomyomata are dependent upon a common causal factor. Nevertheless, myomectomy has, in terms of subsequent pregnancies, produced good results in infertile women and it is difficult to deny the possibility that large submucous leiomyomata could obstruct sperm passage or impair successful implantation of the blastocyst or that their presence may cause vascular disturbances in the uterus.

Cervical factors

The functions of the cervix are mediated largely by the mucus secreted by the endocervical cells. The mucus plays a major role in sperm transport and acts as a biological valve, facilitating sperm entry at the time of ovulation and interfering with entry at other stages of the cycle. The mucus also protects the sperm against the hostile environment of the vagina, filters off abnormal or poorly motile sperm and may also play a role in initiating sperm capacitation. Abnormalities or disease of the cervix may clearly interfere with those vital physiological functions, whilst the cervix is also the probable site at which any immunological reaction against sperm is mounted. It is therefore not surprising that cervical factors are estimated to be a causal factor in between 10 per cent and 30 per cent of cases of female infertility.

Structural and mechanical lesions
These may act either by impeding sperm entry and passage or by reducing the amount of mucus-secreting epithelium. However, the importance of purely mechanical factors has almost certainly been overstated in the past and all are rare causes of infertility. Occasionally, a fixed retroversion and retroflexion of the uterus may result in a malpositioning of the cervix against the anterior vaginal wall, thus impeding sperm access to the os. A prolapse may lead to the ejaculate being deposited in the fornices, well above the level of the os, the sperm then being exposed to the highly unfavourable milieu of the vaginal secretions. Stenosis of the cervical canal, whether congenital in nature or acquired as a result of sclerosis following curettage, infection, criminal abortion or trauma during delivery, is an uncommon cause of infertility. The amount of mucus-secreting epithelium can be reduced below a critical level by cervical amputation, overenthusiastic cauterization or excessively deep cone biopsy. Endocervical polypi and varicosities may be contributory factors to infertility, but cervical ectopy plays no role in reducing reproductive capacity.

Abnormalities of mucus secretion
Cervical mucus is a complex hydrogel and two major varieties are recognized: E-type mucus (actually formed of two subgroups known as E_1 and E_2) is of watery consistency and is secreted by the oestrogenically stimulated cervix, whilst G-type mucus is produced in response to progesterone. E-type mucus increases in amount during the preovulatory stage of the cycle and reaches a peak, forming 97 per cent of the total, at ovulation. G-type mucus predominates during the luteal phase. The long flexible macromolecules, or high viscosity component, of the mucus form elongated linear micellar bundles between which are channels containing the low viscosity, largely aqueous, component. Sperm ascend through the water-containing channels, which in E-type mucus are large and allow for easy passage. In G-type mucus, because of progesterone-induced binding between glycoprotein molecules, these channels form a meshwork which is too narrow for sperm passage.

A deficiency of cervical mucus secretion is due either to a lack of oestrogenic stimulation or to an end organ insensitivity to oestrogen effect and is commonly associated with a hypoplastic cervix. A thick viscid-type of mucus tends to be secreted in chronic infections of the cervix; this is made up partly of Q-type mucus, which does not have a uniform constitution but is formed of subunits or partial components, the range of which varies with the nature, degree and duration of the inflammatory process. A further factor complicating mucus production in the chronically inflamed cervix is that a number of secretory cells become hormone insensitive and autonomously secrete either E- or G-type mucus. Thus, the mucus produced under such conditions tends to be a mixture of Q, E and G types which is resistant to the free passage of sperm.

Immunological abnormalities
Antisperm antibodies are thought to play an important role in some cases of infertility but attempts to correlate the presence of serum antisperm antibodies with infertility in females have proved inconclusive. Attention has therefore recently focused on the possibility that antibodies locally synthesized by, and secreted into, the female genital tract could, because of their more direct contact with sperm, be of greater significance than those found in serum. There is now good evidence that the uterine cervix, but no other site in the female genital tract, possesses a local, secretory, IgA-dependent immune system which is qualitatively (but not quantitatively) identical to that found at other mucosal surfaces, such as the

gastrointestinal tract or upper respiratory tract, and that secretory type IgA is the major immunoglobulin component of cervical mucus. It has been shown that the cervices of many infertile women contain an increased number of IgA-secreting plasma cells and locally secreted sperm-agglutinating or immobilizing antibodies are present in the cervical mucus of a high proportion of infertile women. No correlation exists between the presence of serum antibodies and cervical mucus antibodies and only the locally secreted antibodies tend to be associated with a poor postcoital test and with sperm immobilization within cervical mucus. It has been shown that as soon as sperm come into contact with cervical mucus containing antisperm antibodies they change their forward movement into a static shaking or vibrating pattern. This phenomenon, which is complement independent and mediated by IgA antibody, has been attributed to antisperm antibodies causing a cross-linking between sperm and the glycoprotein micelles of the mucus, this cross-linking being due to sticking of the Fc fragment to the glycoprotein and binding of the Fab fragment with the sperm. Because the micelles are movable only to a limited extent, the spermatazoa undergo jerking movements and are thus effectively immobilized.

Whether the relatively good, but by no means absolute, relationship between the presence of locally secreted antibodies and female infertility is due solely to sperm immobilization within cervical mucus, or whether such antibodies play other roles, such as exertion of an antiembryo effect or impairment of sperm capacitation, is currently open to question.

Endometriosis

Between 30 and 40 per cent of women with endometriosis are infertile. The mechanisms by which this disease reduces reproductive capacity are enigmatic; for even a minimal degree of endometriosis is associated with a significant incidence of infertility. Tubal kinking, deformity or obstruction, because of either perisalpingeal adhesions or fibrosis of intramural endometriotic foci, is the exception rather than the rule, most women with endometriosis having fully patent tubes. Furthermore, although tubo–ovarian adhesions may cause fimbrial fixation and thus impair access of the ovum to the tube, these are relatively uncommon findings. A disturbance of tubal motility has been invoked as a causal factor in reducing fertility, this being variously attributed to muscle spasm secondary to dyspareunia or pelvic irritation, perisalpingeal adhesions or the secretion of prostaglandins by ectopic foci of endometrium, whilst endosalpingitis may be a factor in a small proportion of women. An excess of peritoneal macrophages, which have an increased ability to ingest spermatozoa, has been noted in women with endometriosis.

This failure to find an obvious mechanical factor responsible for reducing fertility in women suffering from endometriosis has, in recent years, directed attention to the possibility of ovarian malfunction in this disease. There is little doubt that virtually all women with endometriosis show normal cyclical changes in their endometria, though luteal phase insufficiency is sometimes recorded, and it has been suggested that many who are infertile suffer from the 'luteinized unruptured follicle syndrome' (see section on ovarian factors), which is probably due to a defect in the mechanism of follicular rupture. However, this abnormality has been found to occur no more frequently in women with endometriosis than in those not suffering from this disease. Most recently an autoimmune hypothesis has been invoked, it being argued that ectopic foci of endometrium expose the body to tissue antigens, which are normally lost during menstruation, with consequent formation of anti-endometrial antibodies. Whether an auto-immune endometritis actually exists in cases of endometriosis, and the possible relationship of such an endometritis to infertility, are questions still being explored.

Key references

Ayers J W T, Birenbaum D L and Menon K M J. (1987) Luteal phase dysfunction in endometriosis: elevated progesterone levels in peripheral and ovarian veins during the follicular phase. *Fertility and Sterility* **47**, 925–9.

Gondos B and Riddick D H (eds). (1987) *Pathology of Infertility*. Thieme Medical Publishers, New York.

Honore L H. (1987) Pathology of infertility. In: *Haines and Taylor, Obstetrical and Gynaecological Pathology, 3rd edn.* pp. 778–817. Edited by H Fox, Churchill Livingstone, Edinburgh.

Insler V and Lunenfeld B (eds). (1986) *Infertility. Male and Female*. Churchill Livingstone, Edinburgh.

Morrison J C, Givens J R, Wiser W L and Fish S A. (1975) Mumps oophoritis: a cause of premature menopause. *Fertility and Sterility* **26**, 655–9.

Sief M W, Aplin J D, Buckley C H. (1989) Luteal phase defect: the possibility of an immunohistochemical diagnosis. *Fertility and Sterility* **51**, 273–9.

15
Ectopic pregnancy

An ectopic gestation, that is nidation of a conceptus in a site other than in the uterine cavity, occurs in about 1 per cent of all recognized pregnancies. Gestation may occur in extrauterine sites, such as the fallopian tube, ovary, peritoneal cavity or broad ligament, or in an abnormal intrauterine site, such as within the myometrium or in the cervix. In practice, approximately 95 per cent of all ectopic pregnancies occur in the tube. All ectopic sites share a common inability to respond fully to hormonal stimulation, to develop an adequate decidua and vascular bed and, with the exception of the peritoneal cavity, to expand to accommodate the developing fetus. Hence, ectopic pregnancies almost always result in early fetal death. Exceptionally, however, a pregnancy in the broad ligament, abdominal cavity or tube may proceed to term.

The aetiology of ectopic pregnancy varies in the different sites and therefore each will be considered in turn, in an order which reflects their relative frequencies.

Fallopian tube

The timing of tubal transport of the fertilized ovum is of critical importance for the conceptus must arrive in the uterine cavity at the optimal time for implantation. Should tubal transport be unduly prolonged or delayed the ovum may still be in the fallopian tube at the specific stage of development which is optimal for implantation.

Abnormalities of tubal transport occur in cases of congenital tubal deformity, congenital diverticula, following reconstructive surgery, salpingitis isthmica nodosa, following failed tubal sterilization, in women using low dosage progestagen-only oral contraceptives, after treatment for tubal tuberculosis and in bilharzial salpingitis. However, the most important factor leading to delayed tubal transport is non-specific chronic salpingitis, which not only causes deciliation and fusion of the plicae but also damages the tubal musculature.

In a proportion of tubal pregnancies the tubes appear fully normal and it has been argued that in such cases conception had occurred during a cycle in which there has been delayed ovulation and a short inadequate luteal phase. Hence, when the fertilized ovum reached the uterine cavity it had not yet developed to a stage when it was secreting enough hCG to prevent decay of the corpus luteum and was, during the subsequent menstrual bleeding, flushed back into the tube by a reflux of menstrual blood. This hypothesis is supported by the fact that it is by no means exceptional for the corpus luteum of pregnancy to be on the contralateral side to the tube containing the pregnancy. However, this latter phenomenon could also be due to transuterine or transperitoneal migration of the fertilized ovum into the contralateral tube where, because of its relatively advanced state of development, it implants.

The relationship between IUCD usage and tubal pregnancy has been discussed in Chapter 13.

It has recently become apparent that embryos replaced after *in vitro* fertilization implant unduly commonly in the tube.

Within the tube, implantation occurs most commonly in the ampulla (Fig. 15.1) with the isthmus and

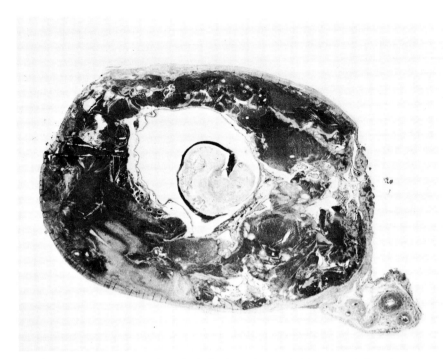

Fig. 15.1 A transverse section of a fallopian tube containing a gestational sac complete with fetus. The patient had bilateral follicular salpingitis (H. & E. × 4.8).

fimbria less common sites. Implantation may be plical, with no establishment of contact with the wall of the tube; plicomural, in which the ovum implants between two plicae and is partially in contact with the wall; and mural, in which implantation is directly into the wall of the tube. Plical implantations rapidly abort, largely because of the lack of an adequate surface for placentation to occur, but in mural implantations the process of placentation occurs in exactly the same manner as it does in the uterus. However, the thinness of the tubal wall, the relative inability of the tube to undergo decidual change, the absence of specific haemostatis mechanisms and the limited distensibility of the tube all contribute to tubal pregnancies being of usually short duration.

It is probable that asymptomatic complete resorption without tubal damage is common, although the frequency of this favourable outcome can not be estimated with any degree of certainty.

Other possible outcomes include separation of the placental tissue with the development of a haematosalpinx and haemoperitoneum, partial separation of the placenta with the formation of a haemorrhagic mass of placental tissue and organized blood clot, abortion into the uterine cavity, abortion into the peritoneal cavity with exceptional instances of reimplantation on the peritoneum, intratubal mummification of the fetus or tubal rupture. This last event occurs in at least 50 per cent of tubal pregnancies and is usually acute, with an associated dramatic clinical picture. Less commonly there is a slow leakage of tubal contents and blood into the peritoneal cavity to form a gradually enlarging extratubal haematoma which binds the tube down to adjacent structures and can even lead to ureteric obstruction. Despite all these tribulations which may befall a tubal gestation there have been nearly 100 reported instances of such pregnancies proceeding to, or almost to, term.

The symptoms attributable to a tubal pregnancy are diverse but, most commonly, the patient complains of abdominal pain and vaginal bleeding. Examination of the abdominal cavity in a tubal pregnancy usually reveals blood in the pouch of Douglas and the pelvis. The involved tube is usually distended,

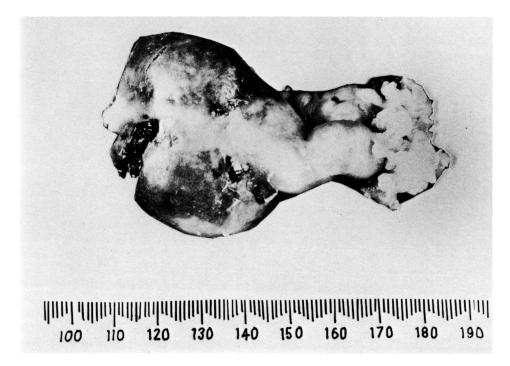

Fig. 15.2   Tubal ectopic gestation. A fallopian tube removed from a patient with 6 weeks amenorrhoea. The tube is distended and congested proximally and blood clot protrudes through a mural rupture.

congested and often covered by blood clot or by an exudate which may be serosanguineous or fibrinous in nature. The fimbrial ostium may be occluded by blood clot but if it is still patent blood may be seen oozing from the fimbrial end of the tube. If rupture has occurred blood clot and placental tissue may be seen protruding through the rupture site and the blood clot may envelop the tube (Fig.15.2). On opening the tube a complete amniotic sac and fetus may be seen, but more commonly the lumen appears to contain only fresh and old blood clot.

Histological examination of a gravid tube usually shows occasional placental villi embedded in blood clot sometimes, but not invariably, with embryonic tissue. Less commonly, obvious placental tissue with an attachment to the tube wall is seen (Fig. 15.3). If tubal rupture or abortion has occurred some time previously there may be no residual trophoblastic or fetal tissue, the only detectable abnormality being the presence of inflammatory debris. However, in such cases an implantation site can usually be identified, with extravillous trophoblastic tissue infiltrating the muscle of the tubal wall and invading the vascular spaces.

Peritoneal cavity

Primary peritoneal implantation does occasionally occur and is defined by the presence of entirely normal tubes and ovaries, the absence of a uteroabdominal fistula and the isolated nature of the placental site. In most cases of apparent peritoneal implantation the pregnancy is a complication of tubal or ovarian nidation, either because of dislodgement from the primary site of implantation with the conceptus seeking a secondary refuge on the peritoneum or because of direct extension of the placental site.

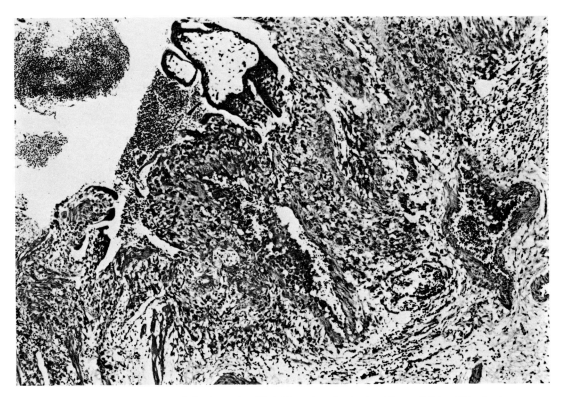

Fig. 15.3 Ectopic gestation in a fallopian tube. First trimester chorionic villi are visible within the lumen (upper left) and the three dilated vessels within the wall (centre and right) contain invading extraplacental trophoblast (H. & E. × 45).

Implantation may be at any site in the peritoneal cavity and reported locations include the broad ligament, mesocolon, omentum, small bowel mesentery, ileum and lesser peritoneal cavity. There have been a few instances of implantation on to the liver or spleen. However, the most common site is the cul-de-sac with implantation on either the posterior surface of the uterus or anterior aspect of the rectosigmoid.

A gestation within the abdominal cavity is not subject to the same restraints of space as a tubal pregnancy and the limiting factor determining whether the pregnancy aborts is the ability of the placenta to establish an adequate blood supply. As many as 25 per cent of such pregnancies do achieve adequate placentation and progress to an advanced stage.

Interstitial pregnancy

Implantation in the interstitial portion of the tube is rare and because of the thickness of the surrounding muscle, does not tend to rupture until a relatively late stage (ten to sixteen weeks). Rupture may be into either the broad ligament or the peritoneal cavity and this form of ectopic gestation has a particular tendency to be associated with massive, sometimes fatal, haemorrhage. Interstitial implantation may occur even after excision of the ipsilateral tube.

It has been suggested that intramyometrial implantation in other areas of the myometrium may be the result of nidation in a focus of adenomyosis.

Uterine cervix

Cervical implantation is extremely rare and usually presents as a spontaneous abortion, although one often accompanied by unusually severe bleeding. A clinical suspicion of cervical pregnancy may be aroused by the finding of an expanded cervix in the presence of a normally sized uterine cavity.

A cervical pregnancy may be due to unusually rapid transport of the fertilized ovum which therefore reaches the endocervical canal before having matured to a stage when it is capable of implantation.

Ovary

Ovarian implantation is exceedingly uncommon but an ovarian gestation is unduly common in women using an IUCD. This is not because IUCDs cause ovarian pregnancy but simply because they fail to prevent an ovarian pregnancy, whilst inhibiting intrauterine and tubal implantation.

An ovarian pregnancy may be primary or secondary. A primary ovarian pregnancy occurs if the ovum is fertilized whilst still within the follicle or if an ovum, fertilized outside the tube, primarily implants on the ovary. A secondary ovarian pregnancy occurs when fertilization takes place within the tube and the conceptus is regurgitated to implant on the ovary.

The clinical features of an ovarian pregnancy are very similar to those of a tubal pregnancy and hence the correct diagnosis is rarely made before operative intervention. To sustain a diagnosis of an ovarian gestation, the tube must be normal and separate from the ovary, the gestational sac must occupy the normal site of the ovary and be attached to the uterus by the ovarian ligament and ovarian tissue must be identified histologically in the wall of the gestational sac.

Ovarian pregnancies usually abort during the first trimester but there have been a few instances of such gestations proceeding to term.

Post-hysterectomy pregnancy

The disconcerting development of a pregnancy after hysterectomy may be due to the presence of an unsuspected tubal or ovarian gestation at the time of uterine removal, to canalization of the vault tissues which allows for fertilization or to fertilization of an ovum in a prolapsed tube.

Endometrial changes in ectopic pregnancy

The endometrium can, but does not necessarily, undergo the changes seen in a normal intrauterine pregnancy. An Arias–Stella change is seen in many (60–75 per cent) cases although this is, of course, in no way diagnostic of extrauterine nidation. The endometrial changes are due to the secretion of chorionic gonadotrophin by the trophoblast developing in its ectopic site and, with the death or abortion of an ectopic fetus, the fall in gonadotrophin levels results in shedding of the endometrium and vaginal bleeding. The clinical resemblance of this phenomenon to the spontaneous abortion of an intrauterine pregnancy makes a search for trophoblast in the uterine contents a mandatory exercise in order to exclude, as far as possible, an ectopic gestation. However, an absence of villous tissue from the uterine contents does not necessarily indicate an ectopic pregnancy for an intrauterine conceptus may already have been fully shed before curettage. In contrast, an absence of any evidence of a placental site reaction strongly suggests that nidation has not occurred in the uterus. Conversely, the finding of placental villi in uterine curettings does not absolutely exclude an ectopic pregnancy; a tubal gestation may well abort into the uterus. Such a possibility has to be considered if villous tissue, but not a placental site reaction, is found.

A final, somewhat esoteric but real, possibility to be borne in mind is that a woman may have concurrent intrauterine and ectopic gestations. Histological or ultrasonic proof of an intrauterine gestation does not completely negate a clinical diagnosis of an ectopic pregnancy.

Key References

Barnes A B, Wennberg C N and Barnes B A. (1983) Ectopic pregnancy: incidence and review of determinant factors. *Obstetrical and Gynecological Survey* **38**, 345–56.

Budowick M, Johnson T R B, Genadry R, Parmley T H and Woodruff J D. (1980) The histopathology of the developing tubal ectopic pregnancy. *Fertility and Sterility* **34**, 1169–71.

Delke I, Veridiano N P and Tanger M L. (1982) Abdominal pregnancy: review of current management and addition of 10 cases. *Obstetrics and Gynecology* **60**, 200–4.

Fox H, Buckley C H and Randall S. (1987) Ectopic pregnancy. In: *Haines and Taylor, Obstetrical and Gynaecological Pathology, 3rd edn.* pp. 818–38. Edited by H Fox, Churchill Livingstone, Edinburgh.

Green L K and Knott M L. (1989) Histopathologic findings in ectopic tubal pregnancy. *International Journal of Gynecological Pathology* **8**, 285–62.

Grimes H C, Nosal R A and Gallagher J C. (1983) Ovarian pregnancy: a review of 24 cases. *Obstetrics and Gynecology* **61**, 174–80.

Honore L H. (1978) Tubal ectopic pregnancy with contralateral corpus luteum: a report of five cases. *Journal of Reproductive Medicine* **21**, 269–71.

Honore L M and Nickerson K H. (1977) Combined intrauterine and tubal ectopic pregnancy: a possible cause of superfetation. *American Journal of Obstetrics and Gynecology* **127**, 885–7.

Iffy I. (1963) The role of premenstrual, post-mid cycle conception in the aetiology of ectopic pregnancy. *Journal of Obstetrics and Gynaecology of the British Commonwealth* **70**, 996–1000.

Kouyoundjian A J. (1984) Cervical pregnancy: case report and literature review. *Journal of the National Medical Association* **76**, 791–6.

Macafee C A J. (1982) Ectopic pregnancy. *British Journal of Hospital Medicine* **28**, 246–9.

Ory H W. (1981) Ectopic pregnancy and intrauterine contraceptive devices: new perspectives. *Obstetrics and Gynecology* **57**, 137–43.

Pauerstein, C J, Croxatto H B, Eddy C A, Ramzy I and Walters M D. (1986) Anatomy and pathology of tubal pregnancy. *Obstetrics and Gynecology* **67**, 301–8.

Randall S, Buckley C H and Fox H. (1987) Placentation in the Fallopian tube. *International Journal of Gynecological Pathology* **6**, 132–9.

Westrom I, Bengtsson L P and Mardh P-A. (1981) Incidence, trend and risks of ectopic pregnancy in a population of women. *British Medical Journal* **285**, 15–18.

Zolli A and Rocko J M. (1982) Ectopic pregnancy months and years after hysterectomy. *Archives of*

16

Pathology of spontaneous abortion

Any pregnancy terminating before the fetus is viable is classed as an abortion. In practice, this applies to all gestations which end before their twentieth week. About 15 per cent of recognized pregnancies abort but these represent only the tip of an iceberg of pregnancy wastage; over 40 per cent of pregnancies fail to develop beyond the first few weeks after fertilization, usually without the woman being made aware that she is, or has been, pregnant.

The causes, and mechanisms, of abortion are still largely unknown but a number of factors are clearly associated with an increased incidence of early pregnancy loss. Amongst these, fetal chromosomal abnormality is the most important, an abnormal fetal karyotype being present in 30–50 per cent of all abortions and in 40–60 per cent of those occurring during the first trimester. The most common abnormal karyotypes found in aborted fetuses are autosomal trisomy, triploidy, tetraploidy and XO monosomy. The incidence of congenital malformations is also much higher in aborted fetuses than in full term infants. Thus neural tube defects are found up to 40 times more often in spontaneously aborted fetuses than in newborn infants and even relatively minor malformations, such as cleft palate or polydactyly, are found unduly commonly in aborted fetuses.

Abortion can occur as a non-specific complication of any severe systemic maternal infection but some infections, e.g. rubella, syphilis, toxoplasmosis and listeriosis, are often associated with abortion, possibly because of transplacental fetal infection, even in the absence of any systemic maternal symptoms. Uterine abnormalities, particularly submucous leiomyomata, fixed retroversion, cervical incompetence and congenital uterine malformations (even of a minor degree) are accompanied by a high incidence of abortion, most notably during the second trimester.

Immunological factors almost certainly play a role in some abortions. During a normal pregnancy the mother develops a blocking antibody which prevents her lymphocytes recognizing paternal antigens on the trophoblastic surface. In some cases of recurrent abortion there is an unusual degree of sharing of HLA antigens between mother and father and the mother thus fails to recognize, in immunological terms, that she is pregnant, does not develop blocking antibodies and aborts. Immunological factors are almost certainly of importance in the high incidence of abortion in women suffering from systemic lupus erythematosus.

Psychological stress, occupational exposure to toxins, maternal ingestion of alcohol and maternal hormonal dysfunction have all been implicated as factors related to abortion but their importance in this respect is still highly debatable.

Anatomical classification of aborted material

The tissue from an abortion which is presented for pathological appraisal may range from a complete fetus and placenta to a few scanty curettings. It is of value to have a macroscopic anatomical classification of such material and amongst various proposed classifications, the following is the most useful:

1. *Incomplete specimen*:
   (a) villi only
   (b) villi and decidua
   (c) decidua and trophoblastic cells
   (d) decidua only
2. *Intact empty sac*
3. *Ruptured empty sac*:
   (a) with cord stump
   (b) without cord stump
4. *Fetus present*:
   (a) with chorionic sac
   (b) without chorionic sac:
       (i)   normal non-macerated fetus
       (ii) normal macerated fetus
       (iii) grossly disorganized fetus
       (iv) focal abnormality of fetus.

In this classification the term 'focal abnormality' refers to defects such as spina bifida, whilst the expression 'grossly disorganized' is applied to those fetuses which are so ill-formed that they can only be classed as 'nodular' or 'cylindrical'. Most of the other categorizations are self-explanatory, although it should be noted that the term 'blighted ovum' is not used, for this is not only a meaningless expression but one that is open to widely differing interpretations, some restricting its use to cases of empty gestational sac and others also applying it to cases of nodular or cylindrical fetus.

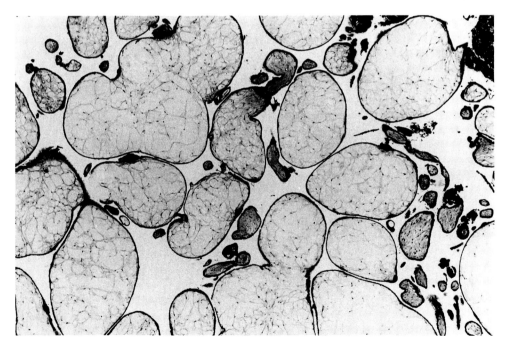

Fig. 16.1   Spontaneous abortion, Group 1 pattern. Villi in a placenta from a hydropic abortion. The villi are swollen and oedematous but there is no trophoblastic hyperplasia (H. & E. × 37).

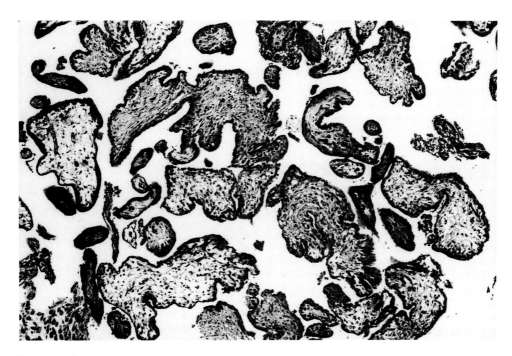

Fig. 16.2 Spontaneous abortion, Group 2 pattern. The villi are fibrosed as a consequence of fetal death (H. & E. × 93).

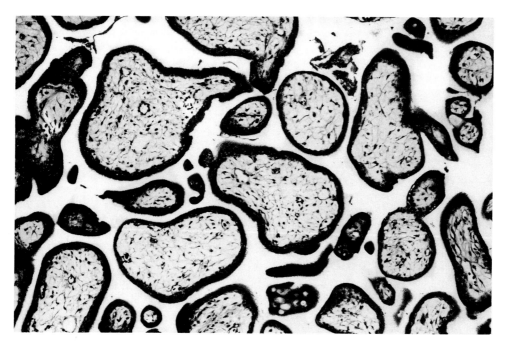

Fig. 16.3 Spontaneous abortion, Group 3 pattern. The villi are of normal first trimester form, there is no evidence of postmortem change (H. & E. × 93).

Histological features of abortion material

A purely anatomical classification of the type outlined above is of value for descriptive and statistical purposes but gives no indication of the possible factors involved in the failure of the pregnancy. It has been proposed that, where possible, abortions be categorized into three groups in terms of the histological appearances of the placental villi.

Group 1. Those in which most, or many, of the villi show hydropic change (Fig. 16.1), the remaining villi being fibrotic. This group corresponds to a 'hydropic abortus', a term which has been much abused but which, when used correctly, refers to the presence of swollen oedematous villi which are rarely sufficiently distended to form macroscopically visible vesicles. Fetal villous vessels are usually absent and the villous trophoblast is attenuated. Trophoblastic hyperplasia is never seen in a hydropic abortus.

Group 2. Those in which the villi show postmortem change but are otherwise normal. Postmortem changes seen in the placental villi include stromal fibrosis, sclerosis and obliteration of fetal vessels and an increased formation of syncytial knots (Fig. 16.2).

Group 3. Those in which the placental villi are normal for the length of the gestational period and show no postmortem changes (Fig. 16.3).

Significance of pathological findings in abortion

Abortion material is usually sent to the pathologist for the positive purposes of confirming that a pregnancy has occurred and for the negative purpose of excluding a hydatidiform mole. The diagnosis of pregnancy is easily confirmed if placental villi are present but if only decidual tissue is present it is necessary to find a placental site reaction before excluding the possibility of an ectopic gestation. A hydatidiform mole is also easy to exclude if the paramount importance of trophoblastic hyperplasia as a diagnostic criterion is borne in mind (see Chapter 17).

The study of aborted material can yield more information than this, particularly in those women who habitually abort. Thus, if the placental villi are of Group 1 type it can be concluded with some confidence that fetal death occurred at a very early stage of gestation, the most likely causes for this being a fetal chromosomal abnormality or a severe anatomical malformation of the fetus. If the placenta has a Group 3 pattern it is probable that the fault lies outside the embryo, the most likely factors involved being either a local abnormality of the uterus or an immunological cause. In Group 2 cases no firm conclusions of this nature can be drawn but in many abortions a histological classification along these lines gives a reasonable indication of the type of investigations which should be undertaken in cases of recurrent abortion.

Key references

Bennett M J and Edmonds D K (eds). (1987) *Spontaneous and Recurrent Abortion*. Blackwell Scientific, Oxford.

Fujikura T, Froenlich L A and Driscoll S G. (1966) A simplified anatomic classification of abortions. *American Journal of Obstetrics and Gynecology* **95**, 902–5.

Huisjes J H. (1984) *Spontaneous Abortion*. Churchill Livingstone, Edinburgh.

Porter J H and Hook E B (eds). (1980) *Human Embryonic and Fetal Death*. Academic Press, New York.

Regan L. (1988) Spontaneous and recurrent abortion: epidemiological and immunological considerations. In: *Implantation, Biological and Clinical Aspects*, pp. 183–95. Edited by M Chapman, G Grudzinskas and T Chard, Springer-Verlag, London.

Rushton D I. (1987) Pathology of abortion. In: *Haines and Taylor, Obstetrical and Gynaecological Pathology*, *3rd edn*. pp. 1117–48. Edited by H Fox, Churchill Livingstone, Edinburgh.

17
Trophoblastic disease

The term 'trophoblastic disease' is, by convention, restricted to hydatidiform moles, choriocarcinomata and placental site trophoblastic tumours, these all being defined in purely morphological terms. By contrast, a diagnosis of 'persistent trophoblastic disease' implies a lack of any morphological diagnosis. This term is applied to the situation in which, after evacuation of a mole, human chorionic gonadotrophin (hCG) levels either remain elevated or continue to increase and a diagnosis of persistent trophoblastic disease does not indicate or presuppose any specific histopathological diagnosis.

Hydatidiform mole

Hydatidiform moles of all types are a form of abortion and are not, as is often implied, trophoblastic neoplasms. The fact that a small proportion of moles invade the myometrium or spread via the bloodstream to distant sites is not an indication of their neoplastic nature; normal placental tissue can behave in an identical fashion.

Within recent years a clear distinction has been drawn, on both morphological and cytogenetic grounds, between complete and partial hydatidiform moles. However, there is now suggestive evidence that this separation of molar pregnancies into two distinct entities may not be as clear cut as had been previously thought.

Complete hydatidiform mole
A complete mole occurs in approximately 1 in 1500 pregnancies in Great Britain and the USA, women aged under 20 or over 40 years of age being at greatest risk. This incidence is considerably lower than that encountered in many parts of Asia, Africa and Latin America and, although there are grounds for believing that the excess incidence in these areas is of lesser magnitude than previously thought, there can be no doubt that a geographical variation exists; this has defied a satisfactory explanation in terms of ethnic susceptibility, socioeconomic status or nutritional deficiency.

A complete mole has a characteristic macroscopic appearance, forming a bulky, multivesicular mass which, when *in situ*, fills and distends the uterine cavity (Fig. 17.1). The total mass of trophoblastic tissue is much greater than would be the case for a normal placenta of the same gestational age, no remnant of a normal placental shape is apparent and the mole has a 'bunch of grapes' appearance as a result of gross distension of the chorionic villi which form clusters of vesicles measuring up to 0.3 cm in diameter. There is no macroscopically normal placental tissue, no gestational sac and no fetus.

Histologically, the villi are markedly distended and oedematous, the entire villous population being abnormal to a greater or lesser extent (Fig. 17.2). The oedematous villi have a generally rounded contour and often show central cavitation. Fetal vessels are usually absent although attenuated vascular vestiges are apparent in a small minority of cases. The villous trophoblast is hyperplastic and indeed, this abnormality is the defining feature of a hydatidiform mole. Trophoblastic proliferation is not usually seen in all the villi, some having a flattened trophoblastic mantle. However, most villi do show

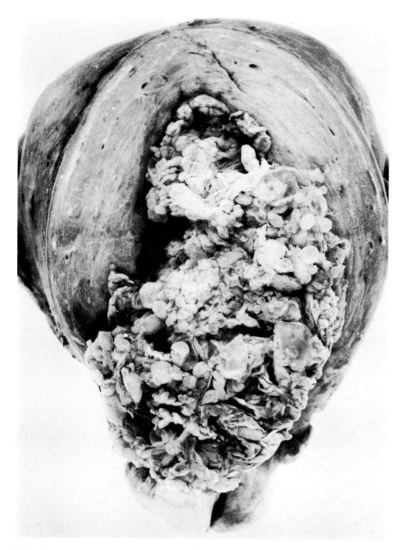

Fig. 17.1   An opened uterus containing a typical complete hydatidiform mole.

trophoblastic hyperplasia and this may be circumferential, multifocal or focal and of slight, moderate or marked degree. It should be noted that the degree of trophoblastic proliferation in a mole can be matched, or even exceeded, in normal first trimester placenta. However, in the normal organ proliferating trophoblast is always at one pole, or along one side of a villus and the circumferential or focal pattern characteristic of a mole is never encountered. A moderate degree of nuclear atypia is usually present in proliferating molar trophoblast, although this is commonly no more marked than the atypia often seen in placentae from normal first trimester pregnancies.

Some light has been shed on the pathogenesis of complete moles by cytogenetic studies. About 90 per cent of complete moles have a 46XX chromosomal constitution, the remainder being 46XY. In all cases the genome is of purely paternal origin and in the majority of XX moles there appears to be fertilization of an 'empty' ovum by a single haploid sperm followed by duplication without cytokinesis; such moles are classed as monospermic or homozygous. All XY moles and a small proportion of XX moles appear

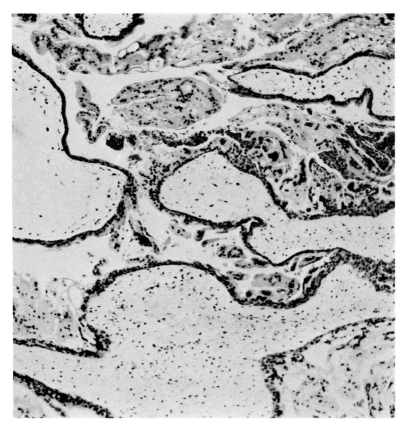

Fig. 17.2 A complete hydatidiform mole. The villi are markedly swollen and there is a moderate degree of trophoblastic hyperplasia (H. & E. × 50).

to result from fertilization of an 'empty' ovum by two haploid sperms which then fuse and replicate, these being classed as dispermic or heterozygous moles.

Approximately 10 per cent of women with a complete hydatidiform mole progress to persistent trophoblastic disease whilst between 3 and 5 per cent will develop a choriocarcinoma. It has been suggested that the risk of eventual development of a choriocarcinoma can be estimated by grading the degree of trophoblastic proliferation, it being argued that the greater the trophoblastic proliferation and atypia the higher the risk of postmolar complications. However, many are unconvinced of the value of such a grading system and, indeed, since all patients with moles should be followed up in the same way, irrespective of the histological appearances of the mole, it is clear that histological grading is now irrelevant. It can, in fact, be argued that any type of grading system for moles is potentially dangerous as, in injudicious hands, it may lead to the unnecessary administration of chemotherapy to some women and to the ill-advised neglect of others.

However, the fact that histological grading of moles is of little value does not mean that a search for prognostic features indicative of an increased propensity for persistent trophoblastic disease or choriocarcinoma should be abandoned. The most significant contribution to our understanding of molar progression has been the demonstration that dispermic (heterozygous) moles are associated with a much higher incidence of subsequent persistent trophoblastic disease than monospermic (homozygous) moles. The biological implications of this finding are far from being understood but are clearly considerable.

Two rather esoteric aspects of hydatidiform mole merit further mention. First, although the vast majority of complete moles complicate an intrauterine gestation, rare instances of molar ectopic pregnancies have been noted, the moles developing in the fallopian tube or ovary. Second, large quantities of hCG are secreted by the hyperplastic molar trophoblast, this hypersecretion of hCG having two side-effects, the production, in many cases, of bilateral ovarian theca lutein cysts (see Chapter 7) and the development, in a small minority of cases, of mild clinical hyperthyroidism, an effect dependent upon the weak thyrotrophic activity of hCG.

Partial hydatidiform mole

A partial hydatidiform mole is one in which only a proportion of the villi show vesicular change, the abnormal villi being admixed with a normal villous population (Fig. 17.3). Hence a partial mole appears macroscopically as an identifiable placenta, of normal size for the gestational period, in which there are scattered vesicular villi, much of the placental tissue appearing normal to the naked eye. A gestational sac and fetus are often, although not invariably, present.

Histologically, villi showing vesicular change are scattered amongst others of normal size (Fig. 17.4). The vesicular villi tend to be smaller than those seen in a complete mole, frequently show central cisternal change and, very characteristically, have an irregular, deeply indented outline(the 'Norwegian fjord' or 'coast of Ireland' appearance) (Fig. 17.5). Cross sectioning of the deep indentations leads to 'trophoblastic inclusions' being seen within the stroma of the vesicular villi. A degree of atypical trophoblastic proliferation is always present in at least some of the vesicular villa, although this is more commonly focal rather than circumferential and is rarely as marked as the proliferation seen in a complete mole.

The vast majority of partial hydatidiform moles have a triploid karyotype, usually 69XXY but occasionally 69XXX or 69XYY. Not all placentae from fetal triploidies take the form of a partial mole and it has been suggested that if the chromosomal load is of maternal origin the gestation will be non-molar, whilst if the extra chromosomal material is of paternal origin a partial mole will result.

The natural history of a partial mole is still not fully defined. However, it is now clear that the incidence of persistent trophoblastic disease following a partial mole is not dissimilar to that encountered after a complete mole, whilst a number of invasive partial moles have now been reported. A choriocarcinoma *can* develop in a patient who has had a partial mole but there is currently no evidence that the incidence of choriocarcinoma after a partial mole is any higher than that found after a normal pregnancy.

The available evidence suggests, therefore, that the potential for complications, certainly those falling short of an obvious choriocarcinoma, after a partial mole is as great as is that after a complete mole and indicates that follow-up after a partial mole should be as mandatory as after a complete mole, although probably for a shorter period.

Relationship between complete and partial moles

Recent flow cytometry studies have led to a blurring of the apparently sharp division of moles into two discrete forms. The use of this technique has shown that some moles which, morphologically, are of the complete form have a triploid chromosomal constitution whilst a proportion of histologically typical partial moles are diploid in nature, this latter observation confirming a previous cytogenetic study of three partial moles with a diploid karyotype. Furthermore, a number of tetraploid moles have now been described, some of these taking the form of a complete mole and others that of a partial mole. It is not yet known whether triploid complete moles are of wholly paternal origin or whether they are mono-, di- or trispermic. The true nature of a diploid partial mole is also obscure. A possibility is that vesicular change in some partial moles is so extensive that they appear to be morphologically complete moles and that there are complete moles in which vesicular change does not affect the entire villous population. Despite these uncertainties it is clear that it is no longer possible to predict with certainty the karyotype

(a)

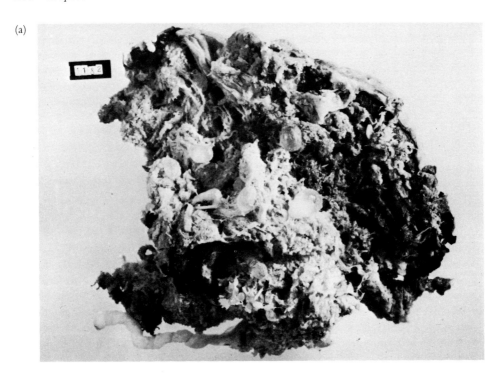

(b)

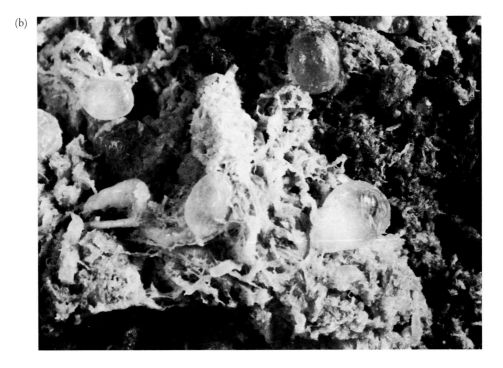

Fig. 17.3.   A partial hydatidiform mole. (a) Vesicular villi are seen scattered throughout macroscopically normal villous tissue. (b) Close-up view of the scattered vesicular villi.

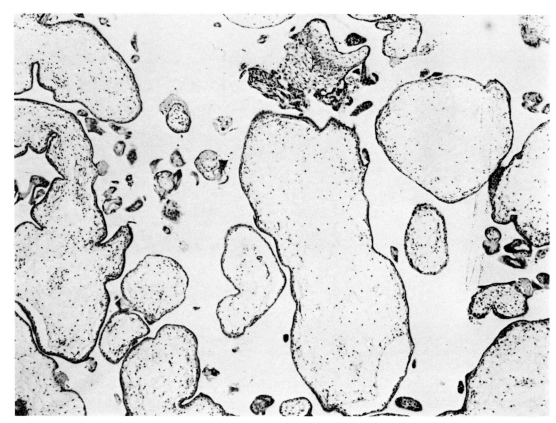

Fig. 17.4 A partial hydatidiform mole from a triploid fetus. Some of the villi show marked vesicular change, whilst others are of normal size. There is a very minor degree of trophoblastic proliferation (H. & E. × 45).

of a hydatidiform mole from its morphological characteristics and this poses the question as to whether moles should be defined in morphological or karyotypic terms. Furthermore, it may no longer be justifiable to distinguish between partial and complete moles in routine practice, for it could be argued that the only valid distinction is between molar and non-molar gestations.

Invasive hydatidiform mole

This term is applied to a hydatidiform mole, complete or partial, in which molar villi penetrate into the myometrium (Fig. 17.6) and its blood vessels. A deeply invasive mole usually becomes clinically evident several weeks after apparently complete evacuation of a mole from the uterus, the patient presenting with a haemorrhage or brownish discharge. If a hysterectomy is performed at this stage the appearances range from, at one extreme, only a small haemorrhagic focus in the myometrium to, at the other end of the spectrum, a large, deeply cavitating haemorrhagic lesion of the uterine wall which mimics a choriocarcinoma. Rarely, a mole may penetrate the full thickness of the myometrium, this leading either to uterine perforation or to extension of the mole into adjacent structures, such as the broad ligament. The histological diagnosis is dependent upon the finding of molar villi within the uterine wall (Fig. 17.7) these being more commonly seen in the myometrial vascular channels than between the myometrial fibres. The vesicular villi are often smaller than those seen in non-invasive mole while their degree of trophoblastic proliferation is very variable and sometimes not conspicuous.

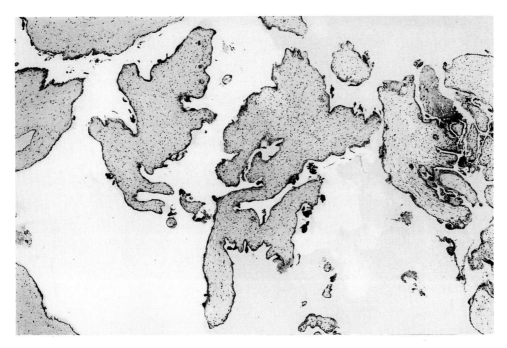

Fig. 17.5   Partial hydatidiform mole. The villi are of irregular outline and are said to resemble the fjords of Norway (H. & E. × 37).

In the past, invasive moles have caused death from uterine haemorrhage or perforation, but their mortality rate is now virtually zero because of the success achieved in their treatment by a limited course of chemotherapy. In fact, the diagnosis of an invasive mole, which can only be made on a hysterectomy specimen, is now almost obsolete for nearly all invasive moles present, and are treated, as cases of persistent trophoblastic disease.

It should be stressed that the invasive capacity of some moles is not an indication of their neoplastic nature. The villi of a normal placenta can penetrate deeply into, and even perforate through, the myometrium to give rise to the conditions of placenta increta and percreta, both of which are the exact non-molar equivalents of an invasive mole.

Molar tissue can be transported via the bloodstream to extrauterine sites, particularly to the vagina and lungs. The transported molar trophoblast can then grow in these sites to form nodules which are either clinically or radiologically detectable. The development of 'metastatic' lesions implies entry of molar trophoblast into uterine vessels and hence their appearance is usually taken as being indicative of the presence of an invasive mole. The 'metastatic' nodules are not usually associated with overt evidence of molar invasion of the myometrium.

The 'metastatic' nodules usually appear several weeks after evacuation of a mole from the uterus but may occur concurrently with a mole or can be the presenting symptom of such a lesion. Vaginal lesions form haemorrhagic, submucous, dome-shaped nodules and their true nature is only apparent when biopsy reveals the presence of villous structures, a finding which rules out a diagnosis of choriocarcinoma. Pulmonary lesions may cause haemoptysis but are usually an asymptomatic radiological finding. Histological examination again reveals their content of villi.

The extrauterine lesions of a mole may resolve spontaneously but are commonly treated with limited chemotherapy which achieves excellent results. The transportation of molar trophoblast to extrauterine sites is not an indication of neoplastic behaviour; in every normal pregnancy trophoblast enters the

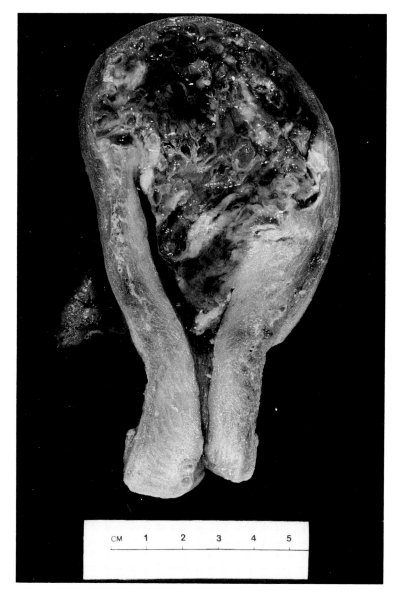

Fig. 17.6 Invasive mole. The uterus is occupied by hydatidiform mole which is invading deeply into the myometrium. At one point mole infiltrates almost to the serosa.

maternal bloodstream and is transported to distant sites, this transported trophoblast only giving rise to detectable lesions if it is molar in nature.

Choriocarcinoma

Choriocarcinoma is rare in Western countries, complicating approximately 1 in 50 000 gestations: 50 per cent follow a molar pregnancy, 30 per cent occur after an abortion and 20 per cent follow an apparently

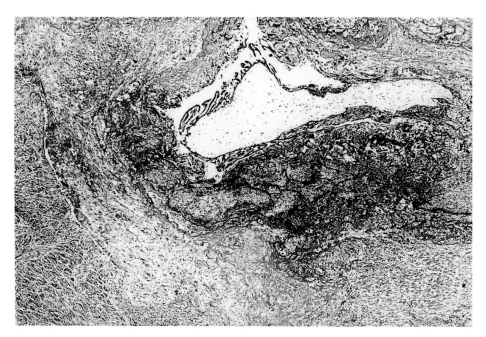

Fig. 17.7   Invasive mole. A molar villus extends deeply into the wall of the uterus. The specimen is from a young woman who continued to bleed heavily despite chemotherapy (H. & E. × 37)

normal gestation. The time interval between the antecedent pregnancy and the clinical presentation of a choriocarcinoma is very variable, ranging from a few weeks or months to 15 years and there is a considerable gap in our knowledge as to what has been happening during the intervening period. However, there is an assumption, which is not based on any factual evidence, that retained trophoblastic tissue eventually, after a latent period, undergoes neoplastic change. Choriocarcinomas can develop as small, often tiny and commonly overlooked, foci within otherwise normal third trimester placentae. Most choriocarcinomas following a normal pregnancy are apparent within four months of delivery and this suggests that these arise from an intramyometrial metastasis of an unnoticed intraplacental choriocarcinoma. However, an alternative possibility of some gestations being choriocarcinomatous *ab initio* can not be excluded.

A study of intraplacental choriocarcinomas also confirms the belief, long held on the grounds of the tumour's capacity to secrete hCG, that choriocarcinomas are derived from villous trophoblast, because in these lesions a transition can be traced from villi with a mantle of neoplastic trophoblast to a true non-villous choriocarcinoma.

Within the uterus (Fig. 17.8) a choriocarcinoma forms single or multiple haemorrhagic nodules which range in size from 0.5 to 5 cm in diameter. These are often accompanied by local metastases to the cervix and vagina. The neoplastic masses are quite often sharply circumscribed and consist of a central area of haemorrhagic necrosis and, although not invariably, a peripheral rim of viable tumour tissue. This central, sometimes complete, necrosis of a neoplastic tissue is a reflection of the fact that a choriocarcinoma has no intrinsic blood supply, relying on its ability to invade and permeate the maternal blood vessels for its oxygenation and nutrition. It is therefore only the growing edge of the tumour which is adequately oxygenated, the remainder undergoing ischaemic necrosis.

Histologically, a choriocarcinoma has a bilaminar structure which recapitulates, sometimes to a remarkable degree, that of the trophoblast of the normal implanting blastocyst, central sheets, or cores, of cytotrophoblastic cells being 'capped' by a peripheral rim of syncytiotrophoblast (Fig. 17.9). The

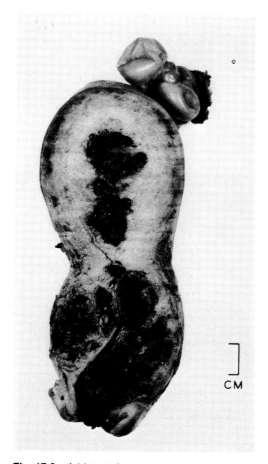

Fig. 17.8 A bisected uterus containing multiple nodules of haemorrhagic choriocarcinoma.

trophoblastic cells in a choriocarcinoma commonly show no greater degree of atypia and mitotic activity than is seen in an implanting blastocyst. Villi are *never* present in a extraplacental choriocarcinoma and indeed, the presence of villous structures negates a diagnosis of choriocarcinoma.

Because of its need to obtain an oxygen supply a choriocarcinoma is avariciously invasive of maternal vascular channels in the myometrium, although it should be noticed that normal trophoblast also invades these vessels. The tumour cells tend to form solid plugs within the myometrial vasculature and although there is often extravascular extension, the malignant trophoblast tends to infiltrate between the muscle fibres with little destruction. The propensity for vascular invasion explains the predominantly haematogenous dissemination of a choriocarcinoma with metastasis to sites such as the lungs, brain, liver, kidney and gastrointestinal tract. Large tumour emboli may impact within the pulmonary arteries. Lymph node deposits of a choriocarcinoma are usually tertiary metastases from a major extrauterine lesion.

In the past a choriocarcinoma was a lethal neoplasm, 90 per cent of the patients succumbing to their tumour, usually in months rather than years. Modern chemotherapy has transformed this gloomy prognosis with a current overall survival rate of over 80 per cent, this figure falling, however, to 70 per cent for patients with metastatic disease. Poor prognostic features include advanced disease at the time of initial diagnosis, cerebral, hepatic or gastrointestinal metastases and a very high pretreatment hCG level.

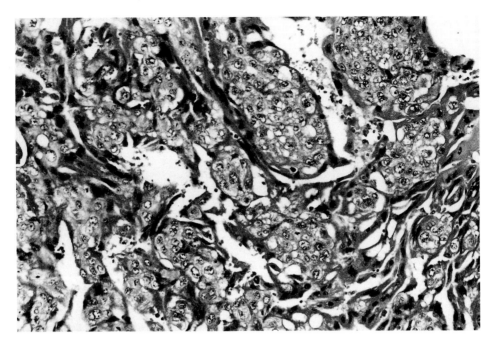

Fig. 17.9   Choriocarcinoma. The tumour consists of masses of pleomorphic cytotrophoblast surrounded by multinucleated syncytiotrophoblast. There is a definite resemblance to implanting blastocyst (H. & E. × 186).

For reasons which are currently obscure those choriocarcinomas which follow a normal pregnancy have a worse prognosis than do those which develop after a molar gestation.

Placental site trophoblastic tumour

This is a rare tumour which is derived from the extraplacental trophoblast of the placental bed. In the vast majority of cases the neoplasm develops after a normal term pregnancy, only 5 per cent occurring after a molar gestation. Patients present, at anything from a few weeks to 18 months after the antecedent pregnancy, with a complaint of either irregular vaginal bleeding or, perhaps more commonly, amenorrhoea. A small proportion of patients develop a nephrotic syndrome which can be an initial symptom. The uterus is commonly enlarged and a pregnancy test is positive in approximately one-third of patients, this combination of signs and symptoms often leading to a diagnosis of pregnancy rather than to one of neoplasia.

Macroscopically, the tumour tends to form a tan, white or yellow mass within the myometrium which may be sharply defined but is not uncommonly poorly circumscribed. The neoplasm often protrudes into the uterine cavity, sometimes forming a polypoidal mass. Rarely, the uterus is diffusely enlarged by infiltrating tumour without there being any discrete neoplastic mass.

Histologically, this neoplasm tends to recapitulate the appearances seen in the normal placental bed. The tumour is formed principally of mononuclear cytotrophoblastic cells with an irregular, and inconsistent, admixture of multinucleated cells (Fig. 17.10). The latter resemble the multinucleated cells of the placental bed rather than true syncytiotrophoblast and the typical bilaminar pattern of choriocarcinoma is not seen. The cytotrophoblastic cells of the tumour infiltrate between, and dissect, the myometrial fibres as cords and sheets with a striking absence of necrosis and haemorrhage. Invasion

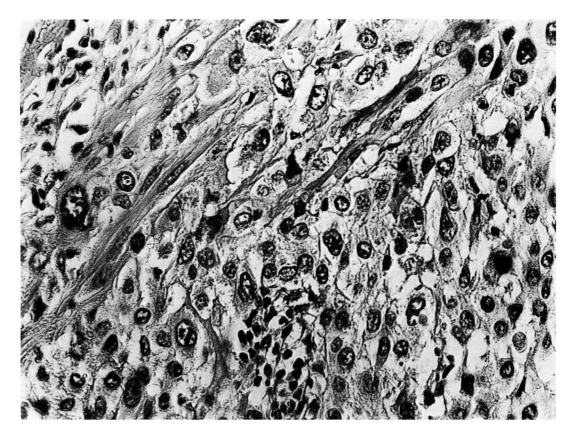

Fig. 17.10 A placental site trophoblastic tumour. The myometrium is massively infiltrated by cytotrophoblastic cells. The cells are infiltrating between the muscle fibres and there is no necrosis or haemorrhage (H. & E. × 405).

of vessels by tumour cells is commonly seen but the massive intravascular growth which characterizes a choriocarcinoma is absent and some vessels within the tumour are surrounded, but not invaded, by neoplastic cells. Non-infiltrated vessels often show fibrinoid necrosis of their walls whilst a pseudodecidual change, and occasionally an Arias–Stella reaction, may be apparent in the adjacent endometrium.

The diagnosis of a placental site trophoblastic tumour in curettage material is often far from easy, the major difficulty being in attempting to distinguish between a neoplasm and an exaggerated, but non-neoplastic, placental site reaction. Assessment of the degree of malignancy of a placental site trophoblastic tumour is also difficult for it is now recognized that about 10–15 per cent of these neoplasms behave in a malignant fashion. It has been suggested that tumours with a mitotic count of less than 2 per 10 high power microscopic fields pursue a benign course but, nevertheless, a few tumours with only 2 mitotic figures per 10 high power fields have behaved in a highly malignant fashion and proved fatal. There is little doubt that a placental site trophoblastic tumour with a high mitotic count should be regarded as being at least potentially malignant, but a sense of security should not necessarily be engendered by a low count. Whether or not the degree of atypia within a neoplasm of this type is of prognostic importance is currently undecided.

The management of a placental site trophoblastic tumour is essentially surgical, because these tumours differ from choriocarcinoma in their lack of response to any form of chemotherapy. In monitoring the follow-up of a woman after removal of the neoplasm the serum levels of human placental lactogenic hormone (hPL) are of more value than those of hCG. This is because the principal secretory product of extravillous, as opposed to villous, trophoblast is hPL rather than hCG.

Key References

Bagshawe K D. (1976) Risk and prognostic factors in trophoblastic neoplasia. *Cancer* **38**, 1373–85.

Driscoll S G. (1963) Choriocarcinoma: an 'incidental finding' within a term placenta. *Obstetrics and Gynecology* **21**, 96–101.

Eckstein R P, Paradinas F J and Bagshawe K D. (1982) Placental site trophoblastic tumour (trophoblastic pseudotumour): a study of four cases requiring hysterectomy, including one fatal case. *Histopathology* **6**, 221–6.

Elston C W. (1987) Gestational trophoblastic disease. In: *Haines and Taylor, Obstetrical and Gynaecological Pathology, 3rd edn.* pp. 1045–78. Edited by H Fox, Churchill Livingstone, Edinburgh.

Fox H and Laurini R N. (1988) Intraplacental choriocarcinoma: a report of two cases. *Journal of Clinical Pathology* **41**, 1085–8.

Gaear L W, Bedline B W, Mostoufi-Zadeh M and Driscoll S G (1986) Invasive partial mole. *American Journal of Clinical Pathology* **85**, 722–4.

Hemming J D, Quirke P, Womack C, Wells M and Elston C W (1987) Diagnosis of molar pregnancy and persistent trophoblastic disease by flow cytometry. *Journal of Clinical Pathology* **40**, 615–20.

Jacobs P A, Szulman A E, Funkmouska J, Maatsura J S and Wilson C C (1982) Human triploidy: relationship between paternal origin of the additional haploid complement and development of partial hydatidiform mole. *Annals of Human Genetics* **46**, 223–31.

Jacobs P A, Wilson C M, Sprenkle J A, Rosenhein N B and Migeon B R. (1980) Mechanism of origin of complete hydatidiform mole. *Nature* **286**, 714–6.

Kajii T and Okama K. (1977) Androgenetic origin of hydatidiform mole. *Nature* **268**, 633–4.

Lage J, Weinberg D, Yawner D and Bieber F. (1988) Tetraploid hydatidiform mole. *Modern Pathology* **1**, 52a.

Lawler S D, Fisher R A, Pickhall V J, Povey S and Evans M W. (1982) Genetic studies on hydatidiform moles. I. The origin of partial moles. *Cancer Genetics and Cytogenetics* **5**, 309–20.

Mostoufi-Zadeh M, Berkowitz R S and Driscoll S G. (1987) Persistence of partial mole. *American Journal of Clinical Pathology* **87**, 377–80.

Surti U, Sulzman A E, Wagner K, Leppert M and O'Brien S J. (1986) Tetraploid partial hydatidiform moles: two cases with a triple paternal contribution and a 92XXXY karyotype. *Human Genetics* **72**, 15–21.

Szulman A E and Surti U. (1978) The syndromes of hydatidiform mole. I. Cytogenetic and morphologic correlations. *American Journal of Obstetrics and Gynecology* **131**, 665–71.

Szulman A E and Surti U. (1978) The syndromes of hydatidiform mole. II. Morphologic evolution of the complete and partial mole. *American Journal of Obstetrics and Gynecology* **132**, 20–7.

Teng N N H and Ballon S C. (1984) Partial hydatidiform mole with diploid karyotype: report of three cases. *American Journal of Obstetrics and Gynecology* **150**, 961–4.

Wake N, Fujino T, Hoshi S, et al. (1987) The propensity to malignancy of dispermic heterozygous moles. *Placenta* **8**, 319–26.

Young R H, Kurman R J and Scully R E. (1988) Proliferations and tumors of the placental site. *Seminars in Diagnostic Pathology* **5**, 223–37.

Young R H and Scully R E. (1984) Placental site trophoblastic tumor: current status. *Clinical Obstetrics and Gynecology* **27**, 248–58.

18

Systemic disease and the female genital tract

Systemic diseases may present with signs and symptoms referable to the female genital tract. These may be important, even presenting, components of the generalized disease or may be only a minor feature of an obviously widespread disorder, and the gynaecologist has to be alert to the possibility that an apparently local lesion may be a manifestation of systemic disease.

Infections

Viral

In a number of viral infections, such as *measles*, there may be a non-specific prodromal vulvovaginitis, whilst involvement of the vulva in the skin rashes of *chicken pox*, *smallpox* and *vaccinia* can occur. Highly uncommon viral infections involving the vulva include *orf*, which is contracted from sheep, and *Coxsackie virus* infection of serotype 16 which produces a vesicular skin rash similar to that seen in hand, foot and mouth disease. *Mumps* can involve the ovary, where it produces a transient oöphoritis.

Bacterial

The rash of *scarlet fever*, due to infection by an erythrogenic strain of Group A beta-haemolytic streptococcus, can involve the vulva and occasionally there may be severe vulvovaginitis. The primary lesion of *diphtheria* is, of course, usually localized to the pharyngeal area and is characterized by the formation of a greyish pseudomembrane. Primary localization of diphtheria in the vulvovaginal area has been described, with formation of a grey pseudomembrane in the vagina which causes bleeding as it is separated. Systemic disturbances are severe and the patient may be left with a serious degree of vaginal scarring. Confirmation of vulvovaginal diphtheria is made from vulval or vaginal cultures and diagnosis by examination of a smear is unreliable, non-pathogenic diphtheroids often being present in the vagina as commensals.

In women with *leprosy*, the vulva is not uncommonly involved and the ovary, uterus and fallopian tubes may also be affected.

Spirochaetal

Primary vulval *yaws* is very uncommon but occasionally a perineal papule is present which develops into a broad-based granulomatous lesion covered by a serous crust. This is seen particularly in babies and young children. Secondary lesions of yaws can appear as small ulcerated or brown crusted papules or nodules at the mucocutaneous junction of the vulva.

Protozoal and metazoal

Intestinal infection with *Entamoeba histolytica* is endemic in many parts of the world and in such areas *amoebiasis* of the anogenital region is well recognized, this usually being secondary to spread from the intestinal tract. In adults, amoebiasis is likely to involve the vagina and cervix and is often not accompanied by intestinal symptoms, whilst in children the infection is likely to be vulval and associated with severe amoebic dysentery. The vulval lesions present as painful serpiginous ulcers with necrotic edges, or as ulcerated masses from which oozes a blood stained discharge. Parasites may be identified histologically or the mobile organisms may be seen in scrapings from the ulcer edge. Amoebiasis of the cervix produces an ulceronecrotic lesion which may spread to involve the uterine body. The appearances may mimic those of a carcinoma but histological examination shows florid granulation tissue formation in which the parasite can usually be identified.

Filariasis can cause vulval oedema if the inguinal lymph nodes are involved. Often the nodes on only one side harbour the parasite and the oedema is asymmetrical.

Enterobius vermicularis, or threadworm, is a common intestinal parasite. Eggs are laid on the perianal and perineal skin at night and inflammation, excoriation and secondary infection can complicate the resulting pruritus. Adult worms may enter the vagina on hatching and this can result in vulvovaginitis. The worms may ascend to the cervix and endometrium where they elicit a chronic inflammatory reaction which may include granulomata, eosinophils and a fibroblastic response. Entry into the tube may similarly provoke a granulomatous response and further outward passage may lead to a perioöphoritis. However, it is perfectly possible for the worms to pass through the tube into the peritoneal cavity without producing any detectable change in the tubal mucosa.

Other inflammatory processes

Anal and perianal lesions are a common accompaniment of intestinal *Crohn's disease* and whilst vulval lesions may be in continuity with these they can also develop separately and independently. Vulval Crohn's disease may present as oedema, indolent ulceration, fistulae, abscesses or perianal tags. There may also be sinuses in the groin and on the anterior abdominal wall. Histological examination reveals non-caseating tuberculoid granulomata and sinuses lined by non-specific granulation tissue. Healing of the lesions tends to be associated with considerable fibrosis and scarring. Vaginal involvement in Crohn's disease is usually a consequence of the development of an ileovaginal or rectovaginal fistula, whilst Crohn's disease can spread to the uterus, fallopian tube (Fig. 18.1) or ovary (Fig. 18.2) directly from the intestine or appendix. The tubal lesions are those of a non-caseating granulomatous salpingitis and this may be accompanied by atypical epithelial hyperplasia. A granulomatous tubo-ovarian mass may result when tubo-ovarian adhesions are dense and granulomata may be seen within the ovarian substance, these indicating the presence of a granulomatous oöphoritis.

Perianal lesions are infrequent in *ulcerative colitis* but occasionally this disease is complicated by pustular lesions in the groins.

Diverticular disease of the large bowel, particularly if accompanied by infection, *intestinal tuberculosis* and *lymphogranuloma venereum* may be complicated by the formation of an intestinovaginal fistula. Extragenital *tuberculosis* and *actinomycosis* may also extend directly from the intestine to involve the genital tract.

Very exceptionally, *sarcoidosis* can involve the genital tract and the typical non-caseating granulomata have been described in the endometrium, myometrium, tube and ovary. It is probable that this diagnosis should not be entertained unless there is definitive evidence of sarcoidosis elsewhere in the body.

Behçet's syndrome begins in early adult life and is characterized by the triad of relapsing vulval ulceration, oral aphthous ulceration and eye lesions such as uveitis or iridocyclitis. Pneumonitis, gastrointestinal

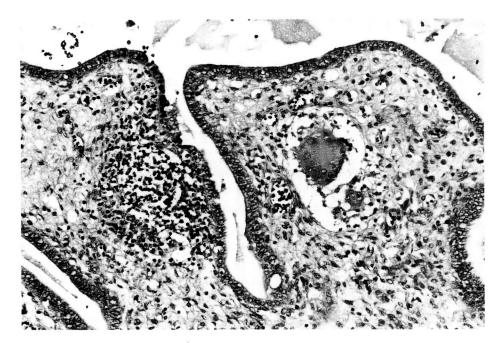

Fig. 18.1 Crohn's disease of the fallopian tube. A sarcoid-like granuloma, with giant cell, is present in the mucosa and there is also a non-specific, chronic inflammatory cell infiltrate. (H. & E. × 186).

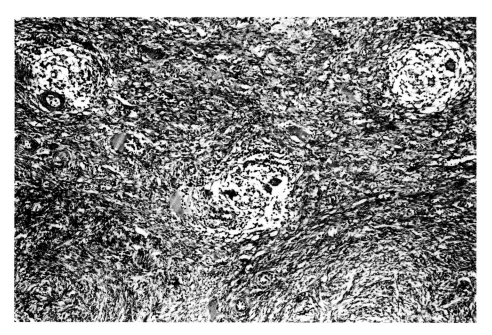

Fig. 18.2 Sarcoid-like granulomata in the ovary of a patient with Crohn's disease (H. & E. × 93).

ulceration, arthralgia and central nervous system abnormalities have all been described as occasional features of this disease. The vulval ulcers are painful, of variable size and usually involve the labia minora; occasionally, painless ulcers also develop in the vagina and on the cervix. Scarring commonly occurs but is not inevitable. Histologically, the ulcers usually present a non-specific appearance but occasionally a necrotizing arteritis or obliterative endarteritis is seen. The aetiology of this disease, although sometimes attributed to a viral infection or an autoimmune process, is unknown and the prognosis is unpredictable.

The vasculature of the cervix, uterus, fallopian tubes and ovaries may be involved in *polyarteritis nodosa*. The medium and small-sized muscular arteries show fibrinoid necrosis, a neutrophil polymorphonuclear infiltrate, microaneurysm formation and associated thrombosis with infarction or haemorrhage. Old healed lesions can be identified by the presence of perivascular fibrosis, intimal thickening and scarring of the vessel wall. The vessels of the genital tract can also be implicated in *giant cell* or *granulomatous arteritis* which may be a local, symptomatic condition limited to the vasculature of the genital tract, or may be associated with temporal arteritis or polymyalgia rheumatica, there being a characteristic, destructive, transmural granulomatous infiltrate with giant cells, epithelioid cells and lymphocytes (Fig. 18.3). Despite the rather dramatic histological appearance of these vascular lesions, symptoms referable to the female genital tract are either mild or absent.

Sjogren's syndrome presents as an immunologically mediated destruction of the salivary and lacrimal glands only, or may be associated with other autoimmune processes, such as systemic lupus erythematosus and may, occasionally, affect the vagina and lead to an acquired vaginal stenosis.

Vaginal and cervical lesions have been described in patients suffering from *ligneous conjunctivitis*. Tissue from areas of induration and ulceration is extensively infiltrated by a homogenous, eosinophilic staining material in which there are non-specific, chronic inflammatory cells.

Metabolic and deficiency diseases

Diabetes mellitus does not specifically affect the female genital tract but is associated with an increased incidence of both bacterial and fungal infections. Delayed menarche or, more commonly, secondary amenorrhoea may also occur in diabetics.

Addison's disease exhibits, as one of its cardinal features, mucocutaneous hyperpigmentation and this is often most marked on the genitalia. Histological examination of pigmented areas shows an increased number of melanocytes and an excess of melanin in the epidermis and upper dermis, this being due to the increase in circulating pituitary melanin-stimulating hormone, which has the same mechanism for synthesis and release as ACTH. An autoimmune oöphoritis associated with premature menopause occurs in a small proportion of patients.

Haemochromatosis, a chronic disease due to excessive absorption and tissue deposition of iron, is also associated with hyperpigmentation of the genital area. In some patients the pigmentation has a bronze tint, due to increased melanin, and in others there is a grey-blue pigmentation due to the presence of haemosiderin.

The skin lesions of *pellagra*, which is due to nicotinic acid deficiency, often involve the genital area, the affected skin being initially erythematous and later thickened and scaly, whilst the red, hyperkeratotic skin lesions of *kwashiorkor*, due to protein–calorie deficiency, can also affect the genital skin.

Riboflavine deficiency may produce an eczematous dermatosis of the vulva and *scurvy* is sometimes complicated by haemorrhagic lesions of the vulva and vagina.

A scaly and pustular or vesicular inflammation known as *acrodermatitis enteropathica* is associated with zinc deficiency. In the infant this may be due to an autosomal recessive inherited absorption defect but in the adult it may be seen following jejunoileal bypass surgery, alcoholism or during treatment of an iron overload by chelating agents.

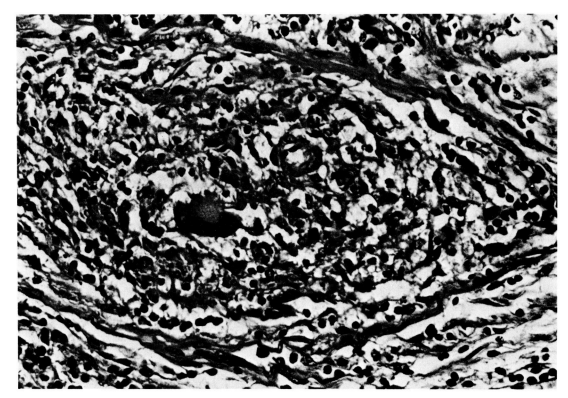

Fig. 18.3   A small muscular artery in the myometrium of a woman with granulomatous vasculitis of the genital tract. There is a destructive granulomatous inflammation of the vessel wall and a giant cell can be seen (H. & E. × 270).

The deposition of *amyloid* in the vulval skin produces yellowish, waxy, rather translucent, pruritic papules or plaques. This may occur in myeloma-associated disease or systemic amyloidosis from other causes.

Isosexual, precocious pseudopuberty has been reported in girls with steroid cell neoplasms of the ovary, ectopic pinealoma and gonadoblastoma. Precocious puberty may also develop in patients with tuberous sclerosis, meningoencephalitis, hydrocephalus, Albright's syndrome and neurofibromatosis.

Hypogonadism has been reported in patients with galactosaemia, even when treatment with a low galactose diet, thought to protect against tissue damage, has been instituted.

Hypercalcaemia, due to a variety of humoral substances, may occur in patients with non-parathyroid malignancy and in the absence of bony metastases in patients with squamous carcinoma of the vulva, small cell carcinoma, steroid cell tumours and teratomata of the ovary, dysgerminoma, adenocarcinoma and adenosquamous carcinoma of the endometrium, and squamous carcinoma of the cervix.

Thyrotoxicosis is a well recognized complication of conditions associated with abnormally high levels of hCG such as occurs in trophoblastic disease and has developed in patients with struma ovarii.

Cushing's syndrome has been reported both in patients in whom steroid cell tumours of the ovary are producing cortisol and due to the ectopic production of ACTH by ovarian neoplasms, including teratomata, and endocrine cell tumours of the cervix.

There have also been reports of *hypoglycaemia* developing in patients with primary small cell carcinomata of the cervix and primary ovarian carcinoid tumours as a consequence of insulin production, and of *Zollinger–Ellison syndrome* due to gastrin-producing mucinous tumours of the ovary.

Systemic hypertension may be caused by the secretion of renin or aldosterone by ovarian Sertoli cell tumours and aldosterone by serous tumours. It is well known that a *carcinoid syndrome* occurs with ovarian carcinoid tumour in the absence of metastases, this being due to the drainage of the ovarian veins directly into the systemic circulation. This syndrome has also been reported in association with carcinoid tumours of the cervix.

Haematological disorders

A wide variety of blood dyscrasias, such as *aplastic anaemia, thrombocytopenic purpura* and *leukaemia*, may result in the development of petechiae on the vulval skin and in the vaginal mucosa. These conditions can also cause severe menorrhagia, whilst patients with uncontrolled *polycythaemia* run an exceptional risk of bleeding. The disordered haemostasis of *hepatocellular failure*, due to vitamin K depletion, can also lead to excessive uterine bleeding, another rare cause of which is *von Willebrand's disease.*

Erythrocytosis may rarely occur in patients with uterine leiomyomata, mature cystic teratoma of the ovary and steroid cell tumours of the ovary. It is attributed to the production of erythropoietin by these neoplasms. *Autoimmune haemolytic anaemia* has been reported in patients with ovarian teratomata and other cystic ovarian neoplasms.

Abnormally large epithelial cells, or megalocytes, may be seen in the cervical epithelium of women who have *megaloblastic anaemia*. It is important that these are not mistaken, in cervical smears, for neoplastic cells.

Dermatological disorders

Skin diseases are of particular importance to the gynaecologist, because the vulva, being both part of the integument and the genital tract, often shares in systemic diseases which, although usually generalized, may occasionally be limited to the vulva. Some of these dermatological disorders are congenital but most are acquired.

Congenital disorders

Epidermolysis bullosa is a complex genetic disorder which may be dominantly or recessively inherited. In the dominant form, the vulval skin shows bullae which heal with mild scarring, but in the recessive form extensive erosions, ulcers and scars are typical. Histological examination shows bulla formation at the dermoepidermal junction.

Darier's disease frequently involves the vulva. Hyperkeratotic dark papules form, these slowly progress and may coalesce to form verrucous lesions. Histologically, there is acantholysis of the suprabasal epithelial cells with the formation of intraepithelial clefts. These are an expression of the genetic defect but the mechanism of this is unknown.

The lesions of *familial benign pemphigus* appear in adolescence and, although they may be limited to the vulva, they also characteristically affect the intertriginous areas. Recurrent clusters of vesicles develop which rupture to form crusted moist papules which later coalesce to form plaques. Histologically, there are intraepidermal bullae and vesicles which form as a result of acantholysis. Persistence of some intracellular bridges prevents complete separation of all of the cells, whilst the basal cells retain their orientation to the basement membrane. The disease is of unknown pathogenesis and, despite its name, a family history of the condition is absent from one-third of cases.

Ehlers–Danlos syndrome takes several forms but all are characterized by a failure of normal collagen synthesis. Hence patients with this defect have tissues which stretch excessively, tear easily and heal poorly. Bleeding tends to be excessive following trauma, and damage during childbirth may be followed by fistulae formation, scarring and stenosis of the vulva or vagina. An inherited disorder of elastic fibres, *pseudoxanthoma elasticum*, has a particular predilection for the genitocrural area, where doughy coalescing papules appear in skin which is soft, lax and wrinkled, and often shows petechiae or telangectasia. Histologically, the lower two-thirds of the dermis contain swollen, irregularly clumped elastic fibres which often undergo calcification.

Acquired bullous diseases

A number of skin disorders, all of which can affect the vulva, are characterized principally by the formation of bullae. The distinction between these various conditions is based largely upon the site of bulla formation, which may be between the dermis and epidermis, in the lower part of the epidermis or in the upper epidermis. Predominant amongst this group of skin disorders is *pemphigus*, which usually develops in middle age and has a particular tendency to involve the skin of the genital area. Mucous membranes, including those of the vagina, vulva and cervix, can also be involved. The disease exists in two forms, *pemphigus vulgaris* and *pemphigus vegetans*, the latter occurring in individuals who have an increased resistance to the disease. In the vulgaris form, painful, flaccid intraepidermal bullae form, these rupture easily to leave red, denuded areas that tend to increase progressively in size. Histological examination reveals suprabasal bullae associated with epidermal acantholysis. In the vegetans variety of the disease, the denuded areas heal, although with verrucous vegetations rather than normal skin. The primary abnormality in pemphigus is a dissolution of intercellular cement within the epidermis, and specific IgG autoantibodies directed against intercellular substance are present in the serum of patients with the disease. A significant association with HLA A10 suggests that there may well be an underlying genetic factor.

Bullous pemphigoid involves only the skin and differs further from pemphigus in that the bullae are subepidermal rather than intraepidermal; when the bullae rupture the denuded areas show little tendency to extend. Specific IgG antibodies which bind to the basement membrane of the epidermis have been detected in some patients with this condition. A form of this disease, *benign mucous membrane pemphigoid* (*cicatricial pemphigoid*), does involve the mucous membranes, including those of the vulva and vagina. The bullae tend to heal with scarring and the disease can cause a vaginal stenosis. Juvenile pemphigoid tends to involve the vulval skin and usually appears in girls aged 3 to 4 years. It is a self-limiting condition and heals without scarring.

In the rare condition of *subcorneal pustular dermatosis*, recurrent crops of pus-filled bullae occur in the epidermis immediately below the stratum corneum.

Bullous erythema multiforme produces a vesiculo-bullous vaginal epithelial lesion which results in scarring and vaginal stenosis.

Acquired non-bullous diseases

Lichen sclerosus comprises lesions known previously as kraurosis, primary atrophy of the vulva or atrophic leukoplakia, but is a specific dermatopathological entity affecting any area of the skin in both men and women. Although it most commonly affects the anogenital area of middle-aged women it occurs in all age groups, from childhood to old age. About 20 per cent of patients will have lesions elsewhere on their bodies. The affected areas show low, flat-topped, white, maculopapules which coalesce to form well defined plaques bearing comedo-like plugs or pits. Affected areas are often bilateral and symmetrical and in long-standing cases the skin may be parchment-like. Additional features include oedema, bulla formation in the active phase, atrophy of the labia minora, splitting of the skin, fissures in the natural

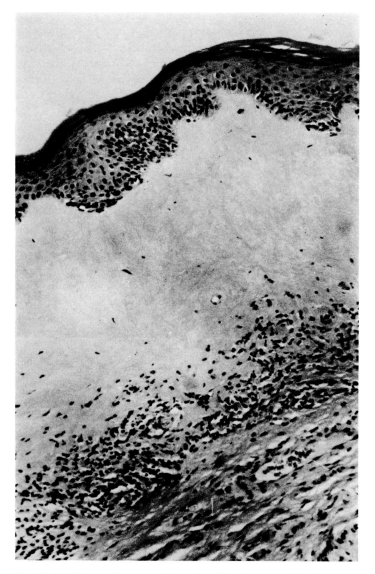

Fig. 18.4   Lichen sclerosus of the vulva. The characteristic features are loss of epithelial rete ridges, thinning of the malpighian layer and hyperkeratosis with superficial dermal hyalinization, deep to which there is chronic inflammation (H. & E. × 108).

folds and the formation of synechiae which may obscure the clitoris. Histologically, (Fig. 18.4) the malpighian layer of the epidermis is thin, rete ridges are flattened or absent and there is often a degree of liquefaction degeneration of the basal layer which may lead to the formation of subepidermal bullae particularly in children; hyperkeratosis is often present. The upper dermis is oedematous in the active phase or hyalinized in late disease. Lichen sclerosus can be arrested or sometimes reversed by topical therapy and, in children, not infrequently resolves spontaneously.

Psoriasis is a common skin disease characterized by small, discrete, erythematous patches covered with silvery scales, removal of which causes fine punctate bleeding. The lesions are often symmetrical and in the vulva the lateral surfaces of the labia majora are the site of predilection. At this site the lesions tend to have a smooth, glazed red surface and lack the scales characteristic of the disease in dry skin. Histologically there is parakeratosis, elongation of the rete ridges with thickening of their lower portion, thinning of the suprapapillary epithelium and microabscess-like collections of neutrophil polymorphs in the epidermis. The dermal papillae are clubbed, elongated and contain dilated capillaries. There is a mild to moderate chronic inflammatory cell infiltration of the upper dermis.

Lichen planus affects both the skin and mucous membranes but in some patients only the mouth and vulva, or occasionally the vagina, are involved. The characteristic lesion in the skin is a small, flat-topped, red or violaceous papule with a shiny surface on which there are whitish streaks, whilst on mucosal surfaces there are small erosions and white papules which fuse to form a lattice. Histologically, there is hyperkeratosis together with irregular acanthosis and liquefactive degeneration of the basal layer of the epidermis. The dermoepidermal junction has a serrated appearance due to the pointed shape of the rete ridges but the junction may be blurred by a band-like chronic inflammatory cell infiltrate in the upper dermis (Fig. 18.5).

The term *eczema* is often used synonymously with dermatitis but should be restricted to cases of atopic skin disease to which there is a genetically determined predisposition. It is often associated with other atopic disorders such as hay fever or asthma. The skin shows areas of erythema, scaling and thickening and there may be crusting and oozing. The histological picture is that of a chronic dermatitis showing variable degrees of acanthosis, hyperkeratosis and parakeratosis, together with a dermal chronic inflammatory cell infiltrate.

Erythema multiforme is a self-limiting, acute disease with a tendency to periodic recurrence in some patients and, as the name implies, a variable appearance. The disease may be idiopathic, drug-induced or associated with an infection and the clinical spectrum ranges from a few inconsequential skin lesions to a severe systemic disturbance. The most serious form of the disease are the *Stevens–Johnson syndrome* and *toxic epidermal necrolysis*, which tend to affect particularly mucous membranes. In Stevens–Johnson syndrome the lesions may be papular, macular, vesicular or bullous, whilst in toxic epidermal necrolysis a blotchy, painful erythema is followed by the formation of subepidermal bullae and detachment of the epidermis. The histological features are very variable but include subepidermal bullae, a perivascular inflammatory cell infiltrate in the dermis, epidermal necrosis and hydropic degeneration of the basic layers of the epidermis

Genital neoplasms and tumour-like conditions developing in systemic disease

The genital tract is a common site of metastases from extragenital neoplasms. These arise most frequently in the gastrointestinal tract, kidney and urinary tract, breast and lung. The genital tract may also be involved in systemic lymphomata, the ovary being the most common site of involvement.

There is an increased risk of vulval, anal, vaginal and cervical carcinomata in women who have had a *renal transplant.*

Women with *Peutz–Jeghers syndrome*, a non-sex-linked autosomal dominant disorder characterized by gastrointestinal hamartomatous polyps also develop ovarian sex cord-stromal tumours with annular tubules and also, in a small proportion of cases, minimal deviation adenocarcinoma of the cervix. Juvenile granulosa cell tumours of the ovary have been reported in girls suffering from *Ollier's disease* (*enchondromatosis*) and *Maffucci's syndrome* (enchondromatosis with subcutaneous haemangiomata). Vulval and, very occasionally, ovarian neurofibromata have been described in patients with *von Recklinghausen's disease* (*neurofibromatosis*). Other rare inherited disorders in which genital tract neoplasms may develop are *von Hippel–Lindau disease* (intraovarian haemangioma and papillary cystadenoma of the mesosalpinx

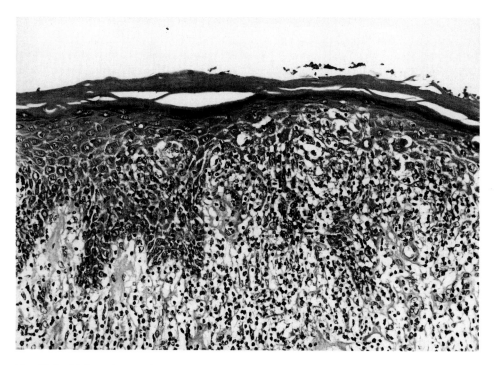

Fig. 18.5 Lichen planus of the vulva. The inflammatory cell infiltrate at the dermoepidermal junction and the typical serrated appearance of the rete ridges can be seen (H. & E. × 186).

resembling an adnexal tumour of wolffian origin), *ataxia-telangiectasia* (dysgerminoma and endodermal sinus tumour of the ovary and gonadoblastoma), *Torre-Muir syndrome* (endometrial carcinoma and, less commonly, ovarian and vulval neoplasms), *Cowden's disease* (early development of ovarian or endometrial carcinoma and vulval apocrine cystadenoma), *Lynch syndrome II* (endometrial and ovarian carcinomata) and *Gorlin's syndrome* (ovarian fibromata). A familial association between thyroid adenomata, Sertoli–Leydig cell tumours of the ovary and ovarian mucinous cystadenoma has also been described.

Retroperitoneal fibrosis, an infiltrative fibromatosis which typically envelops the abdominal aorta and ureters, may extend into the uterus, bladder and vagina. It is characterized by ill-defined masses of fibrous tissue, infiltrated by lymphocytes, plasma cells and eosinophils, in which there may be foci of necrosis, phlebitis and arteritis. These latter features suggest that it may be an inflammatory condition rather than a neoplasm, although its aetiology is uncertain.

Patients with *eosinophilic granuloma* may develop vulval pruritus, irritation, pain and ulceration and yellow-brown papular lesions may form in the vaginal mucosa. Similar, though paler lesions also occur in the cervix.

Key references

Axiotis C A, Lippes H A, Merino M J, deLanerolle N C, Stewart A F and Kinder B. (1987) Corticotroph cell pituitary adenoma within an ovarian teratoma. A new cause of Cushing's syndrome. *American Journal of Surgical Pathology* **11**, 218–24.

Buckley C H. (1987) Interrelationships of non-gynaecological and gynaecological disease. In: *Haines and Taylor, Obstetrical and Gynaecological Pathology, 3rd edn.* pp. 893–905. Edited by H Fox, Churchill Livingstone, Edinburgh.

Korzets A, Nouriel H, Steiner Z, Griffel B, Kraus L, Freund U and Klajman A. (1986) Resistant hypertension associated with a renin-producing ovarian Sertoli cell tumor. *American Journal of Clinical Pathology* **85**, 242–7.

Lojek M A, Fer M F, Kasselberg A G *et al.* (1980) Cushing's syndrome with small cell carcinoma of the uterine cervix. *American Journal of Medicine* **69**, 140–4.

Morgello S, Schwartz E, Horwith M, King M E, Gorden P and Alonso D R. (1988) Ectopic insulin production by a primary ovarian carcinoid. *Cancer* **61**, 800–5.

Ribeiro G, Hughesdon P and Wiltshaw E. (1988) Squamous carcinoma arising in dermoid cysts and associated with hypercalcaemia: a clinicopathologic study of six cases. *Gynecologic Oncology* **29**, 222–30.

Ridley C M. (1988) General dermatological conditions and dermatoses of the vulva. In: *The Vulva.* pp. 138–211. Edited by C M Ridley, Churchill Livingstone, Edinburgh.

Stockdale A D, Leader M, Phillips R H and Henry K. (1986) The carcinoid syndrome and multiple hormone secretion associated with a carcinoid tumour of the uterine cervix. *British Journal of Obstetrics and Gynaecology* **93**, 397–401.

Young R H and Scully R E. (1987) Ovarian steroid cell tumors associated with Cushing's syndrome: a report of three cases. *International Journal of Gynecological Pathology* **6**, 40–8.

Index